PHYSICAL APPRAISAL METHODS IN NURSING PRACTICE

Physical Appraisal Methods in Nursing Practice

Edited by
Josephine M. Sana, R.N., M.A.
Professor of Nursing, University of Michigan
School of Nursing, Ann Arbor

Richard D. Judge, M.D.
Clinical Professor of Postgraduate Medicine
The University of Michigan Medical School, Ann Arbor

Little, Brown and Company
Boston

Library of Congress catalog card No. 74-20224

ISBN 0-316-76995-9 (C)
ISBN 0-316-76996-7 (P)

Printed in the United States of America

Dedicated to students preparing for the practice of nursing
and
nurses committed to the continued expansion
of their knowledge and clinical competence

PREFACE

Societal attitudes and expectations regarding health and health care delivery have changed greatly during the last decade. Problems of adequate access to needed services, their availability, and rising costs are continuing public and professional concerns. These concerns, coupled with the demands of a rapidly expanding science and technology, press the health professions to examine and modify their independent and partnership patterns of practice. Responsive to these forces for change, nursing continues to seek more efficient and effective ways of providing nursing care. From these efforts, new and varied roles and responsibilities for nurses have emerged, generating the need for new and varied knowledge and skills.

Increasingly, nurses find they must employ more precise physical appraisal methods in the clinical assessment of patients. Students preparing for the practice of nursing are expected to develop and use these skills as an integral part of the nursing process. Nurses unprepared or inexperienced in this aspect of clinical practice will need to develop or improve these competencies. The preparation of this book was motivated by this need and designed to provide a useful resource for students and practicing nurses alike.

The book is intended to provide a broad reference base, and the content is organized in three sections to facilitate its use. The chapters in Section I present four distinct and significant perspectives for the reader's consideration of the physical appraisal process. Combined, these chapters provide an introductory contextual framework for Sections II and III. Section II includes the chapters dealing with the specific approaches and methods utilized by the nurse in assessing the adult. Considerations unique and important to the physical appraisal of the very young, the adolescent, and the aged are presented in the chapters in Section III.

No attempt was made to cover extensively the knowledge base underlying normal or abnormal findings, nor was nursing intervention elaborated. For some readers, the content may be too detailed. It is our hope that the organization of the book will facilitate its selective use. For readers desiring more information, the references and suggested readings at the end of each chapter should be helpful guides. Editorial decisions were made in an effort to preserve the focus primarily upon the physical appraisal aspects of the assessment process. Consequently, the reader will need to utilize other resources for guidance in the planning and management aspects of nursing care.

The assistance and encouragement of the contributing authors is acknowledged with deep appreciation. Without their commitment and effort this book would not have been possible. We wish to thank the Director of the Medical and Biological Illustration Unit of the University of Michigan, Professor Gerald P.

Hodge, and staff artists Judith K. Simon and Nick G. H. Tan for the illustrations they prepared for the book. We are grateful for the secretarial assistance of Ms. Bernice E. Gittens, and Ms. Kathryn Richards. Acknowledgments would be incomplete without expressing special thanks to Christopher R. Campbell, Editor, Little, Brown and Company, for his ready help and counsel.

J. M. S.
R. D. J.

CONTENTS

CONTRIBUTING AUTHORS

CANDACE M. BURNS, R.N., M.S.
Assistant Professor of Nursing (Co-ordinator Undergraduate Medical-Surgical),
University of Michigan School of Nursing, Ann Arbor

PATRICIA MITCHELL BUTLER, R.N., M.S.
Assistant Professor of Medical-Surgical Nursing, University of Michigan School
of Nursing, Ann Arbor

JOYCE CRANE, R.N., M.S.N.
Associate Professor of Nursing, University of Michigan School of Nursing,
Ann Arbor

JO WAYLAN DENTON, R.N., M.S.
Assistant Professor of Medical-Surgical Nursing, University of Michigan School
of Nursing, Ann Arbor

ELISA A. DIEHL, R.N., M.S.
Assistant Professor of Nursing and Acting Director, Continuing Education
Service for Nurses, University of Michigan School of Nursing, Ann Arbor

CAROL GILBERT, R.N., M.S.N.
Assistant Professor of Medical-Surgical Nursing, University of Michigan School
of Nursing, Ann Arbor

MARJORIE M. JACKSON, R.N., M.S.
Associate Professor of Nursing, University of Michigan School of Nursing, and
Clinical Director, Surgical Nursing, University Hospital, Ann Arbor

JUDY M. JUDD, R.N., M.A.
Professor of Parent-Child Nursing, University of Michigan School of Nursing,
Ann Arbor

ALICE MARSDEN, R.N., M.A.
Associate Professor of Psychiatric Nursing, University of Michigan School of
Nursing, Ann Arbor

PHYLLIS COINDREAU PATTERSON, R.N., M.S.
Clinical Nursing Specialist, Hematology, University Hospital, The University of
Michigan, Ann Arbor

SUSAN MENGEL PINNEY, R.N., M.S.
Assistant Professor of Nursing, University of Cincinnati College of Nursing
and Health, Cincinnati

BARBARA A. SACHS, R.N., M.S.N.
Assistant Professor of Nursing and Co-director, Pediatric Nurse Practioner
Program, University of Michigan School of Nursing, Ann Arbor

JOSEPHINE M. SANA, R.N., M.A.
Professor of Nursing, University of Michigan School of Nursing, Ann Arbor

SAMUEL SCHULTZ II, Ph.D.
Professor and Chairman of Research Area, University of Michigan School
of Nursing, Ann Arbor

ANNE L. SHARPE, R.N., M.N. Ed.
Clinical Specialist, Pediatric Nursing, C. S. Mott Children's Hospital and University
Hospital, The University of Michigan, Ann Arbor

CAROLYN P. STOLL, R.N., M.N. Ed.
Assistant Professor of Nursing, University of Michigan School of Nursinq, and
Clinical Director, Pediatric Nursing, C. S. Mott Children's Hospital and University
Hospital, Ann Arbor

LINDA TANNER STRODTMAN, R.N., M.S.
Clinical Nursing Specialist, Endocrinology and Metabolism, University Hospital,
The University of Michigan, Ann Arbor

MARGIE J. VAN METER, R.N., M.S.
Assistant Professor of Nursing, University of Michigan School of Nursing, and
Clinical Nursing Specialist, University Hospital, Ann Arbor

PHYSICAL APPRAISAL
PERSPECTIVES

I

EXPANDED NURSING PRACTICE 1

Marjorie M. Jackson

A popular phrase in nursing parlance today is the "expanded role of the nurse." Ever so quickly, like a burst of Chinese firecrackers, the phrase has caught the fancy of the nursing profession. In haste, it has been rejected or endorsed in its embryonic stage without being seriously studied, completely understood, and fully tested in practice. *Expanded role* is a term that means whatever the user wishes it to mean. It is used interchangeably with "extended role" or to characterize a variety of new nursing roles: nurse practitioner, nurse clinician, or clinical nurse specialist. A selective use of the term emphasizes changing role and function; a wider and richer perspective focuses on changing nursing practice. The position presented here is that true expansion of nursing practice will be achieved when nurses assume greater responsibility and accountability for patient cure and restoration in acute, chronic, and preventive health care settings.

Expanded role has had its roots in the management concept of job enlargement, which grew out of an orientation toward and concern for the development of human resources in organizations. The enlargement concept includes a triad: (1) variety of knowledge and skills in doing a job; (2) a better utilization of the worker's total skills and abilities; and (3) responsibility and freedom in the performances of the job. True job enlargement is not the addition of the same kinds of tasks but an expansion of job content with a wider variety of tasks and an increased freedom of methods.

EXTENDED ROLE VERSUS EXPANDED ROLE

Murphy [7] provides an important conceptual distinction between the job enlargement of the nurse who is a role extender and the nurse who is a role expander. She describes role extension as a unilateral lengthening, an additive process, and role expansion as a spreading out, a process of diffusion. With expansion, by definition, there is a richer mix both in the variety of tasks and in the new relationships among the tasks. The very nature of nursing practice is dynamically changed. With extension, by definition, there is continued addition of similar tasks and techniques, so that the nature of nursing practice is essentially unchanged. Nurses have always been in an extended role for, like it or not, a substantial portion of clinical nursing practice has and continues primarily to be inherited medical practice. Many of the major clinical functions in nursing are predominantly medical orders translated into action. This is strikingly evident in hospitals, which constitute the professional center of the health care

3

world. Historically, nurses have been the physicians' assistants, implementing medical regimens and applying medical technology. The current controversy about roles and role alignments was ignited by the advent of a new breed, the physician's assistant, and is significantly influenced by the women's liberation movement's emphasis on equity and autonomy. This controversy revolves around the scope of nursing practice as distinct from medical practice.

THE NATURE OF NURSING PRACTICE

Definitions of nursing abound, and while there is no consensus, there is consistent recognition of its nature as human service and assistance. The primary goal of nursing is to assist persons to attain and maintain optimal physical, psychological, and social functioning. The assistance ranges along the entire health-illness continuum from birth to death and is offered in a variety of health care settings, including the home. This helping role of nursing encompasses both instrumental and expressive functions. These evolve from the needs of patients and from the needs of medical practice and of the medical practitioner. The persistent dilemma of nursing is the proper marriage of instrumental and expressive functions, and this conflict is intensified by the acceleration in the technology of therapy and the escalating demand for health care.

To care and comfort is said to be the special province of the nurse. To cure and restore is said to be the special province of the physician. Murphy has superimposed the extender-expander role concepts on this cure-care model in terms of physician-nurse responsibilities. When viewed in Murphy's juxtaposition, the nurse who takes on primarily the cure functions of medicine becomes an extender of cure, while the nurse who undertakes the care function becomes an expander of care. Yet does it not distort the reality of the bedside, neighborhood clinic, or of the family the public health nurse assists to distinguish care and comfort from treatment and cure? To say that cure is a secondary function of the nurse is to ignore the paradoxes that often occur at times when nurses find it impossible to secure patient comfort and preserve personal integrity because they are responsible for the very procedures that produce the discomfort or demean the patient's personal dignity.

Compounding these dilemmas is the growing complexity in the delivery of health services. Kelly [6] contends that the nurse's clinical role is shrinking and dwindling to coordinator and traffic director as more and more of the tasks central to patient care are reallocated to others: the clinical pharmacist, the inhalation therapist, the IV team. She comments that "The role is shrinking because the nurse is incapable of controlling the care situation or exerting instrumental influence over her work."

Not only is the content of nursing practice changing daily, but the emphasis and the context of practice are also rapidly shifting. Social forces and education are orienting the modern nurse to health rather than illness, to prevention rather than crises, to a holistic rather than a technical approach, to the community rather than the hospital. The National Commission for the Study of Nursing and Nursing Education [8] and the Department of Health, Education, and Welfare [3] document the urgent need for a refocusing and redefinition of roles and practice. Both their reports underline the complementary roles of physician and nurse in a new professional realignment in the vast area of primary health care and in acute and chronic health care settings. It is beyond the province of this chapter to consider the urgent issues of role and function raised by these reports, but the reports are commended as essential resources.

The development of congruent roles of the physician and the nurse can resolve many current functional and jurisdictional disputes in scope of practice. Only through mutual understanding and agreement will a synthesis occur in the two divergent perceptions about nurses' roles, i.e., the nurse as a caretaker or the nurse as an assistant to the overburdened physician.

CLINICAL DECISION-MAKING

Basic to the expansion of practice and central to the complementary roles of nurse and physician is clinical decision-making. Cleland [1] has defined the role extender and role expander in terms of decision-making and has identified the number and quality of cues each uses in clinical judgment. On the basis of the range of cues brought to bear in clinical judgments, Cleland has postulated that critical distinctions can be made between levels of practice and among roles. She states:

At the first level of nursing there are general nurses and nurse practitioners, at the second level there are nurse specialists and nurse clinicians. General nurses and nurse specialists work in structured and defined settings, and with narrow ranges of cues involved in the decision-making and with the dimension of time extending through the patient's current hospitalization, and often extending only through the current 8 hour day. Nurse practitioners and nurse clinicians utilize data gathered from many sources to plan a broad program of patient care with a space focus which also involves the family, and a time dimension which includes the entire course of the illness [1].

Within Cleland's important framework, the crucial question is no longer whether or not the best direction in which to expand the practice of nursing is toward the assumption of more of the tasks of medicine. Rather, the crucial question is how the nurse and physician may become a decision-making team in the diagnostic and therapeutic problems of clinical care. Despite the performance of the nurse as a diagnostician and therapist in the past decade of coronary care and, more recently, in respiratory care, physicians and some nurses have been reluctant to see the nurse as a diagnostician. My use of *team* and *diagnosis* here recognizes that insofar as accuracy and validity of clinical observations and scope and continuity of management are relevant to diagnosis and treatment, and insofar as the nurse accurately validates observations and adds scope and continuity in management, the nurse and physician are interdependent, responsible, and authoritative. They are both clinicians in assessing the clinical variables at the bedside, in the clinic, or in the home and in making clinical judgments about the therapeutic management of patient care. Imperative in the concept of role expansion based on clinical decision-making is the acknowledgment that the nurse in expanded practice prescribes nursing care as independently as the medical clinician prescribes medical therapy. The fundamental strategies for this expansion must be derived from direct clinical experience with patients and from enhanced competencies in the methods and techniques of precise and objective clinical appraisal.

Defining expanding nursing practice as expansion in the scope and methodologies of clinical decision-making turns our attention to the complexities of clinical judgments. How does the nurse acquire the clinical evidence to support her clinical judgments? One of the reasons for the selective ignorance practiced by nurses in restricting their clinical judgments has been the failure to distinguish between the different types of observational data and to understand the rigor of the reasoning processes that characterize the total diagnostic procedure. Feinstein [4] has examined the nature of clinical judgments and has identified the kinds of clinical data and relationships among them that constitute the intellectual technology of decision-making. There are data that describe disease in impersonal terms (morphologic, clinical, microbiologic, and physiologic), data that describe the host in whom disease occurs, and data that describe the interaction between the disease and its host. Feinstein has proposed that the first be referred to as the evaluation of the disease, the second as evaluation of the patient as a person, and the last, as the evaluation of illness, i.e., the consequences of pathological processes in the patient.

Nurses tend to make gestalt observations and inferences and also to couch their observations and judgments in guarded and tentative language. "A good day," "usual night," "seems anxious" typify the all too familiar subjective and unsubstantiated documentation of patient response. The ability to make objective and measurable observations and to process them through systematic reasoning will distinguish the nurse in expanded practice. In processing clinical information and in making clinical decisions, important distinctions must be made between pure description, designation, and diagnosis. Feinstein [4] defines description as an account of an observed sensation, substance, or phenomenon. In designation, a name or classification is given to the observed entity. In diagnosis, the anatomic or other abnormality that is responsible for the observed entity is indicated.

The Nature of Clinical Judgment

Within Feinstein's perspective, the clinician makes two types of decisions: explanatory decisions and management decisions. Explanatory decisions are the name, mechanisms, and causes of disease or disability. Management decisions are therapeutic and environmental: the choosing and evaluating of the modes and technology of therapy, and the environmental strategies that enable the patient to adapt to the burdens of ailment and treatment. Feinstein [5] says the following about managerial decisions:

Physicians have developed a splendid clinical science for explanatory decision, mechanisms of disease, etiology and pathogenetic inquiry decisions, and a magnificent technologic armamentarium of therapy, but our managerial decisions generally continue to be made as doctrinaire dogmas immersed in dissension and doubt.

As these conflicting decisions in therapeutic management inevitably merge when nurses implement medical therapy, nursing has a significant opportunity to develop and enrich the clinical decision base of expanded practice. Nursing can and does contribute to the orderly evaluation of therapy and to the management decisions about the clinical and environmental variables observed in therapy. Donabedian [2] notes that a cursory review of the nursing literature suggests that nurses are much more systematic and self-conscious than physicians in developing quality criteria of patient care. "In contrast to studies of physician care that focus on purely technical performance, there is also greater attention to social and psychological aspects of patient management."

Increasingly utilized, Lawrence Weed's [10] approach to patient record-keeping, in which medical and nursing observations and plans of care are integrated, illustrates only one methodology, but an important one, for making conjoint diagnostic and therapeutic decisions operational. For 20 years, nursing education has emphasized the problem-solving approach in nursing care, but its effectiveness has been limited by the traditional medical record and the reliance of both physicians and nurses on spoken communication. The precise skills called for in a problem-oriented system of care are specifically those required for expanded clinical judgments.

Let me amplify my definition of expanded practice. Expanded practice within a framework of patient problems and solutions demands increased skill in clinical description, in reporting observations in objective terms, in designation of observed entities, and the development of explanatory and managerial decisions that result in significant patient care outcomes. I mean, significant in that the patient and his family will know he has benefited from nursing care as well as medical care. Rather than describing isolated symptoms or signs, or isolated behavior on the part of the patient, the nurse in the expanded perspective will designate the patient's functional and clinical status, such as ability to walk, feed himself, maintain excretory continence, participate in activities of daily living, comply with therapeutic regimens, work at a chosen occupation, and make intellectual decisions. The severity of a symptom will be indicated by an account of its concomitant effect on the patient's total function.

Even more important than developing skills in accumulating the quantitative and qualitative data base for clinical judgment is the ability to make managerial decisions, i.e., to plan and carry out care in environmental and therapeutic decisions such as how the mode and agent of therapy should be managed or modified for this particular patient in his particular situation. In addition to analyzing historical and current information about a patient's functional status, the ability to predict future clinical or environmental events will become a necessary and new skill in expanded practice. Therefore, anticipation and forecasting based on knowledge of the natural history of health and illness, growth and development, and the aging process, as well as on understanding ethnic and cultural variations, will become part of expanded clinical judgment.

PHYSICAL APPRAISAL SKILLS

At nursing's present stage of development, it will be difficult for nurses themselves, and for physicians, to accept the ultimate imperative of the concept of expanded nursing practice. For the new focus will demand a new order of interdependence and temporary dependence on physicians while the nurse learns (1) how to use diagnostic tools and reasoning and (2) the therapeutic measures to function in the decisions of cure and restoration. The dependence on the physician will occur as the nurse masters the techniques of physical examination, interview, inspection, palpation, percussion, and auscultation. The nurse moving into expanded practice will need instruction, verification, and confirmation from the physician until she appreciates the wide range of normal, understands the significance of negative data, and develops the ability to characterize symptoms specifically by the seven dimensions of bodily location, quality, quantity, chronology, setting, aggravating and alleviating factors, and associated manifestations. When problems of testing reliability of clinical observation and standardization of physical appraisal performance are resolved, the nurse will move from dependence to interdependence in physical appraisal skills.

THE NURSING PROCESS

Two challenges confront the nurse in gaining competence and mastery in expanded practice. The first challenge, the development of sound clinical judgment based on objective clinical evidence, has been discussed; the second resides in the ability to optimize the nursing process as a vehicle for expanded practice. The challenge is to transcend definitions that confine the nursing process to interpersonal or communication models. The nursing process is all these, but more. The nursing process is diagnostic and therapeutic clinical decision-making, resulting in clinical judgments that explain clinical evidence and delineate the plan and management of treatment and care.

The current debate over issues of role and function, that is, the distinction between medical and nursing practice, power, and authority, is not addressed here. The thesis here is that true expansion in nursing practice will occur within the legal definition of nursing through validated clinical judgment and in the management of therapy. The nurse as clinician will not trespass into the licensed precincts of medicine. Rather, the heretofore supporting role will become a complementary relationship consistent with the concept of the nurse "carrying out treatment and medications prescribed by the licensed physicians" and "rendering care consistent with clinical orientation, training, and experience [9]."

Meaningful expansion of nursing practice in any health-care setting is rooted in a common focus: decision-making in patient cure and care. Expanded practice demands a critical concern with clinical judgment — the ways in which decisions are made, alternative decisions are proposed, and the consequences of decisions are examined and weighed in the balance of therapeutic accomplishment and human benefit.

REFERENCES

1. Cleland V. *Nurse Clinicians and Nurse Specialists: An Overview,* In *Three Challenges to the Nursing Profession — Selected Papers from the 1972 ANA Convention.* New York: American Nurses Association, 1972.
2. Donabedian, A.   Part II. Some issues in evaluating the quality of nursing care. *Am. J. Public Health* 59:1834, 1969.
3. Extending the Scope of Nursing Practice, a Report of the Secretary's Committee to Study Extended Roles for Nurses. Washington, D.C.: Deaprtment of Health, Education, and Welfare. November 1972, p. 22.
4. Feinstein, A. R. *Clinical Judgment* Baltimore: Williams & Wilkins, 1967.
5. Feinstein, A. R.   What kind of basic science for clinical medicine? *N. Engl. J. Med.* 283:849, 1970.
6. Kelly, N. S.   The nurse's role: Is it expanding or shrinking? *Nurs. Outlook* 21:236, 1973.
7. Murphy, J.   Role expansion and role extension: Some conceptual differences. *Nurs. Forum* 9:380, 1970.
8. National Commission for the Study of Nursing and Nursing Education.   *An Abstract for Action.* New York: McGraw-Hill, 1970.
9. *Regan Report on Nursing Law* (vol. 14, No. 1)   Providence, R.I.: Medical Press, 1973.
10. Weed, L. L.   Medical records that guide and teach. *N. Engl. J. Med.* 278:593, 1968.

PHYSICAL APPRAISAL: AN ASPECT OF THE NURSING ASSESSMENT

2

Joyce Crane

A decade has passed since the concept of nursing by assessment was introduced by McCain [9]. While considered innovative in 1965, systematic nursing assessment is widely recognized and implemented today as a vital, integral part of the nursing process. There are few who would deny that systematic assessment is essential to the practice of professional nursing; that nursing is, in fact, a problem-solving process which incorporates assessment in its modus operandi. This is certainly a basic tenet in the development of new nursing roles. Yet, as nursing practice continues to expand, there is considerable discussion and debate about the depth and scope of the assessment process appropriate to nursing practice. Does expanding nursing practice dictate the need for expanded assessment skills? To what extent should physical appraisal be incorporated into the nursing role? What are the skills needed by the nurse who is engaged in physical appraisal activities? How do these skills relate to others required for systematic nursing assessment? Such questions must be contemplated and answered by those teaching and learning appraisal skills, as well as by those who employ and collaborate with this "new breed" of nurse.

WHY PHYSICAL APPRAISAL SKILLS FOR NURSES?

Increasing numbers of nurses are learning physical appraisal skills today — not only those who are preparing for nurse practitioner roles but also students enrolled in undergraduate and graduate nursing programs, the faculties in these programs, and nurses already practicing in a variety of roles and settings. With increasing regularity, nursing literature is emphasizing physical assessment. In its broadest context, the literature suggests that physical appraisal skills serve to enrich the data base from which nursing judgments are made and therefore belong in the repertoire of practicing nurses. Some authors, however, caution against placing disproportionate value on physical assessment skills themselves [8].

Physical appraisal skills are not new to nursing. Certainly, nurses working in intensive care areas have relied on physical appraisal methods to monitor alterations in patients' conditions and determine the need for nurse or physician intervention. Similarly, these skills have been utilized by nurses in a variety of other settings and to a limited extent have been a component of the nursing assessment from its inception. There is little question, however, that the trend toward expanding nursing practice has accentuated the need for expanded nursing skills for nurses in general, and particularly for those already engaged in physical assessment. Lynaugh and Bates [8] highlight several uses of these skills in nursing practice:

— to confirm hypotheses growing out of the assessment interview;
— to enhance the investigation of nursing problems;
— to increase the nurse's capacity for decision-making;
— to enable nursing management of a greater range of patient care problems.

Physical appraisal skills are requisite to those functions now recognized as inherent in the nurse's expanded role. Included among these functions are: entering people into the health care system on the basis of an assessment of health status; referral to other health care professionals; monitoring the patient's condition to detect changes or trends in his health-illness status; assessing functional abilities and assisting the patient in making necessary adaptations in his life-style; and making independent and interdependent judgments about patient care management.

To the extent that nurses use these skills to make more reasoned nursing judgments, there is justification for their inclusion within expanding nursing practice. Physical appraisal skills have rational uses for nurses if they are incorporated within the context of nursing and are not used primarily to substitute for the physician's role in physical diagnosis.

PHYSICAL APPRAISAL: AN INTEGRAL PART OF SYSTEMATIC NURSING ASSESSMENT

Systematic nursing assessment is a deliberate, problem-solving process comprising the diagnostic component of the nursing process and serving as the essential first step to its other three components: planning, implementing, and evaluating patient care. McCain [9] has defined nursing assessment as an orderly and precise collection of data about the physiologic, psychological, and social behavior (or functional abilities) of a patient. Activities inherent in this process are those of analysis and synthesis. Analysis involves the classification of and distinction between differences in data, while synthesis includes establishing relationships among data, deriving trends, and performing deductive and inductive analysis [3, 11]. The assessment process, with its subprocesses of data collection, analysis, and synthesis, culminates in the identification of functional disabilities that require nursing therapy as well as recognition of the patient's most significant functional abilities. This assessment process begins as soon as possible after the patient is admitted to the agency or on an initial home visit.

and continues as the nurse assesses and evaluates on an ongoing basis, modifying the plan of care as the patient's behavior or functional abilities change.

The process of systematic assessment places all of nursing practice on a consciously planned, problem-solving basis. In addition, it:

1. Provides a format which assures consistency in data collection.
2. Individualizes nursing care.
3. Maximizes the amount and quality of information that one can obtain from the patient in a short period of time.
4. Provides baseline information about the patient's functional abilities which can be utilized later to identify changes over time in functional status, as well as to evaluate the effectiveness of care.
5. Facilitates the establishment of an early relationship with the patient.
6. Provides a basis for decision-making regarding management of nursing care.

The primary resource for collecting data for the nursing assessment is the patient. When the patient is unable to respond or communicate, or when he is an unreliable historian, the data may be supplemented through the use of secondary resources. Secondary resources for data collection are the family or others significant to the patient, health team members, and the patient's records. The particular use of secondary resources is to validate the data collected from the primary resource [10].

The skills required by the nurse in collecting data for the nursing assessment include interviewing, observation, and the physical appraisal skills, namely, inspection, auscultation, palpation, and percussion. In early references to the process of systematic nursing assessment, data collection by the nurse was largely dependent on the use of such techniques as interviewing, direct observation, and inspection. Physical appraisal per se was primarily the physician's responsibility and generally outside the realm of nursing practice. Today, physical appraisal skills are increasingly found in the nurse's repertoire and are looked on as providing a mechanism for enriching the data base from which clinical judgments are made [6]. Physical appraisal, when incorporated as an integral part of the nursing assessment, gives credence to the nurse's hypotheses about the patient's functional abilities and disabilities; it enables the nurse to validate observations and to make reasoned judgments about patient care problems and their management. In addition, physical appraisal skills provide a dimension that enhances the evaluation of the effectiveness of nursing care through the monitoring of physiologic outcomes of care.

The prominent place that systematic assessment, including physical assessment, holds in the practice of nursing is exemplified in the flow chart in Figure 2-1, which illustrates the nurse practitioner's role in the patient-care process. Bates and Lynaugh [2] describe the patient care process as:

. . .familiar to nursing as well as medicine. Given her basic professional knowledge, the nurse gathers data, makes hypotheses, identifies problems, implements management, and evaluates the results. In the expanded role of the medical nurse practitioner, the basic process is the same, but the scope of practice and decision-making is greater.

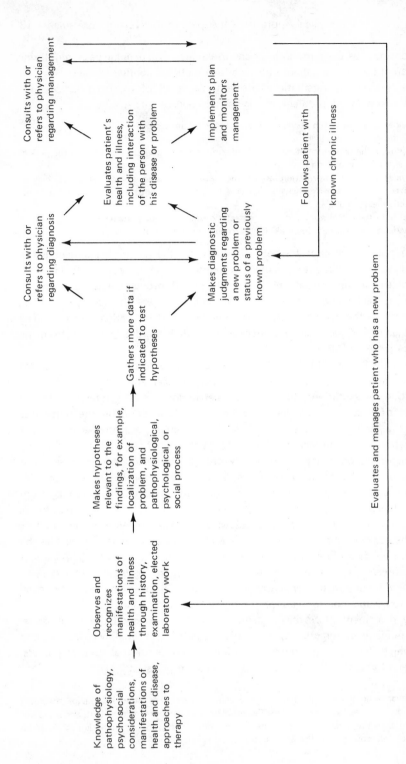

FIGURE 2-1. The nurse practitioner's role in the patient care process. (Copyright August 1973, The American Journal of Nursing Company. Reproduced with permission from the *American Journal of Nursing*, and Bates and Lynaugh [2].)

The process depicted in Figure 2-1 is one of continual interplay between systematic assessment and analysis and nursing action. Note the significant role of physical appraisal in the overall process. These authors add that their reasons for the nurse's extensive involvement in new patient assessments are as follows:

First, the process of interview and physical examination helps the nurse to establish an early relationship with the patient. The team is thus able to avoid the "separation anxiety" and dissatisfactions that both patient and physician may feel when the patient is transferred to the nurse.

Second, significant initial involvement by both professionals helps to broaden the data base and the perception of patient problems.

Third, where medical services are scarce, the physician is the bottleneck at the entry point into the system. Nursing involvement enhances access to health care [2].

SKILLS REQUISITE FOR PHYSICAL APPRAISAL

The physical appraisal examination usually follows the assessment interview and history-taking activities and consists of systematically examining the patient for physical evidence of functional abilities, or disabilities, or both. It enables the appraiser to explore hypotheses derived from the data collected during the interview, as well as to uncover new physical data.

The appraiser must be systematically thorough and deliberate in conducting the examination to assure complete and accurate data collection. Each nurse performing physical appraisal will develop her own systematic approach and should attempt to follow this procedure as closely as possible with each examination, while allowing flexibility in order to meet the patient's particular needs. In many situations it will be a new experience for the patient to have a nurse perform a physical examination. If this is the case, the patient might well find it confusing without an explanation (particularly if the physician also performs an examination). Generally speaking the appraiser should be prepared to tell the patient that the physical appraisal will be used by the nurse as the basis for planning nursing care and will be shared with the physician as it relates to the patient's need for health care within a broader context.

To become successful at physical appraisal, the nurse must not only be well versed in distinguishing normal from abnormal findings, but she must also be able to discriminate variations in normal among patients as well as ranges of normal in a given patient. In addition, Judge and Zuidema [4] refer to two irrevocably interdependent elements required for accurate and complete data collecting: the sensory or perceptual act and the conceptual process. The first step involves perceiving the sensory stimuli, while the second relates the sensory stimuli to some relevant knowledge or past experience. Performing the mechanics of physical appraisal is a relatively simple task, but relating the finding to the decision-making process that follows demands knowledge as well as rigorous training and experience.

Skills pertinent to problem-solving in general are already within the repertoire of nurses who base their practice on the process of systematic nursing assessment. Skills requisite for physical appraisal that are new to many nurses include inspection, palpation, percussion, and auscultation. Their general characteristics are described here. Other chapters of the book will discuss their specific applications to physical appraisal.

Inspection

Inspection may be defined most simply as the visual examination of the patient for detection of significant physical features. It involves detailed and focused observations coupled with comparison of the findings with established standards or norms. Critical examination should note both the general appearance of the area being inspected and its specific characteristics: the presence or absence of usual or unusual landmarks and color, texture, location, position, temperature, size, vital signs, type and degree of movement, symmetry, and comparison with the opposite side of the body. Inspection requires the nurse to discern what is normal, what is unusual but within normal range, and what is abnormal and needing attention.

While seemingly the least complex physical appraisal skill, inspection demands of the appraiser an adequate knowledge base and skill in observing. It may well be the most important technique used in the physical appraisal of a patient. Alexander and Brown [1] suggest that one should never underestimate the value of the naked eye coupled with the perceiving mind as a physical assessment tool.

Preliminary inspection begins during history-taking. However, inspection is most profitable in yielding pertinent assessment data when the appraiser gives full concentration and careful scrutiny to what is being observed. Like other techniques used in examination, inspection should be conducted in a routine, systematic fashion. While initially used alone, it is often combined with the use of other physical appraisal skills throughout the examination. Inspection and palpation are often best conducted together.

Palpation

Palpation is the process of examining the body through the use of tactile senses for the purpose of determining the characteristics of tissues or organs. More simply stated, palpation uses the sense of touch to detect physical signs. This physical appraisal technique not only involves the senses of touch and temperature but also the perception of movement (e.g., vibration), position, consistency, and form. Palpation is used to examine all accessible parts of the body, including organs, glands, blood vessels, skin, muscles, and bones. By palpation one can appraise the presence or absence of masses, pulsatility, organ enlargement, tenderness or pain, swelling, muscular spasm or rigidity, elasticity, vibration of voice sounds, crepitus, moisture, and differences in texture. Frequently, this assessment is used in conjunction with inspection.

In appraisal by palpation, it is essential that the patient be relaxed and positioned comfortably; muscular tension during the examination may interfere with the appraiser's ability to use this technique effectively or may even distort findings. Deep breathing through the mouth may enhance the patient's ability to relax during deep palpation. Tender areas should be palpated last. To maximize data collection, the appraiser should progress in a systematic manner, using a bilateral and symmetrical pattern, so that similar areas on opposing sides of the body can be compared with each other.

Tactile pressure should be applied with warm hands, in a slow, gentle, deliberate manner, first using light palpation and then progressing to deeper palpation. Different parts of the appraiser's hands are used during palpation, depending on what is being evaluated. For fine tactile discriminations, such as texture of the skin and size of lymph nodes, the tips of the fingers are used because they are the most sensitive area of the hand. For temperature, the dorsa of the hands and fingers are used because on the dorsa the skin is thinner and therefore more sensitive to temperature differences. The palmar aspects of the metacarpophalangeal joints are most sensitive to vibration. For position and consistency, the grasping action of the fingers is used. To determine rebound tenderness, ballottement is used, in which pressure is exerted on the organ and then rapidly released to assess the impact on rebound. When palpating the abdomen, particularly when using deep palpation, a bimanual technique is used. In this case, both hands are used, with a passive or "sensing" hand placed against the abdomen and the other serving as an active hand, applying pressure to the sensing hand. In this case, palpation is accomplished with the cushions and palmar surface of the sensing hand.

The successful use of palpation as a physical appraisal technique depends not only on the palpatory skills of the appraiser but also on the appraiser's ability to discriminate and interpret the significance of what is being sensed.

Percussion

Percussion is the striking or tapping of the body surface, lightly but sharply, to produce sounds that enable the appraiser to determine the position, size, and density of an underlying structure. The effect of percussion is both heard and felt by the appraiser. The quality of the sounds obtained vary according to the density of the underlying tissue. Percussion is particularly valuable in determining the relative amount of air or solid material in the underlying lung and the boundaries of organs or parts of the body that differ in structural density. Borders of certain organs, such as the heart, can be mapped out by gradually comparing densities in the organ with surrounding tissues. Percussion can also be used to ascertain if there is a change from normal density; for example, when a solid mass exists within a hollow organ.

Methods of Percussion.   There are two methods of percussing: direct and indirect. *Direct or immediate percussion* is performed by striking the body surface directly with the fingers, either with one finger, usually the middle or ring finger, or with several partly bent fingers held close together. This technique is particularly valuable in percussing over the clavicle or for defining the cardiac border. *Indirect or mediate percussion* is more often an appropriate appraisal tool. This technique is performed by placing the index or middle finger (which becomes the *pleximeter,* i.e., the object receiving the blow) against the body surface and with the palm and fingers remaining off the skin, using the tip of the middle finger of the other hand (which becomes the *plexor,* i.e., the object striking the blow) to strike the base of the distal phalanx of the pleximeter finger. To execute this movement properly, strike a quick, sharp stroke with the middle finger, holding the forearm stationary and making the striking motion, using the wrist. If the blow is not sharp, the sound will be damped. The plexor is withdrawn immediately to prevent attenuation of vibrations. The lightest blow that produces the desired sound is preferred. Both the sound elicited and the sense of resistance and vibration underneath the finger are evaluated. Percuss gently though firmly, making a special effort to apply equal force at all points (Fig. 2-2). It will be necessary to percuss more firmly in heavy individuals.

Percussing the thorax is much like playing staccato notes on the piano, and, as in playing the piano, practice makes perfect. Practice on another person is essential in learning percussion skills, but you can begin practice with a few simple exercises done by yourself. Practice flexing the wrist while keeping the

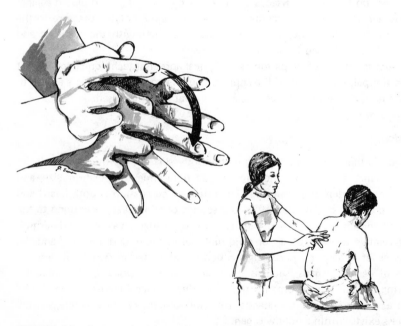

FIGURE 2-2.   Basic method for mediate percussion of the chest. (Modified from Judge and Zuidema [4].)

forearm stationary by placing your hand and forearm on a table and striking the surface of the table with the tip of your middle finger. Use individual blows so that you are sure you are quickly rebounding to the flexed wrist position. You might want to also practice percussing your thigh and other parts of the body, such as the thorax and abdomen, to become familiar with percussion of a less firm surface and to compare differences in sounds elicited.

There are several common errors of percussion which should be avoided:

1. Make sure that only the distal phalanx of the pleximeter is resting on the body surface.
2. The pleximeter must be firmly placed on the skin; if not, the vibrations will be poorly transmitted.
3. Use a very short blow and rebound immediately. If the blow is not sharp, muffling of vibration may occur due to sustained pressure on the plexor.
4. Do not use too forceful a blow. Your pleximeter finger will soon become sore. More important, you should concentrate on characteristics of the sound other than loudness — pitch, duration and quality — for which lighter percussion is often superior.
5. Keep the forearm stationary and try to deliver strokes with equal force. If the motion comes only from the wrist, the momentum of the hand will generally produce strokes of equal force.
6. Do not thump repeatedly in one area. Two or three staccato blows should be all that are needed before moving the pleximeter on to another area to compare sounds.

Percussion Tones.   The tones of percussion have intensity, pitch, quality, and duration. *Intensity* of tone is determined by the amplitude of the vibration; loud tones such as those produced over the lung have a greater amplitude than soft tones heard over the heart. The *pitch,* or frequency, refers to the number of vibrations per second. The greater the number of vibrations, the higher the pitch (for example, over a consolidated lung); the fewer the number of vibrations, the lower the pitch (for example, over the normal lung). *Duration* is determined by the time period of the vibrations and is the length of time the sound lasts. *Quality* is a purely subjective characteristic but serves to distinguish the source of the sound; it varies in relation to the density of the underlying tissue. *Sonorous percussion* is used to determine the density of a specific tissue; over low-density tissue as lung, one hears a resonant sound, while over moderately dense tissue like the heart, a dull sound occurs. A flat sound, without resonance, is heard over such high-density tissue as the thigh. *Definitive percussion* is used to distinguish between two structures with markedly differing densities, for example, the heart and lungs.

Percussion Notes.   Percussion notes are most difficult to describe with words and can actually be comprehended only after hearing them. They are classified into the following qualities that reveal certain acoustic characteristics of tone:

Resonance.   *Resonance* is the clear hollow note which is the normal sound in lung percussion. It is low-pitched, well sustained, and, although not loud, is heard with ease. The resonant note is always longer than the flat note and has a more definite and lower pitch.

Tympany.   The word *tympany* comes from tympanum, or kettle drum, and the sound is truly like the sound resulting from softly beating this instrument. It is somewhat high-pitched, musical with rich overtones, clear, hollow, and well sustained. A like sound can be produced by filling the cheek with air and tapping it lightly with a finger. Tympany is higher-pitched than resonance. This seems to defy the rule that the less dense the underlying area, the lower the percussion note. However, in the stomach, the tympanic note is formed when the air in that closed chamber vibrates in unison with its elastic wall. Adding more air to the stomach is analogous to tightening the drum head — it causes greater tension and a higher pitch.

Hyperresonance.   Like resonance, hyperresonance is a well-sustained, intense sound and can be described as a cross between resonance and tympany. Hyperresonance has a lower pitch than normal resonance, since it is due to an area with greater air/solid ratio, or less density. It therefore indicates an increased amount of air, or decreased amount of tissue, or both. Hyperresonance is accompanied by a distinct feeling of vibration sensed by the pleximeter finger. It is usually pathological in origin.

Dullness.   Dullness occurs with increased density and solidity. The sound is high-pitched, short, soft, and thudding. The pleximeter finger does not receive a vibrating sensation as with resonance or hyperresonance. Variations between resonance and dullness are often termed "impaired resonance" or "slight dullness."

Flatness.   Flatness is absolute dullness, a very short, high-pitched sound which is nonmusical in quality. It has no resonance or vibration and is normally obtained when percussing over solid tissue such as the thigh.

You can demonstrate most of the percussion sounds for yourself on any normal person. First, listen to resonance by percussing the lung at the right anterior third interspace. Then have your subject exhale as completely as possible and percuss again — the note you hear should be impaired resonance. Next, have him inhale as deeply as possible, and the note should become more resonant, perhaps slightly hyperresonant. Now move down to the fourth right interspace. Here, the resonant note should be slightly impaired, due to the underlying liver. The note will become more dull as the fifth and sixth interspaces are percussed. Percussing the seventh interspace should elicit a flat note, because only the liver is present underneath.

Auscultation

Auscultation is the process of listening to sounds produced by various organs of the body for the purpose of detecting variations and deviations from their usual characteristics. This physical appraisal skill is particularly demanding for the learner since abnormal sounds are distinguishable only after the appraiser has developed a clear appreciation of the normal variations in sounds arising from body structures. In addition, the listener must understand the basic facts of sound production within the body, including the distinguishing characteristics of sounds arising in each body structure and the location in which they can be heard most clearly. Auscultation is a useful tool in appraising sounds arising from the heart, lungs, and abdomen and from bruits or murmurs in the neck and abdomen. The techniques of auscultation and the nature of the sounds specific to each of these will be discussed in detail in subsequent chapters.

Characteristics of Sounds. Regardless of location, there are four characteristics of sound to consider in auscultation: frequency (pitch), intensity (loudness), quality (timbre), and duration. These characteristics, as defined by Lehmann [5], follow.

Frequency. The frequency of a vibration is the number of wave cycles generated per second by the vibrating body. Frequency determines the pitch of the sound; the higher the frequency, the higher is the pitch of a particular sound. Low frequency vibrations produce low-pitched sounds.

Intensity. The intensity of sound is related to the height or amplitude of the sound wave produced by the vibrating object. Vibrations of high energy produce waves of high amplitude and are heard as loud sounds, for example the clanging of cymbals. A low energy system produces waves of low amplitude which are heard as soft sounds, such as the light tapping of one's fingertips on a table.

Quality. Two sounds with the same degree of loudness and the same pitch, but coming from different sources, are distinguished by their quality [timbre]. Sounds of equal loudness and pitch from different organs, such as the heart and the lungs, can be differentiated.

Duration. Duration refers to the number of continuous vibrations. As the energy given to the vibrating system is diminished by frictional resistance, the duration of the vibration is reduced. When this occurs it is known as damping. Vibrations coming from the internal organs of the body are damped by the soft tissue that cover these organs.

Types of Stethoscopes. As with percussion, auscultation can be achieved by the direct or indirect method. In the *direct, or immediate, method,* the ear is applied directly to the body surface. While this technique may be used if necessary, it is not the procedure of choice. *Indirect, or mediate, auscultation* is accomplished with the use of a stethoscope. The selection of a stethoscope is crucial to effective auscultation; many nurses will choose to purchase their own to assure adequacy of the instrument to meet their particular purposes. Stethoscopes are equipped with one or both of two general types of pickups or chestpieces: the open bell and the closed diaphragm (Fig. 2-3).

Littman [7] has described in detail the characteristics of each type of stethoscope, highlighting their inherent advantages and disadvantages. He compares the open bell chestpiece to the old-fashioned trumpet-type hearing aid. It consists of a short, cone- or funnel-shaped bell joined to a binaural headset and eartips by flexible tubing, and conducts sounds with practically no distortion. The diameter of the bell does not usually exceed one inch, therefore limiting the volume of sound it can accumulate. A larger-width bell would be unlikely to conform to the surface of the body, and the resulting leaks would minimize the air pressure vibrations within the stethoscope; these are pressure variations that are essential for the perception of sound. With the bell-shaped stethoscope, it is necessary to obtain a perfect seal with the skin, which acts as the stethoscope's diaphragm.

The closed diaphragm chestpiece is usually the preferred instrument. It is larger than the open-bell type and is sealed by its own diaphragm to form a closed system; a perfect seal with the skin is not necessary. Its larger diameter permits it to accumulate a greater quantity of sound. For this reason, it is more sensitive to faint noises. The diaphragm filters out low-frequency vibrations, so that sounds appear of higher pitch.

Combination stethoscopes with at least two chestpieces are commonly used by those who need them for precise discrimination among various abnormal sounds. The open bell is more effective for the perception of certain low-pitched sounds such as diastolic murmurs and some gallop rhythms. The closed diaphragm type is used for most screening and general purposes and, especially for the detection of high-pitched sounds, including the first and second heart sounds. It can be used to pick up most heart and lung sounds and is convenient for placement under blood pressure cuffs [7].

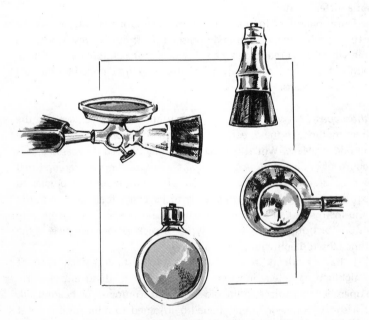

FIGURE 2-3.   The stethoscope. (Modified from Judge and Zuidema [4].)

Use of the Stethoscope. Each appraiser will develop his own procedure and sequence of steps as he learns to perform auscultation. All areas should be covered systematically and symmetrically. The room and the stethoscope should be warm, and the patient relaxed, so that involuntary muscle contractions will not occur and mask findings. Before beginning to auscultate the chest, make sure that you are in a quiet room. The level of background noise may not seem high, but very little noise is necessary to interfere with the low-intensity sounds which are important to detect on auscultation. It is important to eliminate as many extraneous sounds as possible. If the entire rim of the chestpiece does not touch the skin and a leak occurs, extraneous noise in the form of a roaring sound will be heard by the appraiser. Also, if the chestpiece is not held firmly, sounds of respiratory excursion (such as movement of intercostal muscles, joints, or skin) will be heard and may mimic a friction rub. Movement of the chestpiece over hair can produce a factitious sound that resembles rales. This can be eliminated by wetting the hair. Breathing on the tubing or sliding one's fingers over the chestpiece may also cause confusing sounds. The appraiser should purposely produce all these sounds and become familiar with them, so that they can be recognized and eliminated during the examination.

The key to successful auscultation lies in listening to one thing at a time and concentrating on what one is hearing. Auscultation is the most complex of the physical appraisal skills. To be successful in utilizing this assessment technique, the learner will need to concentrate first on normal sounds and be able to achieve the first level of discrimination in auscultation — detecting abnormal from normal sounds — before progressing to the level of discerning the nature and significance of abnormal ausculatory findings.

Recording of Data

Competency in performing the technical skills inherent in inspection, palpation, percussion and auscultation is only made manifest as it is reflected in the problem-solving process that follows. Just as the nurse must be systematically thorough and deliberate in collecting complete and accurate data, similar rigor must be employed in data analysis and synthesis. The data collected through physical appraisal must be classified and distinctions made as to what is functional versus dysfunctional as well as significant and nonsignificant. Instances where data are incomplete become evident and send the appraiser back to collect more information.

At this point, decisions must be made relative to recording these data in a logical, orderly pattern, one which condenses and concentrates the relevant findings into a usable, problem-solving form. The Weed method, described in Chapter 3, provides one such logical approach to record-keeping. Regardless of the recording format, however, the synthesis of data will be facilitated if it is kept in logical sequence and suitably condensed so as to eliminate nonessential and lengthy detail.

Analysis and synthesis of assessment data culminate in the identification of functional disabilities which require nursing action as well as those which merit referral to the physician. In addition, particular attention should also be given to the person's most significant functional abilities, those that should be maintained and fostered throughout implementation of prescribed health care regimen.

Physical appraisal findings, when incorporated within the context of a complete nursing assessment, enable the nurse to make more enlightened decisions about the individual's health care needs.

REFERENCES

1. Alexander, M., and Brown, M. Physical examination: The why and how of examination. *Nursing '73* 3:25, 1973.
2. Bates, B., and Lynaugh, J. E. Laying the foundations for medical nursing practice. *Am. J. Nurs.* 73:1375, 1973.
3. Carrieri, V. K., and Sitzman, J. Components of the nursing process. *Nurs. Clin. North Am.* 6:115, 1971.
4. Judge, R. D., and Zuidema, G. D. (Eds.) *Methods of Clinical Examination: A Physiologic Approach* (3rd ed.). Boston: Little, Brown, 1974.
5. Lehmann, J. Auscultation of heart sounds. *Am. J. Nurs.* 72:1242, 1972.
6. Lewis, E. (Ed.) A rolè by any name. *Nurs. Outlook* 22:89, 1974.
7. Littmann, D. Stethoscopes and auscultation. *Am. J. Nurs.* 65:82, 1965.
8. Lynaugh, J. E., and Bates, B. Physical diagnosis: A skill for all nurses? *Am. J. Nurs.* 74:58, 1974.
9. McCain, R. F. Nursing by assessment — not intuition. *Am. J. Nurs.* 65:82, 1965.
10. McCain, R. F., et al. Systematic Nursing Assessment. Unpublished materials developed at The University of Michigan School of Nursing, Ann Arbor, Michigan.
11. Parker, J. C., and Rubin, L. J. *Process as Content: Curriculum Design and the Application of Knowledge.* Chicago: Rand McNally, 1966.

SUGGESTED READINGS

Alexander, M., and Brown, M. Physical examination: History-taking. *Nursing '73* 3:35, 1973

Alexander, M., and Brown, M. *Pediatric Physical Diagnosis for Nurses.* New York: McGraw-Hill, 1974.

Bates, B. D. *A Guide to Physical Examination.* Philadelphia: Lippincott, 1974.

Fowkes, W. C., and Hunn, V. K. *Clinical Assessment for the Nurse Practitioner.* St. Louis: Mosby, 1973.

Traver, G. A. Assessment of thorax and lungs. *Am. J. Nurs.* 73:466, 1973.

PROBLEM-ORIENTED DOCUMENTATION OF NURSING CARE   3

Margie J. Van Meter

Historically, the nursing records of patient care have been a chronological narrative of somewhat random observations about the patient and the effects of medications and treatments, activities of the nurse, monitoring data for medical decisions, and legally pertinent facts. The nursing plan of care, the independent actions of the nurse, and the results of nursing intervention have not been consistently in evidence on the patient's permanent records. The identification of patient care problems, the degree to which they can be resolved, and the activities needed to achieve this resolution have been recorded in pencil on the Kardex and erased when no longer current. Data, then, are not available for measuring the nurse's contribution to patient welfare, comparing outcomes of various nursing interventions, or developing research programs.

The concept and role of the professional nurse is changing. The psychological and intellectual dependency of nurses is beginning to be replaced by the building of interdependent relations among health team members. This change is being reflected in the nursing records of professional nurse practitioners who want to facilitate patient care, publicly document evidence of their contributions, and leave sufficient permanency for accountability, peer review, and clinical nursing research. The nurse's records are showing evidence of the whole of the nursing process: assessment, formulation of problems, formulation of solutions, intervention, and evaluation. Nurses recognize that only as trends and patterns in patient outcomes are identified will it be possible to have objective delineation of nursing care approaches that have high probability for success [3].

A medical record system that is being widely adapted by a variety of health care settings is Weed's problem-oriented medical record system. [4]. Nurses reading current nursing and medical journals will be familiar with this documented problem-solving process. It guides the practitioner in his approach to the patient and the patient's discrete problems. The process teaches others in the health care disciplines who read the record, because clinical judgments, rationale, and results are readily discernible. This process and record system consists of four main components.

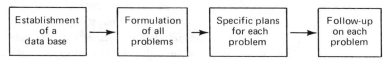

The initial data base should be as significant and complete as possible. It should include a profile of the patient's way of life, subjective symptoms, and objective findings. The compiling of the data is begun on the initial contact with the patient. The data base is standardized so that the type and quantity of data are the same for all patients, regardless of the extent of their presenting complaints.

The data provide the identification of the patient's problems. Each problem must be supported by data and stated at the level that it is understood at the time. An abnormal laboratory value or frequent crying episodes may be the levels at which problems are initially identified. There are no leaps to probable diagnoses, "rule-outs," or question marks. All the known problems are listed and given a title and number. The problem list is updated as more information is obtained: Problem titles are changed as the diagnosis evolves; new problems are identified and added; and problems are terminated when they are resolved.

A separate sheet on the front of the record lists all the problems and the number assigned each problem. This problem list serves as a dynamic table of contents to the patient's record and a summary of all the identified past and current problems. The date of identification and resolution of problems is indicated on this list.

The plan for each problem states specifically how the care planner is going to approach the problem in regard to (1) diagnostic plan, (2) therapeutic measures, and (3) patient education.

All plans, orders, subsequent data, and progress notes are recorded under the numbered and titled problem in the record. This makes it possible to determine from the record the reason for the test, the treatment, and so on.

The periodic progress notes are a record of the follow-up of the problems and the patient's responses to the planned program. The progress notes consist of narrative notes, flow sheets, and final summaries of problems. Narrative data about a problem are recorded in a structured format. SOAP is the acronym for the format.

S — subjective observations (the patient's point of view).
O — objective findings.
A — analysis of the observations. For example: Has the status of the problem changed? On what criteria?
P — plan for continued treatment, diagnosis, and patient education.

Problems with multiple and interrelated variables may be more easily followed by the creation and use of flow sheets on which values are recorded in time sequence and in relationship to therapy. Not only does this facilitate the use of the data but may avoid voluminous progress notes.

In Weed's concept, all disciplines of a health care delivery system contribute to one record and problem list. The departments of medicine, nursing, social work, and dietetics may all be assisting the patients with aspects of the same problem. With a single record and problem list, the contributions of each is seen, and redundancy of recording and effort is prevented.

A combined record is dependent on all disciplines' being in agreement with the adoption of the system, the creation of appropriate record forms, and the reorganizing of such processes as patient admission. Because of these requirements, much delay in the initiating of this effective approach will occur in some health care settings. Nurses can facilitate patient care and upgrade the quality of their documentation of care by using the process individually until the entire health care team accepts the idea of a common record and problem list. This is actually desirable for nursing because in this way nurses can learn much about their independent functions and become accustomed to public documentation of their nursing judgments, plans, and outcomes. Nurses can become as aware of and effective in their independent role as in their dependent role and make uniquely nursing contributions to the patient care process and record, beyond obtaining and recording data needed for medical decisions. Using the problem-oriented method, nurses also learn the nature of the data base needed to make nursing decisions and gain skills in obtaining and describing these data objectively. As a result of these skills, nurses will be able to contribute data of substance and significance to the common record and problem list.

The examples in the literature provide limited evidence of the nature of the data the nurse collects, how she identifies problems, and what her nursing contributions are. Elaboration of the nurse's contribution is best illustrated by an example of an experimental approach used by a nursing staff. The nursing record of a patient in one hospital setting from admission through the first few days of hospitalization is shown in Figures 3-1 to 3-6. It is presented and discussed as one useful model and as a stimulus and generator of ideas for nurses who wish to adapt the process to their practice and setting. Adaptations were made by the nurses for their particular unit and patient population. Potential users of the record will need to develop the format and process for their particular setting in harmony with their philosophy and needs. Format, use, and revisions were decided on by the staff. The nursing leaders of the unit hoped to achieve two functions by using the nursing record forms that were created. One function was to guide nurses with varying levels of abilities in the use of the process, and the second was to set the expectation that all nurses would contribute to the process.

The patient assessment presented incorporates few data from physical examination (the nurses had not yet developed these skills) and demonstrates that the nurse does not have to have highly developed physical appraisal skills or be in an expanded role to facilitate patient care through the use of the problem-oriented record. The interventions under "Goals and Actions" (Figs. 3-4 and 3-5) are independent functions of nurses, not physician-directed activities.

When the patient is admitted to the nursing unit, nursing assessment is done. "Systematic assessment of the functional abilities of a patient," developed by McCain [2], is used as the approach for data collection. The initial data are recorded on the patient profile and admission nursing assessment forms (Figs. 3-2 and 3-3).

PROBLEM LIST NURSING		1 058 771 GANNON, MARY LOUISE 6132 Riverview Palmroy, Michigan 48176	
No.	Problems (State in Behavioral Terms)	Date Identified	Date Resolved
1	Not checking pacemaker function	8-14-73	
2	Guarded ROM rt. shoulder	8-14-73	
3	Regularly uses laxative	8-14-73	
4	Tenderness of battery pack	8-14-73	
5	Lt. chest muscle twitching	8-14-73	8-17-73
6	Experiencing diagnostic work-up for brain tumor	8-14-73	
7	Vague about self-breast exam	8-14-73	
8	No communication with sons	8-17-73	
9			
10			

FIGURE 3-1. Problem list. Problems identified on admission assessment (Fig. 3-3) and new problems indicated on progress notes (Fig. 3-5) are entered here.

PATIENT PROFILE

(Description of a typical day plus Social Status Information)

Admission:

Date____8/14/73____

Time____2 PM____

    68-yr-old housewife and retired laundromat attendant. Lives with husband in own 2-story house. Bedroom and bath on 1st floor. Retirement forced by MI 2 yrs ago. Used to work from 6:30 AM to 5:30 or 10 PM. Now gets up 7:30 A M and goes to bed at 9 PM. Does housework, embroidery, and is active member of the Community Lady's Aid and Baptist church.

    Husband continues to do odd jobs for local people. He had rt. arm amputated at age 10. Has always had difficulty getting jobs even though described by wife as very capable.

    Both receive Soc. Sec. Has Medicare and Blue Cross insurance. MI and pacemaker insertion 2 yrs. ago. Battery changed 2 months ago. Admitted for first time to University Hospital for work-up for possible brain tumor.

A. Augustine, R. N.

Home phone 313-486-3291

Additions:

Date	
8/16/73	*Husband drove down alone to visit. His 2 sisters from nearby town also in to visit.* *L. Moore, R. N.*

FIGURE 3-2. Patient profile form.

ADMISSION ASSESSMENT NURSING	1 058 771
Date____8-14-73____	GANNON, MARY LOUISE 6132 Riverview Palmroy, Michigan 48176
Time____2 PM____	

Include initial observations about status of functional areas: Respiratory, Circulatory, Motor, Temperature, Nutrition, Elimination, Skin, Mental, Reproductive, Special Senses, Rest and Comfort, Emotional.

Functional Area	Observations: Subjective and Objective
Respiratory	Rate 24 during interview. Uses stairs. No DOE. Sleeps flat with
	1 pillow. Nonsmoker. No cough.
Circulatory	BP sitting Rt $^{110}/76$ Lt $^{112}/80$. Apical, rt. radial, lt. raidal pulses
	full volume, regular rhythm. 70/min.
	Hands and feet warm and pink. No pedal edema now and never
	aware of any at home.
	Pacemaker batteries changed 6/73. Does not know type of
	pacemaker or how to monitor functioning of pacemaker.
	Appointment with cardiologist in 1 month. Has fleeting, sharp,
	midchest pain occasionally, i.e., several days may pass between
	episodes, Just pauses in activity and breathes deeply.
	Several brief dizzy spells accompanied by sights and smells and rt.
	arm twitching "until batteries changed." Taking Dilantin now.
Motor	Ambulates with smooth gait and $\bar{s}$ ataxia. Arthritic pain on rt.
	side in 1968 for which took "orange pills." Rt. shoulder a little
	painful today; attributes to position when sleeping and arthritis.
	Guarded complete active ROM rt. shoulder. Slight ulnar deviation
	of both hands. R > L when closing fists.
	Good strength all extremities.
Temperature	98.6 oral
Nutrition	Regular diet $\bar{s}$ food allergies. Eating pattern 3 meals a day.
	wt 140, Ht 5'4½'' Heaviest wt. distribution around abdomen.
	Upper denture.plate. Lower teeth in good repair.
Elimination	Voids approx 4 x per day. No nocturia. Uses Exlax twice a week.
	Becomes constipated $\bar{s}$ Exlax.
Skin	3-inch incision over rt. chest. Same incision for battery change as
	for original insertion. Well healed. Tender since prone on table
	for brain scan.
Reproductive	No vaginal discharge. Last Pap smear 2 months ago. Checks
	breasts for lumps. Not specific about method or frequency.

FIGURE 3-3.   Admission nursing assessment form.

Special Senses	*Hears conversation s̄ requesting repetition. Can read newsprint*
	and bed numbers at 15 ft. Pupils equal and reactive directly
	and consensually to light.
Rest and Comfort	*Sleeps on rt. side. Supine and lt. lateral positions cause "jumping"*
	of lt. chest wall. Pulsations palpated over lt. chest when in lt.
	lateral position. Can give no possible cause; expressed concern.
Mental	*Aware reason for referral to University Hosp. was because of*
	possible brain tumor. Does not think she has tumor because in-
	formed by physician that brain scan is negative.
Emotional	*"Was pretty worried for a while." Views self as calm, hard-working*
	person. Asks no questions. Independent. Visiting with other
	patients in ward.
	A. Augustine, R.N.

No.	Problems Identified on Assessment (Place on Problem List)	Goals and Actions for Resolving Problems (Place on Kardex)
1.	*Not checking pacemaker function*	*Monitoring pacemaker function*
		Provide patient booklet on pacemakers
		Discuss with cardiology nurse specialist
		Apical pulse check, qid
2.	*Guarded ROM rt. shoulder*	*Comfortable use of rt. arm*
		To ask M.D. for A.S.A. if remains
		painful this P.M.
3.	*Laxative used regularly*	*Bowel movement qod*
		Has M.O.M. ordered. Instructed to
		request PRN
4.	*Tenderness over battery pack*	*Tenderness not aggravated by diagnostic or*
		therapeutic procedures
		Put note on chart front when sending
		to other depts.
5.	*Lt. chest muscle twitching*	*Informed of cause of pulsations*
		Discuss with cardiology nurse
6.	*Experiencing diagnostic work-up*	*Discussing diagnostic studies and their*
	for possible brain tumor	*results*
		Daily contact with A. Augustine
		Each eve inform and teach about next
		days studies
		Neurological ck q. shift
7.	*Vague about self-breast exam*	*Doing self-breast exam with correct*
		technique and intervals
		Assess further for details and teach
		after current brain tumor problem
		resolved.
		A. Augustine, R.N.

FIGURE 3-4. Form for problems identified on assessment, and goals and actions for resolving problems.

	PROGRESS NOTES NURSING		1 058 771 GANNON, MARY LOUISE 6132 Riverview Palmroy, Michigan 48176

Date Time	Number Problem	Observations: Subjective & Objective	Goals & Actions for Resolving Problems (use to update Kardex)
8/15/73	3 Laxative	MOM taken last PM and had B.M.	Pharmacy has nothing com-
		today. Does not like M.O.M.	parable to Exlax. Will discuss
		Causes gagging.	with M.D. possibility of using
			own Exlax.
			L. Moore, R.N.
4-12 PM	6 Brain	No episodes of hallucinatory	
	Tumor	smelling or sights or rt. arm	
	Work-up	twitching. 5 + strength all	
		extremities. Pupils equal and	
		reactive. BP and P continue in	
		same range. Calling nurses by	
		correct names.	
		Focused on negative brain	
		scan in discussion of possible	
		tumor. C. Farner, R.N.	
8/16	2 Rt.shldr.	Moving freely. No pain	
		No A.S.A. taken.	
		A. Augustine R.N.	
8/17	1 Pace-		Booklet given to read and will
9 AM	maker		discuss this afternoon. Cardi-
			ology nurse to visit 8/19. Con-
			sultation with Cardiology nurse
			→ Muscle twitching that occurs
			only in these particular posi-
			tions is probably the conduc-
			tion of the pacemaker impulse
			through the heart apex to the
			chest wall.
		Expressed relief and	Pt. informed
		gratitude for information	To be placed on rt. side when
			necessary to be on stretcher.
			A. Augustine R.N.

FIGURE 3-5. Progress notes form.

Date Time	Number Problem	Observations: Subjective & Objective	Goals & Actions for Resolving Problems (use to update Kardex)
	8 No com-	Two married sons in state.	Goal: Discussing meaning of no
	munication	Rarely visit parents. Once a	contact with sons to her.
	from sons	yr. is shortest interval between	
		visits of 1-2 hr. No letters or	A. Augustine to provide time
		phone calls. Youngest son	each day for her to talk.
		visited during hospitalization	
		for M.I. Oldest son did not	A. Augustine, R.N.
		communicate then. Gives	
		no reasons for sons'	
		alienation.	

FIGURE 3-5 (*Continued*)

TREATMENT ACTIVITIES NURSING															

1 058 771

GANNON, MARY LOUISE
6132 Riverview
Palmroy, Michigan 48176

Treatment ↓ Date →	8-14-73			8/15			8/16			8/17			8/18		
	12-8	8-4	4-12	12-8	8-4	4-12	12-8	8-4	4-12	12-8	8-4	4-12	12-8	8-4	4-12
Jobst stockings off ½ hr q. shift		√	√	√	√	√	√	√	√						
Diagnostic Studies		Brain Scan	EKG	U/A			EEG								
Activity															
Ambulatory-Independent		√	√	√	√	√	√	√	√	√					
Chair															
Bedrest															
Hygiene-Independent					√			√			√				
Nutrition															
Diet-Type Regular		√	√		√	√		√	√		√				
NPO															
Formula (Cal/cc) Amt															
Elimination															
Stools		o		Lg				o			o				
Voiding															

Nurse's Signature: A. Augustine, R.N.; F. Wonder, R.N.; G. Demmer, R.N.; L. Moore, R.N.; C. Farnar R.N.; G. Demmer, R.N.; A. Augustine, R.N.; K. Parker, LPN; F. Wonder, R.N.; A. Augustine, R.N.

FIGURE 3-6. Treatment activities form.

Information that may be helpful in identifying significant others in the patient's life and the nature of family and social problems and concerns and in discharge planning is obtained throughout the patient's hospitalization. For this reason the information is placed together under "Additions" on the patient profile form. This is particularly useful in the setting for which these forms were designed, a setting in which many patients cannot communicate, have extensive problems, or both.

The patient's problems identified from the initial assessment are listed (Fig. 3-4), together with the goals and nursing actions for treating and resolving the problems. The problems are listed next to the plan, so relationships can be readily seen. The problems are also placed on the problem list form (Fig. 3-1), which is the index to the patient's nursing care record.

The problems identified for nursing intervention are stated in terms of specific patient behaviors. Nursing interventions are directed toward assisting patients and families in attaining and maintaining a state of optimal functional ability (behaviors); the physician's goal is to prevent, cure, and alleviate disease. By focusing on patient behaviors, the effect of nursing on the patient's status can be determined.

These forms were designed to guide actions and to set expectations, as shown by such notations as "State in Behavioral Terms," "Place on Problem List," "Place on Kardex," and the functional areas to be assessed are listed.

Follow-up of problems is recorded on the progress notes. Observations are noted in one column and the corresponding care plan in another. This makes nurses aware of when they are recording only observations and not the care plan. The plan is translated into the familiar nursing terminology of "goals and actions." Actions include present activities, future actions, and nursing orders. The progress notes are used for ongoing data collection and evaluation of identified problems, patient data not related to identified problems, and newly identified problems. New problems are identified and recorded by placing the data in the observations column and the title (the analysis) of the problem in the problem column; each problem is also recorded on the problem list (for example, see Figs. 3-1 and 3-5). The plan is indicated under "Goals and Actions." Analysis of previously identified problems is indicated by revised goals and actions, retitled problems on the problem list, or indicating on the problem list that the problem is resolved (see problem 5, Fig. 3-1).

The dependent functions of the nurse can readily be recorded on check sheets and flow sheets; the nursing staff using the forms illustrated were also using a medications form, a fluid balance form, and a vital signs flow sheet. The goal is to avoid repetition in recording, so that available forms that are satisfactory may be retained. The treatment activities nursing form was created for more efficient recording of the services the nurse continually provides for the patient during his hospitalization. Generally, such information tends to be the major content of the nursing record. Using a system such as the one illustrated here makes readily apparent to a nurse whether she is recording only what she has done for the patient or has actually observed and recorded the patient's responses and status.

The treatment activities — nursing form (Fig. 3-6) can be used to quantify patient progress by recording such data as the number of minutes he sat in chair, the number of yards he walked, progress with his diet, or frequency of tracheostomy suctioning. If, rather than a check, these quantities are recorded in the blocks, much can be learned about the patient's status.

In the hospital setting where it is required that the responsible nurse be identified on the record for each 8-hour shift, this can be achieved by providing a convenient place for signatures on the treatment activities sheet like the slanted lines shown in Figure 3-6. The black band at the bottom edge quickly identifies these 8-hour records of each shift.

The area of most difficulty in records of this kind is problem identification. Nurses vary in their ability to see the interrelationships of multiple behaviors of a patient. A problem may have been identified at one level by one nurse, while another nurse with more limited knowledge and experience may identify components of that problem as separate problems. This difficulty is not unique to the setting or to nursing. Goldfinger [1] discusses this in a critique of the problem-oriented record. Redundancy in the problem list is less likely to occur in a primary care setting in which the nurse practitioner works with a case load of patients for whom she alone identified the nursing problems.

This record system does not automatically ensure superb nursing care nor make everyone an excellent practitioner. It is a tool with which comprehensiveness, continuity, and quality can be better achieved and more easily evaluated. Staff development will be needed to help groups of nurses with a variety of abilities to use the record system more effectively for patients' benefit and their own professional and clinical development.

Articulation of problem lists and summaries of acute and long-term problems and hospital and primary care settings are future goals that are essential for patient care continuity. For effective implementation of the nursing care plans that must appear on the problem-oriented record, nurses also must write on the Kardex the plans that others are to follow. Traditionally, this information was written only in "erasable" pencil on the Kardex. With the problem-oriented system the reverse is seen — the plan is entered only on the "permanent" record (under "Goals and Actions" in the records illustrated here) and not placed on the daily working records.

The major benefit of instituting the problem-oriented nursing record forms is that the system will require all nurses to collect and interpret data, develop nursing care plans, evaluate the outcome of the plans, and document their use of the nursing process. It is a dynamic process with ongoing assessment and planning.

In some hospital settings, a decision might be made to set some minimal expectations for all nurses and request the nurse or nurses with the most effective assessment skills and the best clinical judgment to begin the process by doing the initial assessment, problem identification, and plans. All nurses would contribute from that point. Most decisions are then being made by the most competent nurses.

The nurses who developed the nursing care approach described here are experiencing the rewards of writing the data in the "Resolved" column on the problem list, knowing by documented evidence that patients have progressed because of planned nursing intervention, and of being able to follow up problems without dependence on an Olympian memory (problem 7 in Figs. 3-1 and 3-4). Another benefit that is occurring is the potential for examining patient outcomes from the plan of care. The ability to audit nursing records is an important step in making possible the establishment and evaluation of standards of nursing care in terms of patient outcomes and in facilitating clinical nursing research.

REFERENCES

1. Goldfinger, S. E. The problem-oriented record: A critique from a believer. *N. Engl. J. Med.* 288:606, 1973.
2. McCain, R. F. Nursing by assessment, not intuition. *Am. J. Nurs.* 65:82, 1965.
3. Stevens, B. J. Why won't nurses write nursing care plans? *J. Nurs. Adm.* 2:66, 1972.
4. Weed, L. Medical records that guide and teach. *N. Engl. J. Med.* 278:593, 1968.

THE USE OF COMPUTERS AND DECISION THEORY TO ENHANCE AND MEASURE THE EFFECTIVENESS OF NURSING APPRAISAL

4

Samuel Schultz II

As the nursing profession moves more and more into the practice of clinical assessment methods such as physical appraisal, it also will become responsible for both *assessing the accuracy* and *improving the effectiveness* of those methods. The critical nature of these requirements for the profession of nursing is clear when we consider present shortages in health care manpower and ever-increasing health care costs. With the nurse performing physical appraisal, she will be initiating a great many health services, and thus the costs of health care incurred by consumers will depend on the effectiveness of her decisions. If nurses as physical appraisal practitioners are not trained to weigh the costs against the benefits or potential effectiveness of treatments, their appraisals will operate in an economic vacuum and help only to accelerate the costs of health care further. In addition, if nursing is to assess the effectiveness of its appraisal role accurately, it must do so within the full context of the whole health care system. That is, the effectiveness of nursing appraisal is dependent on what happens to the patient, and the decisions made by the nurse about the patient, after the appraisal is made. If the patient does not properly follow the decisions made by the nurse, or if the next health care professional in the patient's path through the health care system does not maximally utilize the decisions made and information gathered by the nurse the effectiveness of those nursing decisions will certainly be reduced. All these requirements for assessing and improving the effectiveness of nurse decision-making then require some technology and some expertise in applying it.

Because of the relative youth of the physical appraisal role as a major role for nursing, one would expect that a whole new area of research need be established to do these things. This is only true to the extent that for nursing per se, research in the area of physical appraisal effectiveness (PAE) is underdeveloped. On the other hand, medicine has been in the business of diagnosis for many years, and humanity has been engaged in decision-making for a much longer period. From these endeavors has developed a vast resource of technology and research in the general area of measuring and improving the effectiveness of decision-making and diagnosis. Drawing on these resources, an attempt will be made here to provide for nursing a review of these tools and how they apply to physical appraisal. These tools include *decision theory, operations research, bayesian models of decision-making, sequential decision-making, multiphasic screening, cost/benefit* and *cost/effectiveness analysis, the psychology of decision-making and information processing in general,* and the most important development of technology, *the computer.* In this chapter, a brief tutorial on the areas of technology will be provided, and their utility to nursing assessment will be interpreted. Finally, relevant research into health care decision-making using these tools will be briefly cited.

COMPUTERS AND THEIR LANGUAGES

In the main, human physical characteristics are virtually universal in their similarity, regardless of geographical location. Thus the material in this book relating to these characteristics should be usable anywhere in the English-speaking world. Unfortunately, computers and their languages (programs or software) are not so universally similar. Though the machines (hardware) are becoming ubiquitous, several of their characteristics, especially their software, prevent any large degree of universality. Just as all Fords are not alike, and all Ford Pintos are not the same, all IBMs and all IBM 360s are not the same. However, the problem with the computer is still worse. While anyone who can drive a Ford Pinto can probably drive *any* Ford Pinto regardless of options, anyone who can use an IBM 360 cannot necessarily use *any* IBM 360. There are many models of the 360 (as there are of its replacement, the 370) none of which are alike (as, for example, are two Pintos that differ only in trim), since their options (peripherals) often are a mix of models and manufacturers make them so different that each behaves like a totally unique machine.

The even greater diversity in software complicates the problem further. An IBM 360 model 50 in Detroit may "speak" a language different from that of the same model in Ann Arbor, only 40 miles away, because it has been programmed differently. (This is greatly oversimplified, since general-purpose computers often use several languages and often do so simultaneously, or in a very short period [microseconds] of time). However, the computer systems used in health care settings usually are not what one would call general purpose systems. The problem is further exacerbated by the fact that computer languages with the same name often have several versions, depending on when they were created, what type of machine they were written for, and the specific local variations in use when they were first written. Even the most universal languages (e.g., FORTRAN) have local variations which can be crucial in some computer applications. All these variations put us in a position analogous to our not being able to drive any other car than our own, even if it looks just like our own, without substantial training. This chapter will not and could not teach you how to use "the computer" (which should now clearly be seen as an imprecise term) for physical appraisal or any other problems. As Judge and Zuidema [12] state: "You cannot learn it in the library. You must do it at the bedside." Just as this book cannot adequately transmit the behavioral skills in physical appraisal, neither can it transmit computer usage skills at the practice level. Rather, the purpose of this chapter is to inform, raise problems, and suggest solutions to the overlap of roles for computers, physical appraisal, and clinical information processing in general and specifically for nursing.

Rather than leave the impression that this chapter will discuss several tools which you cannot use because of the lack of a universal language for computers, one can take comfort in the knowledge that computers are now speaking English or at least a rigid dialect of English. Further, one need not be a highly trained programmer to use a computer. Increasing numbers of applications involve "conversational" programs, ones which allow neophyte users to conduct a dialogue with the computer in English. Once you learn how to turn on the machine or "sign on" the computer (identify yourself to the computer as a valid user), usually taking a minute or so, many computer systems will teach you how to use the program you want to use.

COMPUTER ROLES IN NURSING ASSESSMENT

The computer currently has several primary roles in evaluating and enhancing nurse assessment: computer-assisted instruction in diagnosis and basic processes and functions; computer-aided decision-making (especially diagnosis); computer-aided analysis of research data (e.g., the appraisal process); and finally, computer-aided management of clinical information. The computer also plays a plethora of auxiliary roles that affect the nursing assessment role, and these will be mentioned in passing. It will be noted as well that the functions of the computer in nursing closely follow the research, practice, learning (teaching), and administrative roles of nursing.

Jacquez [11] is the preeminent resource for all readers interested in pursuing in depth the state of the art of research into computer-aided diagnosis. Another book, particularly useful for hospital applications, is that of Lindberg [16]. Finally, the *Journal of Clinical Computing* is a continuous resource of information in this area.

Computer-Aided Data Analysis

Of all the "computer applications" in nursing assessment, computer-aided data analysis is probably the least often applied, since the clinical nursing role has typically involved very little research, formal or otherwise. In the main, only nurse researchers, especially in the academic setting, are likely to use the computer-aided data analysis function. This is unfortunate, since it is precisely this ability of the computer to converse with the nurse (as a neophyte computer user) that makes it a useful tool in applied nursing settings (see Fig. 4-1 for an example of an interaction of this sort). That is, since more data will be generated and available as the computer becomes ubiquitous in various nursing settings, with the expansion of nursing roles such as assessment, it will then become imperative, as well as easier, for nurses to analyze those data in order to monitor and enhance the effectiveness of nursing procedures.

```
GO
MTS (LA01-0036)
WHO ARE YOU?

#           $COPY ◆CCHOURS
#$SIGNON K1U3
#ENTER USER PASSWORD.
?███████████
#JOB-TYPE=TERMINAL, PRIO=NORMAL, CLASS=UNIV/GOVT
#◆◆LAST SIGNON WAS: 14:03.18
# USER "K1U3" SIGNED ON AT  14:10.12 ON FRI AUG 23/74
#$RUN STAT:MIDAS
#EXECUTION BEGINS



 M I D A S
 STATISTICAL RESEARCH LABORATORY
 UNIVERSITY OF MICHIGAN
 14:11.56
 AUG 23, 1974




 COMMAND
?READ INTERNAL FILE=ALL30
 VARIABLES TO READ (E.G., 1-10)
?ALL


 READ OBSERVATIONS
 FROM INTERNAL FILE

    33 CASES READ FOR   96 VARIABLES


 COMMAND
?HISTOGRAM OPTION=HIST%
 VARIABLE(S) FOR HISTOGRAM/FREQUENCY
?8
 INTERVAL EXPRESSION -- #INT:(MIN,MAX)   (MIN,MAX)/WIDTH   #PER/(MIN,MAX)
?/500


 HISTOGRAM/FREQUENCIES

 MIDPOINT   HIST%   COUNT FOR ME9MATP$      (EACH X =1)

  9450.0     3.0     2 +XX
  9950.0     0.      0 +
 10450.      8.0     2 +XX
 10950.     16.0     4 +XXXX
 11450.     12.0     3 +XXX
 11950.     16.0     4 +XXXX
 12450.     20.0     5 +XXXXX
 12950.      8.0     2 +XX
 13450.      4.0     1 +X
 13950.      0.      0 +
 14450.      0.      0 +
 14950.      0.      0 +
 15450.      4.0     1 +X
 15950.      4.0     1 +X

 MISSING             8
 TOTAL              33  ( 500.00   = INTERVAL WIDTH)
```

FIGURE 4-1.   Conversational computer print-out from the University of Michigan Statistical Research Laboratory Midas Program. User's entries are underlined for purposes of illustrations.

The convenience of the computer as a tool further amplifies its utility. A computer terminal* is likely to become *the* essential tool of nursing, more used than charts, Kardex, or stethoscopes, and it will be used multifunctionally, not in just one, but in all of the roles mentioned. Through one terminal, nurses should be able, for example, to retrieve and analyze data, or engage in self-instruction in any area of nursing. More precisely, the nurse should be able to converse with several computer systems, depending on which function or combinations of functions are needed at a particular moment.

Computer-Assisted Instruction

As nursing moves into the appraisal role, a substantial educational effort will have evolved out of the need to develop these skills on a profession-wide basis. This book is obviously one part of that effort. Because most of this training will be in-service, because a great deal of instructional technology is available to help develop appraisal skills, and finally because of the likely availability of the computer at nursing stations and in other nursing environments, the "computer-as-teacher" role can be very useful to nursing.

A computer network for instruction in the health professions which is readily accessible and usable by telephone from anywhere in the United States and elsewhere is the Health Education Network Users Groups (HENUG) of the Association for the Development of Computer-Based Instruction Systems (ADCIS). It links the vast resources of Massachusetts General Hospital (MGH) Computer Science Laboratory and Ohio State University Medical Center to users of the network. Figure 4-2 shows an MGH program for instruction in cardiopulmonary resuscitation, a simulated encounter with a patient who has had cardiopulmonary failure of some sort, a patient who could "die" before you on the computer terminal unless proper action were taken. It is this kind of patient-encounter simulation which typifies the reality orientation of the MGH programs and which makes them so effective instructionally. This technique could certainly be applied to nursing assessment. Most of the programs give either a running account of the effectiveness of an action or a diagnosis or a recapitulation in full detail after the encounter is over. Currently, some nursing assessment programs are being developed by the nursing staff at the MGH Computer Science Laboratory.

The programs at Ohio State University are more numerous and more traditional in subject matter and approach, comprising somewhat less than 100 programs in such basic sciences as pathology and histology, as well as in applied clinical instruction. Some of these programs are more than 10 hours long, allowing users to leave and return days or hours later and begin where they left off. One could easily obtain an extensive education in the health sciences with this resource. Another program on the Ohio State system is CASE, developed at

---

*A computer terminal is essentially just a typewriter-like keyboard and some display device, such as a printer or a video screen, that allows two-way communication between an user and a computer by telephone or other communications line (see Fig. 4-3).

THE PATIENT IS AN 81-YEAR OLD MAN WHO IS 2 DAYS POST CATARACT EX-
TRACTION YOU ARE A STAT CONSULT BECAUSE THE PATIENT DOES NOT LOOK
RIGHT.
     WHAT DO YOU DO FIRST?

1.   TAKE AN EKG
2.   START AN IV
3.   CHECK MAJOR VESSELS FOR PULSES, SEE IF PATIENT IS RESPONSIVE
4.   GIVE A SHOT OF INTRACARDIAC EPINEPHRINE

> 1

     THAT WILL TAKE SEVERAL MINUTES ASSUMING YOU HAVE AN EKG
MACHINE IN THE ROOM AND LONGER IF YOU HAVE TO GET ONE. . . . .
THE PATIENT, IF TRULY ARRESTED, WILL BE BEYOND
RESUSCITATION BY THE TIME YOU DOCUMENT THE FACT.

     THE BICARB IS RUNNING. NOW IT IS TIME TO TRY SOME SPECIFICS.
LET'S TAKE A LOOK AT THE PATIENT'S RHYTHM.

THE RHYTHM STRIP IS SHOWN ON PAGE 6; IS THIS

1.   VENTRICULAR FIBRILLATION
2.   VENTRICULAR TACHYCARDIA
3.   SLOW IDIOVENTRICULAR RHYTHM
4.   ELECTROMECHANICAL DISSOCIATION

> 2

     CORRECT. NOTE THAT IT COULD ALSO BE THE SINE WAVE OF
HYPERKALEMIA, A CHOICE YOU WERE NOT OFFERED.

     THE FIRST SHOCK TOOK YOU FROM V TACH TO VF SO AN
IMMEDIATE RESHOCK IS REASONABLE, IN FACT. . .

     A FEW SECONDS OF ASYSTOLE. . .
THEN GOES TO THE RHYTHM SHOWN ON PAGE 3.
WHAT WOULD YOU LIKE TO DO. . .

1.   DEFIBRILLATE AGAIN
2.   GIVE 1 MG EPINEPHRINE IV, MASSAGE, THEN SHOCK
3.   START A LIDOCAINE DRIP THEN SHOCK

> 3

     THAT MAY WORK, THOUGH IN THE SETTING OF FINE FIBRILLATION MY
FIRST CHOICE WOULD HAVE BEEN EPI. THE XYLOCAINE IS RUNNING AT
4 MG/MIN, SHOCK, AND. . .

FIGURE 4-2.   Three different segments of a student's interaction with the Massachusetts
General Hospital Computer Laboratory cardiopulmonary resuscitation program. User's
entries are underlined for purposes of illustration.

the University of Illinois Medical Center at Chicago, a computer-aided simulation of a patient encounter which allows the user to type in free-format English as though she were speaking normally with the patient. This is currently a useful approach, but the free-format English gives an illusion of reality at the expense of the richness of a real patient encounter. Nevertheless, this is another instructional technique from which nursing appraisal could easily gain.

Few of these programs are designed specifically for nurses, although their content and style certainly make most of them useful for nursing. Also, many other institutions have computer-assisted instruction in the health sciences. Brigham et al. [3] have published a complete compendium of available programs, and those interested should read the volume and contact the relevant institution or Robert Votaw, HENUG coordinator at the University of Connecticut Health Center, Farmington, Conn. 06032 (telephone 203-674-2403).

Computer-Guided Appraisal

The computer can also serve to its maximum potential in nursing assessment as an active aid in the appraisal process, structuring and guiding the appraisal process; helping nurses make decisions about the relative weights (costs, benefits) which should be applied to signs and symptoms; and helping to combine in the most effective way all the information the nurse obtains. There is strong research evidence to show that although humans may be effective in gathering information, their ability to combine that information efficiently is usually biased and conservative — conservative in the sense that they collect more information than is necessary to establish confident estimates about the likelihood of the events, processes, or functions in question. This evidence has tremendous implications for nursing appraisal and for the usefulness of the computer in such appraisal. Nursing can avail itself of the computer in structuring the appraisal process from beginning to end: guiding the collecting of the data; helping combine the data; and producing statistically likely diagnoses with estimates of confidence about those decisions. These programs can be based on the combined opinions of the experts in the different areas of appraisal, or on existing data on the signs and symptoms usually associated with particular diagnoses, or on both. Whichever method is used, it must be made clear to nurses that the computer is a tool, not an obtrusive mechanical monster which will separate the nurse from the patient, patient care, and "true nursing" — a tool which allows the nurse to do a better, less expensive job in appraisal and to spend *more time in direct patient care activities and less in paperwork.*

Computer-Aided Nursing Diagnosis

Computer-aided diagnosis is now probably one of the least frequent yet most promising applications of computer technology in the health professions. Some reasons for its infrequent use are (1) resistance by health professionals, often because of a perceived threat to their professional territory; (2) the failure of many programs to utilize expert opinion based on past experience, in lieu of requiring years of patient data, which usually do not exist; (3) the failure of health professionals to develop a common computer language so that all parties, including the computer, can communicate; and finally, (4) the enormous stresses on the health care delivery system to *deliver* services in times of shortages rather than discovering ways to improve the delivery of those services. Again, the volume by Jacquez [11] is excellent in covering this problem area.

Two programs, each one written by nurses, are good examples of computer-aided nursing assessment. Lagina [15] has written a program which allows nurses to assess the anxiety level of preoperative surgical patients quickly. Goodwin and Edwards [9] have devised an extensive computer-aided nursing assessment program for appraisal of the skin, which conducts a conversational dialogue concerning all aspects of skin pathology and then displays a complete assessment for the patient. Unfortunately, these programs have yet to be fully adopted in any ongoing health care system. The problem seems to be that these programs are developed by nurses in academic settings, and implementing them in any existing health information system (HIS) is difficult. What is needed is a channel of communication between the nurses who write these programs and the people who design and implement HISs. Before readily available computer systems for appraisal, instruction, and so on, are found in most nursing settings, there will probably have to be economic justification for purchasing the expensive equipment needed. As nurses take a more active role in deciding the types, quality, and quantity of care they will also become responsible for these decisions and thus be required to support them empirically.

Health Information Systems

Most of the applications discussed have been somewhat peripheral in terms of their immediate justifiability in reducing the costs of health care. There is, however, one application which stands an excellent chance for such justification, namely, the health information system as implemented in some large setting (e.g., community, hospital) and referred to earlier as "computer-assisted management of clinical information." Barker et al. [1] have prepared an excellent survey of the extent of the role of these systems in many nursing settings which identifies the positive and negative attitudes of nurses toward these systems. This group defined a nursing application as [1]:

. . .a procedure which assists the nurse in decision-making via a systematic collection of data, and summarization of data utilizing electronic data processing as an interface. Development of, is the responsibility of nursing with the assistance of EDP personnel. Nursing applications may fall into any one of five categories; i.e., patient centered, personnel centered, educational, research, and miscellaneous.

Notable is the distinction between personnel- and patient-centered systems — this is surely a sign of the influence of nursing. The earliest systems, often misnamed "health care" systems, were simply accounting systems primarily for bookkeeping (revealing the background of the system designers). Now that nursing is beginning to exert its influence on how these systems are built, we are beginning to see patient-oriented systems, designed to monitor and enhance health rather than fiscal integrity.

Also notable in this report are the new expanded nurse roles mentioned, e.g., "systems analyst nurse," "coordinator, computer nurse." Perhaps the designers of these systems are beginning to realize that the nurse is really at the center of the action and the major source of information about the patient and that, because of this, these systems should be oriented more toward nursing. Some of the advantages of such systems for nursing listed in the survey were [1]:

. . ."more complete and accessible information," "improved nursing assessment," "more time for patient care," "more time at bedside," "reduce non-nursing function," and "improved educational programs."

Some criticisms were [1]:

. . ."extensive training requirements," "adaptation to change," "computer oriented rather than patient oriented," "could limit creativity," "cost of system," "getting nurse away from patient care," and "implementation problems."

Obviously, computers appear to be a mixed blessing, but we can also see some contradictions that might imply that it depends on the specific nurse and the specific computer and how much each can change to work together. This will probably occur by necessity, since these systems appear to be an economic inevitability; therefore, nursing must see that computers perform the way nurses want them to. Wesseling [20] describes the automation of the nursing history and care plan, and Farlee and Goldstein [8] describe a role for nurses in implementing these systems. Both these papers are suggested reading for those who may have to, or want to, perform such a role.

An ongoing system at the El Camino Hospital (453 beds), Mountain View, California, illustrates how one HIS works. Beginning in March, 1971, the directors of the hospital and the Technicon Medical Information Systems Corporation, also of Mountain View, signed a contract which was to design and implement probably the most extensive HIS of any hospital anywhere in the United States. The Technicon system, called MIS-I for *Medical Information System*, consists of eight basic subsystems:

1. *Admissions system* for immediate processing of admission data, including emergencies and outpatients, and patient and bed census data for location and utilization.
2. *Pharmacy system* for automated medications due list, review of past and current medication orders, with the options for unit dose, label generation, prescription records, and billing.

3. *Nursing system* which eliminates manual processing of requisitions, Kardex, charge slips, and most paperwork. It also allows patient care planning and nursing notes, with instant production of patient status, location, history, and so on.
4. *Business office system* for the standard patient billing, accounts receivable, payroll, and other fiscal functions.
5. *Physician system* which allows instant retrieval of current orders and their completion status, test results, prestored personal order sets, and immediate access to patient data in convenient format.
6. *Radiology system* for automatic prep orders, radiologic summary, and provision for reviewing the chart.
7. *Laboratory system* for capturing physician orders, placing results in the record, specimen pickup, recording tests, cumulative test summaries, and so on, and connection to automated laboratory systems.
8. *Ancillary systems* such as diet ordering and hospital diet lists, requisitions, and reporting for ECGs, EEGs, EMGs, pulmonary function tests, and inhalation and physical therapy.

Thus this system attempts to handle most of the information that is processed in this health care system. In doing so it has eliminated the many time-consuming and error-prone manual procedures too well known to health professionals.

The system is especially easy to use (the author has seen and used it) because of Technicon's Video Matrix Terminals. These computer terminals consist of a video display monitor (which resembles a small television set), a standard keyboard, and an attached light pen (see Fig. 4-3). The nurse need simply touch the word that appears on the screen in order to retrieve the information. For example, if the nurse wants the medical record of a particular person, she simply touches the words *patient list* and her particular floor, e.g., *9W,* and a patient list is displayed; she then touches the patient's *name* and *medical record* with the light pen, and the medical record for that person is displayed. If she wants a permanent printed version of that record, she simply again touches the print function word and a nearby printer prints a copy or two at the rate of 250 print characters per second. Figure 4-4 is an example of such a print-out for a patient care plan. Each nursing station has at least one video terminal and one printer, and some have more than one terminal. Terminals are used by both physicians and nurses and are also available at the other health subcenters, such as admissions and pharmacy. The important point is that both the machines (hardware) and the programs (software) have been designed expressly for and by health professionals such as nurses. In El Camino Hospital, a nurse is designated to act as a liaison between the hospital and Technicon to see that the system operates in the way nurses and others desire.

Just to dispel the idea that this could not work in a remote setting outside of a large hospital, the El Camino Hospital *does not* house *any* computer to perform these functions. The computer is located miles away and is used via telephone line connections. Thus it is possible for nurses in any setting (now, with the advent of communications satellites, including the most remote settings) to bring computing power to the patient (with a light portable terminal). Thus, computer-aided nursing appraisal can operate in any setting.

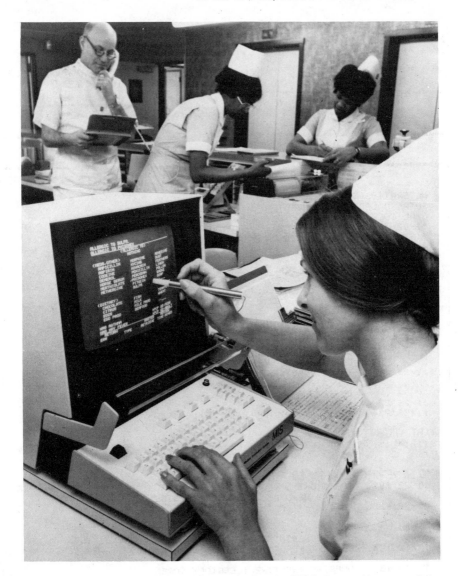

FIGURE 4-3.   Technicon Medical Information System MIS-I in use. (Courtesy of the Technicon Medical Information Systems Corp.)

```
2EAST-9583                   EL CAMINO HOSPITAL
12/5 /73  4:41 AM                    PAGE 001         000  0  0000  00000
                                                      0     0 0    0 0    0
                                                      0    0  0 0000   000
                                                      0    00000 0 0     0
                         M 48 123A                    000 0   0  0  0  00000
  A8-215084  ADM: 11/19/73
                    SERV: MED                             PATIENT CARE PLAN

             FROM  7:00 AM 12/5 /73 TO  3:30 PM 12/5 /73
```

DX:
  ULCERATIVE COLITIS
  TOTAL COLECTOMY PROCTECTOMY WITH ILEOSTOMY
  OTAL COLECTOMY PROCTECTOMY WITH ILEOSTOM,EXPL LAPAROTOMY LYSIS O
  11-02-73:TOTAL COLECTOMY, PROTECTOMY WITH ILEOSTOMY
  11-12-73:EXP. LAP LYSIS OF BOWEL ADHESIONS

VITAL SIGNS:
  11/12 122. V-SIGNS 'TIL STABLE, THEN, Q2H, X6, THEN, Q4H

DIET AND FLUID BALANCE:
  11/2   55. FOLEY CATH, CONNECT TO DRAINAGE
  11/12 125. RECORD I & O
  11/12 137. IV'S....HYPERALIMENT'N SOLN, 1000 ML, Q8H--GIVE AT
              CONSTANT RATE. DO NOT SPED UP OR SLOW DOWN: ADD TO IV
              BOTTLE, KCL-INJ, 20MEQ, IN IV, EACH BOTTLE, NACL-INJ,
              30MEQ,IN IV, EACH BOTTLE, MVI 5CC,IN IV, ONE BOTTLE--
              EACH 24 HRS
  11/23 210. IV'S....HYPERALIMENT'N SOLN: ADD TO IV BOTTLE, .K.
              ACETATE 5 MEQ,IN IV--MORE, EACH BOTTLE------ORDER CHANGE
              BY PHARMACY
  11/28 228. DIET, BLAND
  11/30 234. DIET--PT MAY HAVE TEA AS DESIRED

UNIT TESTS/EXAMS:
  11/14 151. UNIT TESTS: URINE FOR--GLUCOSE AND ACETONE, Q6H--(12-6-
              12-6)

HYGIENE/ACTIVITY/SAFETY:
  11/22 201. POSITIONING--ROLL BED INTO UPRIGHT POSITION SEV. X PER
              DAY AS WELL AS TURN SIDE TO SIDE
  11/28 229. ACTIVITY--UP IN WHEELCHAIR TID.

PROCEDURES:
  11/3   73. SUPPORTS,BINDERS: ANTI-EMBOLISM STOCKING, TOES TO KNEE
  11/12 133. RESTART NURSING:*ROUTINE DECUBITI CARE-----USE GARAMYCIN
              UNGT PRN
  11/12 135. NURSING:*ROUTINE ILEOSTOMY CARE
  11/12 138. WEIGH PATIENT NOW, STRETCHER SCALE QOD
  11/16 158. NURSING:*PT MAY HAVE DRY SHAMPOO
  11/18 166. NURSING:*PASSIVE EXERCISES AND MASSAGE OF LOWER
              EXTREMITIES AND HIPS BID
  11/22 202. NURSING:*COUGHING AND DEEP BREATHING Q 2 HRS DURNG
              WAKING HRS
  11/27 222. NURSING:*DAILY SUBCLAVIAN CATH CARE . CHANGEDSG AND

                              CONTINUED

FIGURE 4-4.   Print-out of patient care plan. (Courtesy of El Camino Hospital, Mountain View, California.)

Another feature is that several facilities could use one central computer, thus lowering the cost. Technicon has utilized a backup system which can take over if the main one fails.

The El Camino system is not the only HIS, although it appears to be unique in attempting to computerize the entire hospital system at one time. In other hospital systems, like that of Massachusetts General, the designers have chosen to go in steps, computerizing one function at a time (starting with a laboratory data system first). The El Camino system is not perfect. As with all new things, it has many flaws (most of them human, by the way), but these appear to be working themselves out with the help of many competent health and computer professionals. In a current HEW project, the performance and impact of the system in Mountain View is being thoroughly examined, and one verdict on this kind of system will be in soon.

Technicon's system is not necessarily devoted to any one diagnostic or assessment method, since MIS-I allows health professionals to tailor their own idiosyncratic systems. Another system, Weed's PROMIS (Problem-Oriented Medical Information System) [19], is based on the problem-oriented method (see Chap. 3). Weed's system is a patient-oriented system, independent of a particular health care configuration or type of computer. I see no particular reason why the Weed system could not be implemented within the Technicon system because of the latter's independence of philosophy. This is, in fact, its main advantage; that as patients, professionals, and health care delivery systems change so can the computer system.

Automated Multiphasic Health Testing

Before turning to the methodology for evaluating the effectiveness of nursing assessment, one final application of computers to the health care system, namely, automated multiphasic health testing (AMHT), should be mentioned. AMHT systems have been in operation for several years and appear to be useful and successful tools. Cononi and Siler [4] discuss the role of nursing with respect to AMHT and conclude that nurses are especially well suited to staff AMHT centers in a supervisory role.

Simply defined, AMHT is the automated (computer-aided) administration of more than one health test to a person or persons. AMHT allows the full range of health data collection — from self-entry of history data by the patient to nurse-assisted entry of vital capacity data, with the computer recording total and 1-second expired volume. The experience of the Kaiser group in California has demonstrated the cost/effectiveness of AMHT, and it has become a major component of the group's health maintenance system. Thus, again, AMHT should not be seen as a professional threat but as a useful tool to aid the nurse in physical appraisal and assessment in general. If nursing now takes an aggressive role in implementing AMHT and other systems, it will serve the profession and its goals well.

Need for a Systematic Approach

In presenting the rationale for his problem-oriented approach, Weed [19] emphasized the need for systematic data collection and processing in medical diagnosis and assessment. In his critique of the traditional system, which lead to the development of the problem-oriented philosophy, he made the following eight points:

1. Physicians, seeing only a random presentation of patients for symptomatic treatment, never felt responsible for, or saw the need for, following up those patients and thus never engaged in preventive medicine.
2. This randomness of patient presentation lead to a randomness in the information recorded by physicians that never clearly defined problems and associated patterns.
3. The randomness of the information recorded prevented a full examination of the effectiveness of patient treatment.
4. The foregoing (1–3) produced an educational and licensure system dependent on a pedagogy of memory, leading to a system in which the physician's entire future performance was predicted by his knowledge at licensure time — a performance-oriented system dependent on memory.
5. It was assumed that the future physician could effectively combine isolated, specialized pockets of knowledge into a comprehensive system for patient treatment.
6. There was an imbalance between the plethora of molecular biologic studies designed to serve future patients and the paucity of useful techniques applicable to existing patients.
7. Future physicians were trained without instruction in the economic realities of the cost/benefit of treatment, which lead to enormous expenditures on the wrong problems at the wrong time, both at the clinical and basic scientific research levels.
8. All the foregoing lead to the present non-system of medical education and practice which defies uniform application of sound decision-making necessary in a world of limited resources for health care.

Weed's assessment of the history of physician education may be more or less accurate, but the importance of his message for all health professionals, including nurses, is that health information processing and decision-making problems have been contained by a complex set of educational, research, and clinical heuristics which have evolved and demand the application of some sound principles and technology. The systematizing effect of Weed's problem-oriented method is one solution which incorporates some of these principles. The computer offers further advantages, including organization, efficiency, and rapid analysis.

Measuring the Effectiveness of Nursing Assessment

One can consider nursing assessment as being composed of several parts: (1) data collection, (2) data screening, (3) data aggregation, (4) data analysis, and (5) decision-making.

Data collection consists in a methodical accumulation of information about the patient. Techniques such as interviewing, observation, auscultation, percussion, palpation, inspection, and measurement are used. The kind of data collected depends heavily on the orientation of the collection process (e.g., problem-oriented, adaptation-oriented, health- or illness-oriented). *Data screening* is the act of eliminating irrelevant signs, symptoms, and cues and increasing the detectability of relevant ones. This, too, depends on one's theoretical bent. *Data aggregation* is the concatenation of all the isolated data into a meaningful, cohesive set. Again, how this is done depends heavily on one's theoretical orientation — "the medium is the message" presents this component's bias well. *Data analysis* is the process by which the ordered collection of data is tested for meaningfulness and significance and is concentrated into a relatively more efficient small set of indicators. Obviously, theory is crucial to this process. Finally, *decision-making* is the act of translating the processed and analyzed data into proposed alternatives for action. Theory's obvious importance cannot be overemphasized. These steps rarely occur in such a neat sequential order but rather appear as both a somewhat random and somewhat orderly chain of steps, occurring as a function of the demands of the particular problem and the sequence in which critical data appear. Nevertheless, this structuring of nursing assessment can allow us to analyze the process to determine the effectiveness of each part of the process and of the process as a whole.

What we have then is a complex of people and models (theories), some who are giving off signs and symptoms, some who are receiving, screening, and processing them, and attempts to relate patterns of them to preexisting matrices or models based on experience and theory. This process then clearly involves the biases of human information processing and judgment to a large extent.

Methods of Reducing Bias.   Much research has been done to demonstrate bias in human information processing and decision-making. The Oregon Research Institute is devoted primarily to the study of that topic, especially as applied to clinical decision-making. Early in the 1960s, researchers at the University of Michigan, Ohio State University, and other academic centers who were studying human behavior in gambling situations began to notice that people underused the information available to them and thus did not risk bets which the odds said they should have. In other words, people are conservative decision-makers (wait for more information than they really need). Further work showed that it is the way in which people aggregate data (put it all together) that is conservative rather than the way in which they perceive the data. That is, people devalue the data not when they collect it but when they aggregate it. However, if they wait too long to make a decision based upon some continuing aggregation of the data, they clearly waste data. What this says for nursing assessment is that, like all human information processors, nurses will be likely to be wasteful (conservative) in their collection of data (appraisal), which costs money.

Edwards [6, 7] has summarized this line of research and delineated these issues and possible solutions to the conservatism problem. He mentions that training has worked to reduce conservatism, but only when the data came from the same source and were of the same nature in both the training and the test situation [7]. Another apparently more reliable solution is one of a series of methods or models proposed by Edwards, namely, probabilistic information processing (PIP). Simply described, PIP is a system in which humans in concert can protect themselves against their own conservatism. Basically, in PIP, several independent information collectors do the data collection and another independent set of human information processors estimate likelihood ratios (LRs); LRs are defined as the ratio of the probability of a symptom S given one disease D_1 to the probability of the same symptom S given another disease D_2; thus

$$LR = \left[\frac{Prob\ (S_1\ given\ D_1)}{Prob\ (S_1\ given\ D_2)}\right]$$

The LRs import is that it directly related the appraiser's evaluation of the diagnostic potential of a symptom — its ability to discriminate two diseases. The PIP model passes on the LRs for each symptom for each pair of diseases to a bayesian processor (e.g., a computer calculating via Bayes theorem). Bayes theorem is a uniquely important statistical rule for combining evidence, especially useful in clinical situations. One of its unique features is the ability to combine "subjective" estimates by expert opinion *and* objective estimates by statistical tallies, and so on, into a numerical (probability) estimate. In one form, Bayes theorem states that the revised estimate (R) of the odds (probability) favoring one hypothesis (diagnosis) over another (the estimate of the odds after considering the latest item of evidence) is equal to the prior estimate (P) of the odds made before considering the new item of evidence, multiplied by the LR of that new item of evidence; that is, R = (P) $\times$ LR. Thus, by using Bayes theorem, probabilities can be revised on the basis of new evidence.

One more fact about the appraisal process which will clarify the relationship between the PIP model, the likelihood ratio, Bayes theorem, and nursing assessment is that the assessment process is a sequential process of hypothesis formation, testing, and rejection, associated with some subjective estimate on the part of the assessor of the odds or probability of each of the various hypotheses. What occurs can be described as a tree of decision-making. An example given by Kleinmuntz [14] (Fig. 4-5) illustrates a health decision tree, in which we can see this sequential process clearly. The picture looks like an inverted tree branch (often many branches of one tree are depicted). In this example, all parts of the tree are binary, with yes or no answers. Often we must attach probabilities to each node of the tree, which reflect the odds of any of the alternatives being true.

Thus, in a PIP method of appraisal, a set of independent health professionals — nurses, physicians, laboratory and radiologic technicians — all collect their independent data. Then another set of health care experts assess the likelihood ratios for each pair of diseases for each symptom. This can often be stored on

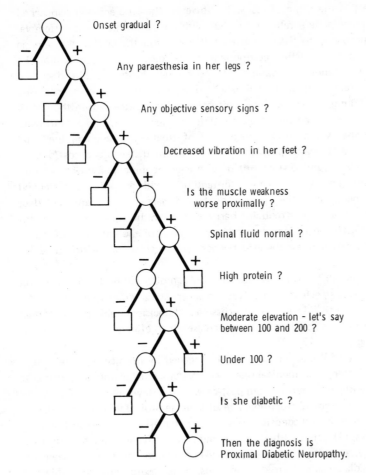

Onset gradual ?

Any paraesthesia in her legs ?

Any objective sensory signs ?

Decreased vibration in her feet ?

Is the muscle weakness worse proximally ?

Spinal fluid normal ?

High protein ?

Moderate elevation - let's say between 100 and 200 ?

Under 100 ?

Is she diabetic ?

Then the diagnosis is Proximal Diabetic Neuropathy.

FIGURE 4-5. Health decision tree.

the computer as a pool of expert opinion or population statistics. Then these data are fed to the computer as they become available for calculation of the bayesian probabilities of each of the diseases. An action-taker (therapeutic agent) then makes a decision on the basis of the probabilities. This process, too, can be put into a PIP formulation to insure that the proper therapeutic action will be taken, given the set of probabilities for the various diseases, again insuring nonconservatism in the entire assessment—therapeutic measure chain. In fact, the larger picture of the health care chain says that we feed the outcomes of each of the treatments back into our treatment model to test the effectiveness of treatment continuously.

The technicalities of the appraisal process and some of the accompanying jargon may at first glance appear to place yet another barrier between nursing and the patient in the name of research. However, they are actually concerned not with the nurse-patient relationship but with cost/benefit and cost/effectiveness. Their purpose is to determine the following: For the cost of the nursing appraisal and of each further component of the health care system that the nursing appraisal sends the patient to, how much health benefit does the patient receive (e.g., increased nonhospital days, days without pain, increased number of productive days) and how effective is the process within the health care system (e.g., reducing the access [in time and distance] of the patient from entrance into the system to the beginning of treatment; reducing the total system cost for that health problem)? Nurse-patient distance and cost/benefit are definitely related, but one cannot be dismissed at the expense of the other. Competent nursing professionals must contend both with the patients' social and psychological needs and the quality of health care patients are provided. Increasing patient contact or reducing barriers between the nurse and the patient alone will not sufficiently increase the health status of the patient. TLC alone will not significantly increase the effectiveness of ineffective or inefficient health care.

Obviously, the PIP model is not the only model of health information processing; nor is it a perfect model. It is, however, one attempt to maximize the effectiveness of health information processing and decision-making. A great deal of other research is underway to increase the effectiveness of human decision-making [5, 13, 17, 18].

The University of Wisconsin is presently engaged in a project to develop and evaluate a computer-aided medical diagnostic system which combines judgments by physicians with information from past cases, using Bayes theorem. Gustafson et al. [10] have presented preliminary results of the project which contrast four methods of arriving at a diagnosis: (1) subjective bayesian, using expert opinion to estimate LRs; (2) actuarial bayesian, using medical record data to form LRs; (3) hybrid bayesian, using (1) and (2); and (4) contemporary standard diagnostic techniques. In diagnosing thyroid conditions, early results show the subjective bayesian method to be superior to the contemporary standard method in percentage of disease entities identified. As more actuarial data become available, it is expected that the hybrid method will prove superior. In this project many kinds of evidence are being gathered, and much of what is being found has to do with how health professionals are trained to assess LRs. So far this project has found several differences, which depend on data clarity and availability and whether a group or individual setting is used. These results should be heeded as training programs for nursing appraisal develop.

The previous discussion encompasses much of decision theory, operations research, cost/benefit theory, and bayesian decision-making. One more important topic is that of utility and value theory in decision-making. This corpus of theories states that one should do or one does (depending on whether you think this theory is prescriptive or descriptive) things which maximize expected utility or value, where value is usually an objective, easily measured quantity, and utility is the subjective valuation of value (value can be measured in dollars, reduced bed days, and so on). There seem to be four theories here, depending on whether the probability associated with an alternative outcome is subjective or objective and whether the outcome is measured by value or utility. The theories state that if we multiply the probability of each alternative outcome by its associated value or utility if it occurs, the alternative with the largest value is the one that should be or is chosen. Figure 4-6 depicts the four theories as a function of their inputs. At this point, we shall not compare the theories, merely give an example of one, namely, the EV theory.

Figure 4-7 shows an example of a decision tree for a case in which the disease is unknown, an example given in Barnoon and Wolfe [2]. The consequences (values) are a loss of lifetime and disability, and a decision must be made to select the best treatment from five. We can see that the calculated probability of one disease, D_1, is .7 and of the other, D_2, is .3. This may have been calculated with bayesian estimates using PIP or by some other method, but we shall assume these values. The six alternative courses of action are treatments 1 through 5 and no treatment. We shall not go through the calculation here, but the alternative with the greatest expected gain (value) in life expectancy and decrease in disability is treatment 4, since it has the highest value. (This is not obvious from Fig. 4-7 but can be calculated from the tree in the figure as in [2].) Thus, not knowing which disease was present, knowing only the likelihood of the presence of each, we are able to establish that treatment which has the greatest payoff or expected gain.

Unfortunately, some of the most difficult decisions in health care decision-making involve ethical issues which are personal and difficult to quantify at best. Edwards [7] has also treated this issue but, as yet, utility theory is of little help in these cases. However, there are a great many health care problems that are quantifiable and are amenable to such analysis. Quality audits should be contrasted with such analyses to see if present decision-making follows any rational pattern such as utility theory. In any case, by putting assessment and other health care issues into such a framework they are open to analysis and quality control rather than protected and masked from an effectiveness audit.

	(Objective) Value	(Subjective) Utility
(Objective) Probability	Expected Value Theory/EV	Expected Utility Theory/EU
(Subjective) Probability	Subjective Expected Value Theory/SEV	Subjective Expected Utility Theory/SEU

FIGURE 4-6. Four decision theories.

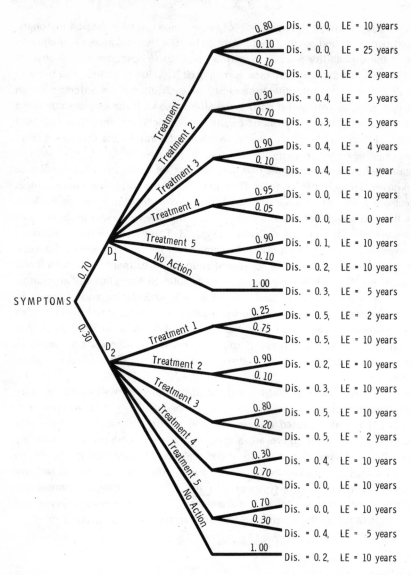

FIGURE 4-7. A decision tree for the case where disease is unknown, consequences are loss of lifetime (lifetime expectancy = LE) and disability (Dis.), and a treatment must be selected from several alternatives. (From Barnoon and Wolfe [2].)

ISSUES FOR NURSING ASSESSMENT

One of the classic problems of nursing and part of its identity problem is the "What is nursing?" issue. Some of the greatest and most informed leaders of nursing have debated this issue, and I shall not attempt to answer it here. In nursing assessment, this problem is translated into "What is nursing assessment?" What is disputed is the just territory of nursing, especially in relation to medicine. The difficulty comes when the profession faces a new role such as nursing assessment, unsure of itself, and worries about whether or not some point in the assessment process is really nursing. For example, it is often thought that nursing can do much assessment but is limited in its therapeutic alternatives. My suggestion for a solution is that nursing be patient-oriented rather than health-professional oriented and that people — nurses, physicians, laboratory technicians — perform in ways in which they are capable and not according to historical role prescriptions. What this says for evaluating the effectiveness and efficiency of the assessment process is that it should be multidisciplinary and patient-centered. It must analyze the nursing assessment role as part of the health care system. This must and can be so, even though there may be dozens of role relationships available to nurses as a function of the type and setting of various health services as they evolve with the whole health care system. The evolution of nursing assessment should not become entangled with the socioemotional role development nursing goes through as new independent nursing roles emerge.

Another issue is the reticence of nursing to examine its own effectiveness. This is changing as the nurse research role develops and as more nurse researchers are educated. Some of the problems are the overburdened state of the whole health care system in addition to the nursing role itself and a lack of perceived competence and perceived sufficient education to conduct evaluative research. *A Ph.D. is not necessary to do research* — only a willingness to solve problems and seek expert advice when it is needed. One major problem, cited by the 1973 Carnegie Commission Report on Women in Higher Education, is that the traditional societal norms have made mathematical analysis, computers, and the like nonfeminine and thus nonfemale roles. This is also changing, albeit slowly. Nursing should use evaluative research not only as a way to assess its own competency but also as a way to enhance the stature of the profession as perceived by other health care professionals. Respect is gained by those who are self-critical and engage in evaluative research.

One final issue is the current philosophical discussion over the difference between nursing as health-oriented and medicine as disease-oriented. The problem seems to be one of efficiency in the assessment process. In trying to adapt, human beings rarely concern themselves with things that work well and proceed as expected, but pay attention to and work on things that do not work well. That is, things are noticed if humans perceive that something is not as expected or not performing properly. This is called *exception orientation*. Most

TV repair technicians and plumbers, for example, work this way and have done so for a long time, probably because it is more efficient to find out what is wrong with a system than to find out what is right with it. In the health care system, physicians have been exception-oriented for good reason — it seemed to be the most efficient way. With the advent of "health" concepts we are left with the task of seeing what is right with the patient and keeping it that way, besides correcting what is wrong. This assumes enormous amounts of assessment and data collection and thus chances for human information processing errors, such as conservatism. If health orientation of nursing is to be successful it seems that only with the help of the computer and modern methods of machine-oriented information processing and decision-making can it become so at minimal cost and error to the patient. What is clearly needed is a self-examination by the nursing profession of its theories of health, health maintenance, and assessment in light of this recent technology. Perhaps both technology and the nursing profession could gain from the experience.

REFERENCES

1. Barker, M., Monroe, J. Mershimer, R., and McNamara, K.   Hospital Information Systems Sharing Group Nursing Application Study Report, 1971-1972. Ohio State University Hospitals, 410 W. 10th Ave., Columbus, Ohio 43210.
2. Barnoon, S., and Wolfe, H.   *Measuring the Effectiveness of Medical Decisions.* Springfield, Ill.: Thomas, 1972.
3. Brigham, C., Kamp, M., and Cross, K.   *A Guide to Computer Assisted Instruction in the Health Sciences* (LHNCBC 73—01). Bethesda, Md.: Lister Hill National Center for Biomedical Communications, December 1972.
4. Cononi, A., and Siler, M.   Automated multiphasic health testing in the hospital situation *J. Nurs. Adm.* 2:80, 1972.
5. Dawes, R. M.   Slitting the Decision Makers' Throat with Occam's Razor: The Superiority of Random Linear Models to Real Judges. *Ore. Res. Inst. Bull.* 12 (13): December 1972.
6. Edwards, W.   Conservatism in Human Information Processing. In B. Kleinmutz (Ed.), *Formal Presentation of Human Judgment* New York: Wiley, 1968. Pp. 17—52.
7. Edwards, W.   N=1: Diagnosis in Unique Cases. In J. Jacquez (Ed.), *Computer Diagnostic Methods.* New York: Wiley, 1972. Pp. 139—151.
8. Farlee, C., and Goldstein, B.   A role for nurses in implementing computerized hospital information systems. *Nurs. Forum* 10 (4):339, 1971.
9. Goodwin, J. O., and Edwards, B. S. A Computer Program to Assist Nursing Decision-Making. *Nurs. Res.* 24 (4):299, 1975.
   Nursing, Ann Arbor, Michigan, May 1974. To be published in *Nurs. Res.*
10. Gustafson, D. H., Ludke, R. L., Glackman, P. J., Larson, F. C., and Greest, J. H. Wisconsin Computer Aided Medical Diagnosis Project — Progress Report. In J. Jacquez (Ed.), *Computer Diagnosis and Diagnostic Methods.* Springfield, Ill.: Thomas, 1972.
11. Jacquez, J. (Ed.).   *Computer Diagnosis and Diagnostic Methods.* Springfield, Ill.: Thomas, 1972.
12. Judge, R. D., and Zuidema, G. D. (Eds.).   *Physical Diagnosis: A Physiologic Approach to the Clinical Examination* (2nd ed.). Boston: Little, Brown, 1968.

13. Kahneman, D., and Tversky, A.   On the Psychology of Prediction. *Psychol. Rev.* 80: 237, 1973.
14. Kleinmuntz, B.   Medical Information Processing by Computer.   In J. Jacquez (Ed.), *Computer Diagnosis and Diagnostic Methods.* Springfield, Ill.: Thomas, 1972.
15. Lagina, S.   A computer program to diagnose anxiety levels. *Nurs. Res.* 20: 484, 1971.
16. Lindberg, D. A. B.   *The Computer and Medical Care.* Springfield, Ill.: Thomas, 1968.
17. Slovic, P., and Lichtenstein, S.   Comparison of Bayesian and Regression Approaches to the Study of Information Processing in Judgment. In *Organ. Behav. Human Perform.* 6: 649–744, 1971.
18. Tversky, A., and Kahneman, D.   Availability: A heuristic for judging frequency and probability. *Ore. Res. Inst. Bull.* 11 (6), June 1972.
19. Weed. L.   Medical Records. In *Medical Education and Patient Care* (The Press of Case Western Reserve University). Chicago: Year Book, 1971.
20. Wesseling, E.   Automating the nursing history and care plan. *J. Nurs. Adm.* 2:34, 1972.

PHYSICAL APPRAISAL OF ADULTS

II

NURSE-PATIENT COMMUNICATION AND RELATIONSHIP IN THE PHYSICAL APPRAISAL PROCESS

5

Alice Marsden
Josephine M. Sana

The conduct of the interview is a basic determinant of the effectiveness of the physical appraisal data-gathering process and will be greatly influenced by the nurse examiner's interactional behavior with the patient. The *communication skill* used to elicit data relevant to immediate appraisal purposes and planning appropriate follow-up health care is but one of three concerns discussed in this chapter.

The nurse's primary objective is to initiate and maintain an open, mutually comfortable exchange of meaningful communication with the patient. This goal will be either notably facilitated or seriously compromised by the nature and tone of the nurse-patient relationship that the nurse establishes by choice or by chance. Our position is that the interaction of the nurse examiner and the individual (whether designated as patient, client, or consumer) for the specific purpose of physical appraisal constitutes the foundation for a *helping* or *nonhelping relationship.* Furthermore, the type of relationship established not only affects the quality of data obtained in the interview itself but also — and more important — has major impact on the process and outcomes of the physical appraisal. Ultimately, the individual's welfare is influenced. The first two major concerns consequently focus on the development of a helping relationship and the communication process as essential aspects of physical appraisal.

When the patient views the nurse examiner as a helper, then a helping relationship is more likely to occur. In this situation, the patient can experience less tension and is more apt to share his thoughts and feelings and be more informative generally. Mutual goals are then more easily identified and more readily established, and cooperative efforts are consequently more quickly realized. *Anxiety* is an additional concept that explains much behavior that the nurse examiner may experience herself, or observe in the patient, or both. It is generally recognized that a high degree of anxiety affects a person's thought processes, perceptual abilities, and physiologic functioning. These alterations can interfere with the nurse examiner's performance, or the nature of patient responses, or both. Because of the implications of an anxious state for both the patient and the nurse examiner, as well as for the establishment of effective communication and a helping relationship, anxiety is the third major topic considered in this chapter.

The environment in which the nurse and patient interact deserves early consideration by the nurse to ascertain its potential effects. Initial attention is therefore directed to the interview setting.

INTERVIEW SETTING

The nature of the place or setting in which the nurse examiner conducts the physical appraisal examination and interview will vary considerably. Although various agency settings such as hospitals, clinics, and nursing homes come immediately to mind, the importance of the home setting cannot be overemphasized. Increasingly, nurses find their practice in this environment and of necessity must adapt their assessment practices to the unique characteristics of each of a highly diversified range of homes. Each setting will provide special opportunities or problematic considerations for the nurse and the patient.

Data-gathering in a home may involve both the patient and family members, minimize the patient's apprehensions and fears, ease the establishment of the relationship, and generally facilitate the appraisal process. Adaptation in this setting may rest primarily with the nurse, challenging her skills and ingenuity often, and in new and different ways. In the hospital or clinic setting the nurse usually has the advantage. She must recognize that the patient's preappraisal experiences and the unfamiliar surroundings and people, as well as a whole range of environmental sensory inputs (often new, uncontrollable, and anxiety-provoking), will affect his responses.

Several guidelines useful to the nurse in selecting a place conducive to the interview and examination are listed below.

1. The room should provide privacy for the patient and nurse examiner.
2. The room must not be noisy or its furnishings and equipment distracting.
3. Room temperature should be comfortable for both patient and nurse.
4. Interruptions are distracting and disruptive to interaction and communication and should be discouraged by adequate planning.
5. Both the patient and nurse examiner should be comfortably seated facing each other and sufficiently close to interact in a relaxed manner.

THE NURSE-PATIENT RELATIONSHIP

A *helping relationship* is any relationship in which one person facilitates the personal development or growth of another; in which he helps the other to become more mature, adaptive, integrated, or open to his own experience (italics added) [1]. Implicit in this definition is the need for the "helper" to collect data about the "helpee" in order to identify need for and facilitate change in the "helpee." For our discussion, the nurse is considered a professional helper. This signifies that she utilizes a body of knowledge and has abilities which assist her in collecting pertinent data and developing a helping relationship at one and the same time.

In recent years, there has been considerable interst in identifying the belief systems that effective helpers have in common. Coombs et al. [6] states that "What we believe to be important inevitably determines the methods we use in dealing with people"; and in their Florida studies of the helping professions, several categories of belief systems that effective helpers have in common were suggested. It was found that effective helpers were person-oriented, holding positive views of people, e.g., considering them worthy, dependable, capable, motivated, and friendly. They tended to view themselves as self-disciplined and trustworthy and felt valued and wanted, as well as adequate. Helpers had a specialized kind of knowledge in which they were well versed; manifested commitment, involvement, and altruism; and were open and revealing about themselves [6].

The nurse committed to establishing a helping relationship will need to examine her own complex of values, beliefs, and biases for their implications for and effect on her practice.

Stages of the Nurse-Patient Relationship

The nurse-patient relationship may be described as having three phases: the initiation or orientation phase, the development or working phase, and the termination or closing phase [2, 3, 10]. Theoretically, each phase is discussed as a separate one, but in actual practice, one phase merges into another.

Initiation or Orientation Phase.   The relationship is initiated when the examining nurse orients the patient to her name, status, purpose of their meeting, and what they will be doing together. The approximate time she will spend with the patient should be indicated. Providing the patient with this information permits him the opportunity to develop realistic expectations [13] regarding the appraisal interview and examination. This phase is a time for exploration and testing of each other, and the nurse needs to be alert to her own and the patient's feelings. It is the time when communication patterns are being formed and the nurse is establishing her role as a helper. The initiation or orientation phase is the crucial preliminary to progression of the relationship.

During this beginning phase, the nurse will need to make the clinical decision to proceed with the primary purpose, the appraisal; or if she observes highly anxious behavior, to reorder priorities and assist the patient in reducing his anxiety so that the appraisal can be done.

Development or Working Phase.   This phase is the substantive body of the interaction, during which all aspects of the physical appraisal are accomplished. The ease and facility with which this phase progresses is largely dependent on the nurse examiner's having skillful interview and examination practices.

Termination or Closing Phase. Preparation for the comfortable closure of the appraisal session is begun during the orientation phase. Abrupt termination is avoided, and the patient is assured of a final opportunity to be informative or to question. Time is made available for discussion of findings and preliminary counsel regarding appropriate future care and referrals. What occurs during this time is very likely to determine the patient's impression of the entire interaction and whether or not he follows through with recommendations made by the nurse.

NURSE-PATIENT COMMUNICATION

Communication is the essence of the helping relationship, and without the use of communication skills, helping relationships could not exist. Communication is generally understood to refer to verbal and nonverbal behavior within a social (human-to-human) context [16]. It includes a message that is sent by one individual and received by another. When the message sent is understood, the sender and receiver have a shared experience, which is fundamental to any relationship. The nurse performing the physical appraisal must develop and demonstrate a working knowledge of the communication process, nonverbal and verbal, to assure and expedite the collection and interpretation of information from and about the patient.

Nonverbal Communication

It is impossible for an individual *not* to communicate nonverbally at all times. Each person communicates by his gestures, facial expressions, body posturing and movement, tone and other characteristics of voice, and even by his mode of dress [7]. The nonverbal message may be accompanied by a verbal message, and these messages may or may not be contradictory. If the verbal and nonverbal messages are congruent, the receiver will respond to the verbal message. However, when the nonverbal message contradicts the verbal one, the receiver will believe the nonverbal rather than the verbal message. An example of this is illustrated by the patient who decides that something is wrong with his heart because the nurse auscultates one area longer or repetitively despite later verbal reassurance to the contrary. Instances of this nature may be avoided or at least minimized by prior alerting of the patient to these possibilities.

Nonverbal communication is directly influenced by the beliefs we hold. An integral part of our personality, beliefs are expressed through our nonverbal as well as our verbal behavior. Becoming aware of beliefs, changing them, and acquiring new ones are part of the ongoing process of living. It is part of becoming the kind of person and professional we aspire to being. If a nurse's beliefs are similar to those of an effective helper, the establishment of helping relationships will be facilitated; if they are not, helping relationships will be more difficult to achieve, even though the nurse is familiar with communication techniques. Unfortunately, people's beliefs are not always in their immediate awareness. However, an experience may trigger into awareness a belief that the nurse never knew she had. Optimally, the nurse possesses sufficient insight into her beliefs and sufficient communication techniques and skills to conduct physical appraisal within the context of the helping relationship.

Listening

No single aspect of the communication process influences its effectiveness and success more than the quality of listening demonstrated by the nurse during the appraisal interaction. Listening is an active rather than a passive phenomenon. It involves the nurse in directing a deliberative attention to hearing and understanding the patient's frame of reference and what he is saying. It is a basic skill, requiring continuous practice to develop expertise, and unless its priority is carefully guarded, active listening may be subjugated to the nurse examiner's pressures of time, interest, or need. When the nurse is an active listener, she demonstrates her interest in the patient, her desire to understand him, and her respect for him as an individual. This approach can be sustained only if the nurse actually has these feelings for the patient.

Silence

Periods of silence are necessary and useful, albeit intolerably uncomfortable at times. Hein [9] elaborates several functions served by silence:

. . . to sift and sort the thoughts we have absorbed and file them for later use.

. . . [gives] us an opportunity to observe our patients unobtrusively.

. . . can be used for the reflection of our thoughts and the formulation of an alternate approach when the interview continues.

. . . [invites] a response . . . conveys an expectation to our patients that they can respond if given the needed time to formulate an answer.

. . . [allows] us to assess the level of anxiety in ourselves and our patients.

Recognizing these values in the use of silence and employing periods of silence in a planned way can do much to enhance communication and allay feelings of discomfort in both patient and nurse.

Skills and Techniques for Facilitating Verbal Communication

Words are the basic tools used in verbal communication. Words are symbols only and can mean different things to different people. Thus it is their meanings which must be understood and shared if successful communication is to occur. When meanings are shared, there is a feeling of understanding and being understood, and verbal exchange is a useful, productive experience.

Questioning. Multiple purposes are met by the use of questions in the appraisal interview. Hein [9] clearly states these purposes as follows:

1. To describe and elaborate perceptions, ideas, and feelings.
2. To clarify perceptions, ideas, and feelings.
3. To validate observations.
4. To substantiate facts.
5. To assess the reliability of the information received.
6. To interpret the meaning of a group of facts.
7. To compare information with some predetermined criteria (e.g., nursing goals).
8. To formulate solutions based upon previous assessments and comparisons.
9. To evaluate the outcome of a plan or action [9] .

How artfully these purposes are realized will be materially influenced by the kinds of questions asked by the nurse. Knowledge of the type of response elicited by different kinds of questions will help the nurse decide what kind of question to use.

Closed and Open-ended Questions. Two of the most common formulations of questions are the closed and open-ended types. A *closed question* asks for specific factual data and can be answered simply by a yes or no with no other information. It is especially useful in eliciting explicit confirmation or negation of a particular point. When a patient needs to conserve strength and energy, answering closed questions is the least tiring. In selective circumstances, the nurse may employ the closed question to direct and circumscribe patient response choices deliberatively. If, as is frequently the case, the nurse overuses the closed question, the patient may see this as a pattern of interaction and offer little or no additional information. A nurse with this approach would have to maintain a large repertoiré of questions.

An *open-ended question* is nonspecific in nature, cues the patient response only in a general way, and elicits expanded descriptive information. The open-ended form, exemplified by beginning a question with "what?", allows the patient to express his thoughts, feelings, opinions, and experiences. The patient has the satisfaction of communicating what he feels is important and of doing so in his own way. The responses may furnish valuable data that otherwise would not have been solicited had the nurse utilized the more confining closed question. The latitude of response that the open-ended question permits provides the nurse with more data and clues to topics for needed exploration.

The nurse can use brief phrases and words to encourage the patient to continue and expand on the descriptive information he is giving. These phrases and words are referred to as *minimal encouragers* [10] . Here are some examples:

> "Go on."
> "Tell me more."
> "Oh?"
> "So?"

"What then?"
"Um . . . m."
"And?"

Minimal encouragers are useful in that they assist the patient responding to an open-ended question to elaborate a given point. They also elicit examples of specific behaviors, helping the nurse to comprehend better what the patient is saying and to influence the direction of the interview.

"Why" Questions.   The nurse should use "why" questions selectively, recognizing that these questions call for formulations of rationale and reasons that the patient may not have worked out in his thought processes or have in mind at the time he is asked. As the patient verbalizes descriptive information during the interview, however, insights into "why" may evolve naturally, in both patient and nurse.

Benjamin [2] suggests that adult usage of the word *why* differs from that of the innocent inquiry of young children seeking information only and conveys learned negative connotations, e.g., disapproval, intimation of wrongdoing, displeasure. He postulates that "whatever the meaning intended by the interviewer, the effect on the interviewee will be predictably negative, for he will most probably have grown up in an environment in which 'why' implied blame and condemnation [2]."

Clarification and Paraphrasing.   Clarification of words and phrases is one of the most effective facilitators of verbal communication. Routinely, the nurse needs to request clarification of ambiguous terms, indefinite pronouns, and vague referents. The use of medical terminology by either patient or nurse can contribute significantly to ineffectual communication, and the user's meanings must be clarified. Identifying clearly "who, what, when, where, and how" will provide useful information and protect against erroneous interpretations.

Paraphrasing is the restatement of another's ideas in your own words. By paraphrasing the patient's words you indicate what you think the patient is saying. This technique may assist the patient in clarifying content that is confusing to him as well as to you and also serves to reassure him that you do, or are trying to, understand what he is saying.

Information-Giving and Feedback.   A patient may request information during the data collection process, and it is appropriate to furnish such information, when possible, to satisfy his need. A satisfied patient is more amenable to continuing with the physical appraisal and can be more cooperative than one kept in the dark and unduly concerned. Lengthy information-giving involvements can cut into the time available to the nurse and compromise the primary purposes and should be avoided. Generally, brief informative statements are all the patient is interested in and will meet his need. The termination phase described earlier allows time for feedback and information-sharing to take place.

Reflection of Feelings

Often during physical appraisal, the patient will manifest verbal and nonverbal behaviors suggestive of particular feeling states, e.g., discouragement, fear, unhappiness, excitement, pleasure, worry, and relief. The tone of voice, an abrupt change in conversation or demeanor, sighing, and inappropriate laughter are a few examples of such verbal and nonverbal behavior. The nurse observing these behaviors must be cognizant that they provide only *clues* to the patient's feelings and that the nature of the feelings must be validated by the patient, since feeling states are private and personal. It is important that this validating be done by the nurse. She must accept what the patient communicates verbally and modify her appraisal approach to work within his frame of reference.

Hazards of Communication

The following are some hazards which may at times constitute definite barriers to communication.

Asking Multiple Questions.   When the nurse asks two or more questions in one sentence, the patient may attempt unsatisfactorily to answer all of them as one or, since the option is his, may select the question he wishes to answer. Valuable interview time may be lost in clarifying avoidable confusions and repeating questions to recoup pertinent data.

Overuse of Open-ended or Closed Questions.   If the nurse depends too heavily on the closed question, it is likely that the interview will assume the character of a one-sided interrogation. This practice usually limits the quality and quantity of useful information obtained and creates considerable discomfort for both the patient and nurse examiner.

Overdependence on the open-ended form of question may leave the control and direction of the interview with the patient rather than the nurse. Time may be lost with extraneous content and irrelevant detail. The inexperienced nurse may find it difficult to obtain the kinds of data needed and may react in a way that the patient views as negative — to the detriment of their relationship and communication.

Responding to Multiple Ideas.   The descriptive information provided in the patient's response to an open-ended question usually encompasses multiple ideas and avenues for the nurse to explore. She may elect to encourage the patient to continue talking, judging that the topic he pursues is important to him and therefore has significance. An alternate course of action for the nurse is to respond to the topic she judges to be most clinically significant, thereby directing the interview to important data. The nurse must be alert to the hazard of not listening actively, or she will have difficulty making a deliberative choice among the options. Responding to the last idea mentioned is the tendency and should be guarded against.

An example illustrating this hazard involves a patient who responded to the nurse's request that she describe "what kinds of activities she engaged in routinely" by saying: "Up until about a year ago, I did a lot of sewing for my teen-age daughter, managed my home, helped with my husband's books, and was very active in my church." The nurse might have inquired about the events of a year ago, or specifics of the patient's home management, or the meaning of helping with the husband's books. Instead, she responded to the last idea and elicited more precise data about the church activities. This information was useful, but more clinically significant data were obtained by later inquiry into what occurred a year ago.

Imposing Values and Providing Sanctions.   Many people have a tendency to nod their heads in approval or say "Good" when another person is talking. This type of response arises from social amenities. When the nurse uses this response, she may view it as encouragement to the patient to continue. The patient, however, may construe this response as approval for what he is saying. Verbal and nonverbal mannerisms conveying approval or disapproval can, and often do, influence the kind of information the patient will share. Purposeful guarding against this is necessary, especially when the patient evidences values differing sharply from those held by the nurse.

FORMAT AND DATA-CATEGORY CONSIDERATIONS

Data collection during the interview and examination must be guided by some predetermined, organized framework to assure that the appraisal will be thorough and the data needed will be obtained. Various formats may be utilized to achieve these purposes and also to provide a systematic framework for recording the data to facilitate analysis and reference use. Format decisions will be influenced by the agency and setting in which the nurse practices and the particular needs of the patient population being served. Some uniform approach should be adopted which allows variable applications; e.g., for complete assessment on initial contact or periodically, or for partial assessment for follow-up purposes and specialized care needs.

The format should accommodate historical data, current findings, and nursing diagnoses. Information about the patient's perceptions of his health status in general and his specific concerns should be incorporated. Data about the patient as a person, his work, education, interests, family, and life-style form a category essential to include. These data permit the nurse to gain insight into the patient's real and potential health problems and the support systems available to him.

The succeeding chapters, which cover areas of system function and functional abilities important in physical appraisal, convey no absolute prescription for format but suggest some of the things nurses need to consider in deciding which format to use for the physical appraisal process. Other useful categories of data to collect and ideas about the overall framework for the interview and examination can be found in varied nursing approaches described by Little and Carnevali [12], Mayers [14], and McCain [15]. Additional helpful perspectives may be gained by examining the medical models detailed in Judge and Zuidema [11] or in Weed's problem-oriented approach [17] (see Chap. 3).

ANXIETY

Numerous theoretical frameworks can be used to aid in understanding and responding to the behavior of individuals. The theoretical concept of anxiety [4, 8, 13] is one of the most appropriate because it is generally useful in explaining much of the behavior the nurse observes. The theoretical concept also includes an operational definition of anxiety which offers additional assistance in determining the presence and level of anxiety.

The following are some specific ways in which an understanding of the concept of anxiety is helpful to the nurse during the process of patient appraisal:

1. Aids in recognizing behavior indicating anxiety in her patients.
2. Aids in recognizing behavior indicating anxiety in herself.
3. Aids determining whether or not the physical findings are more likely to be a manifestation of the patient's anxiety or of an organic condition.
4. Aids recognizing the patient's inability to give accurate data because level of anxiety impairs function, e.g., decreases ability to concentrate and narrows perceptual abilities.
5. Aids in recognizing clues indicating behavior that is used to avoid feeling anxious.

Manaser and Werner's [13] operational definition of anxiety provides a useful guide in determining appropriate nursing actions to reduce severe anxiety. Their operational definition of anxiety states that an individual:

1. Has *expectations.*
2. These *expectations are not met.*
3. Experiences *extreme discomfort.*
4. Behaves in ways to *relieve* discomfort.
5. *Justifies* his behavior verbally.

Expectations

Expectations are expressed in terms of "wants, wishes, hopes, aspirations, and desires" [14]. Many of these are expressed verbally, while others are outside awareness but can be brought into awareness as the need arises. Whether conscious or not, they are operant in our behavior.

Expectations Not Met

Expectations held may or may not be met. When circumstances evolve in harmony with our expectations, no untoward effects on our sense of comfort and well-being are experienced. Impending unmet expectations, however, can be described as a threat to the individual, to his sense of himself as a person of worth, independence, and capability. Many times, unmet expectations are expressed as disguised communications, e.g., statements of inadequacy, uselessness, being unappreciated, or thwarted [13]. Frequently, when illness or the possibility of illness occurs, the patient's expectations of continuing his accustomed life-style are challenged. New questions related to the meaning of his illness, hospitalization, and recovery and their impact on his own and family's way of living press the patient to seek new answers. Questions posed by the patient during the interview must be regarded seriously and answered as truthfully as possible to facilitate his setting realistic expectations. When the patient's expectations are unmet, his anxiety increases, and he experiences extreme discomfort.

The Extreme Discomfort of Anxiety

The extreme discomfort associated with increased anxiety usually is manifested by feelings of helplessness and powerlessness. The patient often complains of weakness, nervousness, fatigue, tension, or apprehension and uneasiness. Other behaviors indicating anxiety which may be observed by the nurse include downcast eyes and difficulty in making eye contact, slowed or rapid speech, tone-of-voice change, purposeless and restless movements, chain smoking, nail-biting, pacing, and tensed posturing.

Physiologic responses to anxiety occur in the autonomic nervous system with varying effects on the body. Figure 5-1 provides an overview of the organs in which functioning may be affected by anxiety. It is imperative that the nurse be alert for behavioral indications that the patient is anxious and that she attempt to alleviate the discomfort during the interview and throughout the appraisal. Since physiologic findings and their interpretations may be manifestations of anxiety rather than of organic dysfunction, these considerations must be incorporated into the nurse's appraisal practices.

As anxiety increases, the patient has greater and greater difficulty in organizing his thought processes and may have trouble remembering, making relationships, and comprehending during the interview [8]. Questions may have to be repeated and rephrased and more time allowed the patient to respond. The very anxious patient may be unable to provide useful data, and the nurse may have to change her priorities from collecting data to therapeutic intervention to reduce the patient's anxiety.

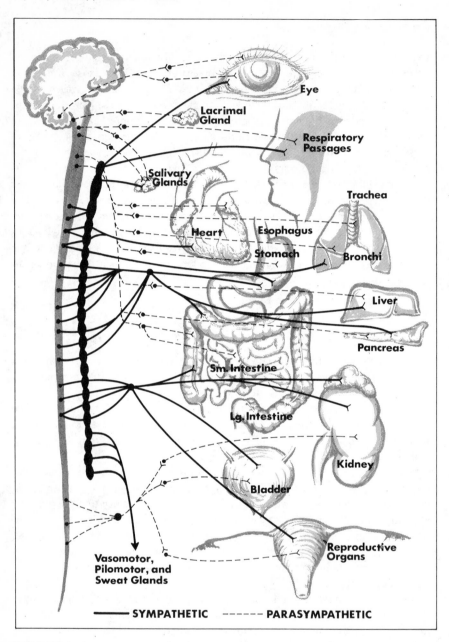

FIGURE 5-1. Organs affected by stimulation of the autonomic nervous system.

Relief Behavior

When a person is unable to reduce his anxiety, his efforts (usually outside of awareness) will be directed toward converting the distressing feelings into other behaviors that make him feel more comfortable. This provides only temporary relief, and when anxiety is reexperienced, this same pattern repeats in cyclical fashion. Some of the more commonly encountered clues to relief behaviors are listed in Table 5-1. Individual instances of relief behavior do not have particular significance. It is the behavioral pattern which is important. Byrne [5] defines behavioral patterns as "a cluster of behaviors that appear to have a common drive or goal . . . " and states that there is "a degree of repetition." It is this clustering of behaviors into discernible repetitive patterns that is significant to note, as it will influence the planning and provision of nursing care.

Table 5-1. Clues to Relief Behaviors

Relief Behavior	Clue
1. Acting out	Anger
	Annoyance
	Irritability
	Demanding
	Crying
	Inappropriate laughter, jokes, sarcasm
	Opposing actions and verbalizations
	Overdramatization and overreaction for the given situation
	Marked changes in patterns of daily activities: sleep, appetite, elimination
	Compulsive attention to details; extreme orderliness
2. Avoidance	Withdrawal, apathy, boredom, and unnaturally timed and prolonged silences
3. Somatization*	Pain syndromes
	Unusual fatigue in view of level of activity
	Headaches
	Paresthesias
	Weakness
	Paralysis
4. Verbalization	Repetitions: Reintroduces same topic repeatedly; asks same questions; gives exaggerated details about an event and/or person
	Significant omissions
	Blaming
	Self-excusing
	Intellectualizations
	Subject-changing

*Somatization is hypothesized if an organic basis is questionable and/or is contradicted by anatomic or physiologic facts, e.g., glove paralysis.

Justification

The last concept in the operational definition of anxiety is justification, exemplified in the patient's effort to give rationale to substantiate his relief behavior. It is important for the examining nurse to recognize this step to avoid becoming involved in discussing this aspect of the patient's behavior with him. This involvement is counterproductive, as no useful outcome is likely, and time is wasted unnecessarily in a misdirected effort. Within the theoretical framework of anxiety presented, nurse efforts are more appropriately concentrated on helping the patient identify the expectations he holds that are compromised. Success in these efforts permits the nurse to help the patient to set more realistic expectations and to avoid the anxiety discomfort precipitating the relief behaviors and the need for their justification.

REFERENCES

1. Barrett-Lennard, G. T.   Significant aspects of a helping relationship. *Ment. Hyg.* 47(2):223, 1963.
2. Benjamin, A. *The Helping Interview.* Boston: Houghton Mifflin, 1969.
3. Brill, N. I. *Working with People.* New York: Lippincott, 1973.
4. Burd, S. F., and Marshall, M. *Some Clinical Approaches to Psychiatric Nursing.* New York: Macmillan, 1963.
5. Byrne, M., and Thompson, L. F. *Key Concepts for the Study and Practice of Nursing.* St. Louis: Mosby, 1972.
6. Coombs, A. W., Avila, D. L., and Purkey, W. W. *Helping Relationships, Basic Concepts for Helping Professions.* Boston: Allyn and Bacon, 1971.
7. Fast, J. *Body Language.* New York: Lippincott, 1970.
8. Hays, D.   Teaching a concept of anxiety. *Nurs. Res.* 10(2):108, 1961.
9. Hein, E. C. *Communication in Nursing Practice.* Boston: Little, Brown, 1973.
10. Ivey, A. E. *Microcounseling: Innovations in Interviewing Training.* Springfield, Ill.: Thomas, 1971.
11. Judge, R. D., and Zuidema, G. D. (Eds.). *Methods of Clinical Examination: A Physiologic Approach* (3rd ed.). Boston: Little, Brown, 1974.
12. Little, D. E., and Carnevali, D. L. *Nursing Care Planning.* Philadelphia: Lippincott, 1969.
13. Manaser, J. C., and Werner, A. M. *Instruments for Study of Nurse-Patient Interaction.* New York: Macmillan, 1964.
14. Mayers, M. G. *A Systematic Approach to the Nursing Care Plan.* New York: Appleton-Century-Crofts, 1972.
15. McCain, R. F.   Nursing by assessment, not intuition. *Am. J. Nurs.* 65:82, 1965.
16. Satir, V. *Conjoint Family Therapy* (revised ed.). Palo Alto, Calif.: Science and Behavior Books, 1967.
17. Weed, L. L.   Medical records that guide and teach. *N. Engl. J. Med.* 278:593, 652, 1968.

SUGGESTED READINGS

Mitchell, P. H. *Concepts Basic to Nursing.* New York: McGraw-Hill, 1973.
Murray, R. L. E. (Ed.).   The concept of body language. *Nurs. Clin. North Am.* 7(4):617, 1972.
Ujhely, G. B. *Determinants of the Nurse-Patient Relationship.* New York: Springer, 1968.

GENERAL APPEARANCE AND SKIN BEHAVIOR

6

Phyllis Coindreau Patterson
Linda Tanner Strodtman

GLOSSARY

alopecia Loss of hair.

canthus Angle at either end of slit between the eyelids.

ecchymosis Extravasation of blood under the skin (i.e., black-and-blue spots).

erythema Redness of skin, produced by capillary congestion.

excoriation Abraded skin area.

hirsutism State of increased amounts of body and facial hair, especially in the female.

induration Area of increased tissue firmness or hardness.

intertriginous Relating to chafing of apposing skin surfaces (i.e., deep fat folds seen under breasts and in obese states).

keloid Fibrous hyperplasia, usually at the site of a scar, rounded, white or pink, and most often seen on upper trunk or face.

melanin Dark brown, insoluble organic compound, produced by the melanocyte, giving the skin its characteristic shades of brown.

nevus In the general sense, a birthmark or mole.

parotid ducts Ducts found in the posterior mucosal surface of the cheek opposite the maxillary second molar.

petechiae Pinpoint-sized hemorrhages.

pruritus Itching, or term for conditions characterized by itching.

purpura Condition characterized by the presence of confluent petechiae or ecchymoses over any part of the body.

stippling Surface irregularities or indentations indicative of normal gingivae.

stomatitis Inflammation of the mouth.

stria Streak or line (e.g., white or colorless striae on abdomen, breasts, or thighs caused by mechanical stretching of skin).

submaxillary ducts Ducts located on the floor of the mouth on either side of the frenulum of the tongue which may be seen as dark spots.

telangiectasia Dilatation of a group of small blood vessels visible through skin, often with form of a medusa's head, spider, or woven mat.

turgor State of normal or other fullness of tissue.

urticaria Smooth, slightly elevated patches which are redder or paler than surrounding skin; often accompanied by severe itching.

*The skin is an ecosystem, with a microscopic
flora and fauna and diverse ecological niches:
the desert of the forearm, the cool woods of the
scalp and the tropical forest of the armpit.*
Mary Marples [2]

Perceptions of human skin and its behavior are often narrowly focused. Skin is usually considered in terms of appearance and comfort, or as a defense mechanism, or both, with little or no attention given to it as a whole. In health it is a discrete world, or ecosystem, with its living and nonliving components all interacting with one another and existing in equilibrium. In bodily disequilibrium or dysfunction, the skin may be the cause or it may reflect the result.

Although the skin is a distinct area to assess, it is only a part of the person and thus the examiner usually forms an impression of the patient's general appearance before skin assessment is made. This composite picture gives a good indication of the individual's level of general health. After this initial impression, the character of the skin and specific areas, such as mucous membranes, scalp, and nails, are examined. It is the intent of this chapter to provide the nurse with the basic physical appraisal knowledge for this examination with the understanding that in-depth knowledge and skill will be developed by each nurse through study and experience.

GENERAL APPEARANCE

General appearance is evaluated by a series of observations. It is not unusual for a nurse to observe a patient and with little or no conversation formulate a statement that sums up his current condition. Some typical summary statements are, "The patient looks ill," "is in no acute distress," or "must be moved nearer the nurses' station as soon as possible" (for closer observation). With experience the general features or characteristics of illness are learned by the nurse. Her ability to correlate these current observations with previous nursing care experiences and knowledge determines the validity of her conclusions. However, the development of acute observational skills augments the nurse's experiential knowledge and adds insight to her current and future practice.

Since observation involves *looking,* one must know how to look and what to look at. Observation is performed in an orderly cephalocaudal direction. Information regarding not only the patient's functional abilities but also social and emotional data can be obtained by thorough visual observation. It is important to interview the patient for more detailed information, but very few questions are necessary during the general inspection. Since general inspection of an individual is all-inclusive, some guidelines for areas and features to observe are shown in the diagram in Figure 6-1. These guidelines are meant to offer a beginning outline for observation and to provide stimulating ideas upon which to expand.

Head and Face

Visual examination of the head will be used as an illustration of the interpretative process that occurs in the first few minutes of observation of a patient.

Beginning at the top of the head, the care of the hair is noted, since it is often indicative not only of personal hygiene but also of the general feeling tone, social status, body image, and identification with a social or age group (e.g., long hair may be associated with the adolescent or young adult group). When feeling ill, many women may fail to continue keeping their hair well groomed. Nurses are aware of the "lipstick sign" and the "beard sign," using them as an indication of medical or emotional improvement — women again become concerned with their appearance and apply cosmetics, and men want to shave. Occasionally, these may be signs of an attempt to mask true feelings and physical appearance. One differentiates between the two uses only by comparison with the baseline data.

When looking at the face in general, one notes its color (pasty, erythemic, pale, cyanotic), lines and wrinkles (age, expression of emotional state), nutrition (fullness of cheeks), complexion (clear, mottled, scarred, moles, hair, lesions, cosmetics), symmetry, ability to use all facial muscles, general expression, and whether or not there is eye contact. The eyes are very expressive and can be evaluated as "dull," "alert," "blank," "active," and so on, to indicate the patient's state of health and emotional state. One notes the position in which the head is held for hearing and whether or not earrings are worn. The nostrils may be flared, indicating respiratory distress. Distinct breath odors (acetone, fetid) should be noted. The condition of the mouth is also viewed as indicative of a person's health, attitudes, and emotional state; e.g., set, smiling, corners down, expressionless. The lips may demonstrate the state of health by their color (pale), texture (fissures, lesions), and movement (quivering, paralysis). Finally, one looks at the chin and observes the quantity of hair and whether the movement is set or trembling. The ability to see and perceive a great deal about a person from looking at his face can be innate, but the subtleties of the face and its expression may be learned with experience.

Continue down the body, observing and interpreting data as you collect them. Of what use is this information to a nurse? Establishment of baseline data on physical impairments as well as reactions to stress are essential for comparison with future observations. These data allow one to anticipate patient behavior and plan his nursing care accordingly. The plan should be flexible, encompassing alternative approaches, which are usually based on past successes, failures, and research findings. In addition, by observing the important aspects of a person's appearance on admission, the nurse can help the patient and his family preserve or adapt to a new body image that may be necessitated by a change in functional ability.

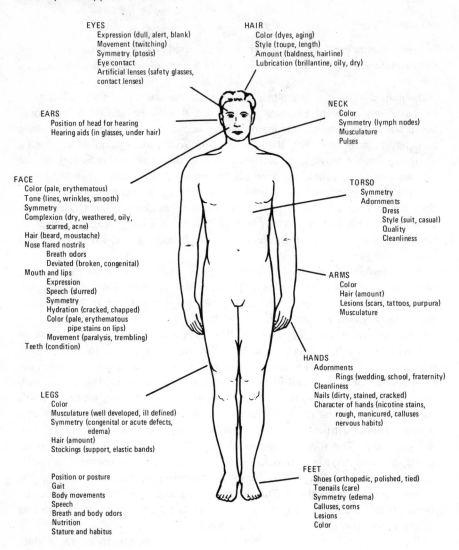

EYES
Expression (dull, alert, blank)
Movement (twitching)
Symmetry (ptosis)
Eye contact
Artificial lenses (safety glasses,
contact lenses)

HAIR
Color (dyes, aging)
Style (toupe, length)
Amount (baldness, hairline)
Lubrication (brillantine, oily, dry)

EARS
Position of head for hearing
Hearing aids (in glasses, under hair)

NECK
Color
Symmetry (lymph nodes)
Musculature
Pulses

FACE
Color (pale, erythematous)
Tone (lines, wrinkles, smooth)
Symmetry
Complexion (dry, weathered, oily,
scarred, acne)
Hair (beard, moustache)
Nose flared nostrils
Breath odors
Deviated (broken, congenital)
Mouth and lips
Expression
Speech (slurred)
Symmetry
Hydration (cracked, chapped)
Color (pale, erythematous
pipe stains on lips)
Movement (paralysis, trembling)
Teeth (condition)

TORSO
Symmetry
Adornments
Dress
Style (suit, casual)
Quality
Cleanliness

ARMS
Color
Hair (amount)
Lesions (scars, tattoos, purpura)
Musculature

HANDS
Adornments
Rings (wedding, school, fraternity)
Cleanliness
Nails (dirty, stained, cracked)
Character of hands (nicotine stains,
rough, manicured, calluses
nervous habits)

LEGS
Color
Musculature (well developed, ill defined)
Symmetry (congenital or acute defects,
edema)
Hair (amount)
Stockings (support, elastic bands)

Position or posture
Gait
Body movements
Speech
Breath and body odors
Nutrition
Stature and habitus

FEET
Shoes (orthopedic, polished, tied)
Toenails (care)
Symmetry (edema)
Calluses, corns
Lesions
Color

FIGURE 6-1. Guidelines for assessment of physical appearance.

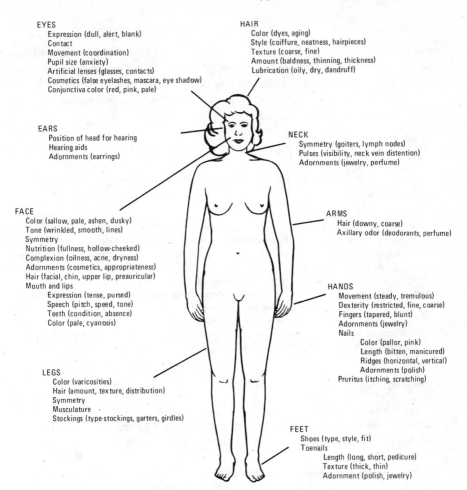

EYES
  Expression (dull, alert, blank)
  Contact
  Movement (coordination)
  Pupil size (anxiety)
  Artificial lenses (glasses, contacts)
  Cosmetics (false eyelashes, mascara, eye shadow)
  Conjunctiva color (red, pink, pale)

EARS
  Position of head for hearing
  Hearing aids
  Adornments (earrings)

FACE
  Color (sallow, pale, ashen, dusky)
  Tone (wrinkled, smooth, lines)
  Symmetry
  Nutrition (fullness, hollow-cheeked)
  Complexion (oilness, acne, dryness)
  Adornments (cosmetics, appropriateness)
  Hair (facial, chin, upper lip, preauricular)
  Mouth and lips
      Expression (tense, pursed)
      Speech (pitch, speed, tone)
      Teeth (condition, absence)
      Color (pale, cyanosis)

LEGS
  Color (varicosities)
  Hair (amount, texture, distribution)
  Symmetry
  Musculature
  Stockings (type-stockings, garters, girdles)

HAIR
  Color (dyes, aging)
  Style (coiffure, neatness, hairpieces)
  Texture (coarse, fine)
  Amount (baldness, thinning, thickness)
  Lubrication (oily, dry, dandruff)

NECK
  Symmetry (goiters, lymph nodes)
  Pulses (visibility, neck vein distention)
  Adornments (jewelry, perfume)

ARMS
  Hair (downy, coarse)
  Axillary odor (deodorants, perfume)

HANDS
  Movement (steady, tremulous)
  Dexterity (restricted, fine, coarse)
  Fingers (tapered, blunt)
  Adornments (jewelry)
  Nails
      Color (pallor, pink)
      Length (bitten, manicured)
      Ridges (horizontal, vertical)
      Adornments (polish)
  Pruritus (itching, scratching)

FEET
  Shoes (type, style, fit)
  Toenails
      Length (long, short, pedicure)
      Texture (thick, thin)
      Adornment (polish, jewelry)

Position or Posture

What type of position does the patient assume? For example, is he stretched out in a relaxed manner, or upright and tense? Does he assume this for physical needs (e.g., curls up in a splinting position to decrease pain or needs to be propped up for easier breathing)? Can he move freely? Is he restless or still, fidgety or tremulous, round-shouldered or barrel-chested?

Gait

In what manner does the patient walk, and with what aids? Possible abnormal gaits are the following:

1. Ataxic — staggering or reeling, resembling the walk of alcohol intoxication.
2. Slapping — walks on broad base with feet wide apart, raises leg high and then slaps feet on the ground. These patients fix their eyes on the ground to observe where they are going and to place their feet (e.g., as in tertiary syphilis).
3. Spastic — jerking uncoordinated movements (e.g., as in multiple sclerosis).
4. Scissors — characterized by walking with thighs close together, because of the rigidity of the abductor muscles (e.g., as in spastic paraplegia).
5. Parkinsonian — walks with the trunk and head bent forward and body held rigid. These patients take short steps with the arms held rigid. They may suddenly run forward (propulsion) or backward (retropulsion).

Body Movements

Body movements may be classified into voluntary (performs normal body activity) and involuntary (body moves in an abnormal pattern in either conscious or unconscious state). Does the patient have any of the following?

1. Tic — habit muscle spasm (usually appears in the eye, face, or neck under stress).
2. Tremor — trembling movement (often due to fatigue, parkinsonism).
3. Convulsive movements — series of violent involuntary contractions, either clonic (intermittent contraction and relaxation) or tonic (sustained contraction).

Speech

Characterizing a patient's voice may be helpful in noting dysfunction (e.g., following laryngectomy) or planning for a change in status (e.g., when administering hormones such as androgens or estrogens). The voice is evaluated in terms of strength (weak or strong, soft or loud), tone (hoarse, whining, squeaky), enunciation, and resonance.

Three basic speech defects may be encountered: (1) *aphonia,* which is a loss of voice; (2) *anarthria* or *dysarthria,* the inability to articulate distinctly (e.g., stammering or stuttering); and (3) *aphasia,* a defect or loss of expressive powers in speech, writing, and/or signs, or of comprehending spoken or written language. In motor aphasia, the patient understands but cannot repeat words or speak spontaneously. Receptive or sensory aphasia is characterized by a lack of understanding of the written or spoken word.

Breath and Body Odors

Offensive breath odors are usually associated with poor oral hygiene, dental caries, and infections in the oral cavity. Putrefactive diseases of the lungs with infected sputum (e.g., lung abscesses, bronchiectasis) may cause accompanying fetid breath. In certain diseases or metabolic disorders accompanied by metabolic acidosis (e.g., diabetes mellitis) the breath may have the characteristic sweet fruity odor of acetone. Alcoholic odor of the breath usually indicates ingestion of alcohol, but one should not overlook the possible ingestion of alcohol-containing drugs. In some uremic patients, ammonia is detectable on the breath, and severe liver disease occasionally will cause a musty breath odor.

Body odors are usually associated with personal hygiene practices but may be dependent on cultural habits. Odors are also characteristic of certain types of conditions, including wound infections, advanced carcinoma, and gastro-intestinal bleeding. It is difficult to describe these odors, but once the nurse has smelled the identified odor, she can easily recognize it on a subsequent occasion.

Nutrition

A person's nutritional state is frequently obvious and is usually evaluated in terms of overweight or underweight, to varying degrees.

Overweight, or obesity, is classified as exogenous or endogenous. The distribution of fat and its metabolic etiologies are the distinguishing character-istics. *Exogenous obesity,* usually caused by excessive caloric intake, is demonstrated by a generalized distribution of the excess fatty tissues. *Endogenous obesity,* a characteristic of certain endocrine diseases (e.g., Cushing's disease) in which fat distribution is localized to certain areas of predilection, commonly the girdle area, is not related to dietary intake.

Obesity should be differentiated from edema. Edema is demonstrated by tissues that pit (indent) when pressed with a finger. This is not present in obesity. Ascites (fluid in the abdominal cavity) can easily be distinguished from fatty tissue by eliciting the fluid wave (for description of techniques, see Chap. 11).

An underweight condition may vary in degree from mild to severe, with the severely underweight person being referred to as cachectic or emaciated. The characteristic facial appearances are sharp nose, sunken eyes, and hollow temples and cheeks. Some people are naturally slender and are not necessarily ill. When one assesses nutrition, the patient's normal body weight and the rate at which he has either lost or gained weight should be ascertained. Weight loss can occur with wasting diseases (e.g., tuberculosis or carcinoma) or as a result of anorexia secondary to the worry syndrome. Be sure to question the patient regarding weight change. The recent weight loss may be intentional and without consequence.

Included in the term *nutrition* is the tissue turgor and tone and volume of skeletal muscle. The volume or mass of the skeletal muscles can be surmised by observation and palpation (Chap 13).

Stature and Habitus

Stature is the height or tallness of a person standing. There are normal variations in height, dependent on age, sex, racial descent, and heredity. Individuals whose height is excessive are referred to as *giants.* Gigantism may be the result of hypersecretion of growth hormone. The physical characteristics of the giant are dependent on whether the hormone oversecretion occurs before or after fusion of the bony epiphysis. The former is referred to as eunuchoid gigantism and the latter, as acromegaly.

Individuals whose height is far below normal for their age and race are called *dwarfs.* Included in this category is the *midget,* who has normal proportions but on a smaller scale. Dwarfism may be the result of systemic or nutritional disorders that occur in childhood. However, a large number of short-statured persons are normal since their parents are also short.

Habitus refers to body type or build. Normalcy covers a wide range of body types. The *asthenic type* is usually slender, active, and wiry and may appear to be underweight. The *sthenic type* is broad-shouldered, deep-chested, and athletic in appearance. The *pyknic type* is heavy, soft, and rounded due to an accumulation of body fat.

Body type is modified by secondary sexual characteristics. The masculine body is usually angular and rugged, with a well-muscled thorax and shoulders wider than hips. The feminine body characteristics are roundness and softness, with relatively more subcutaneous fat, ill-defined muscles, and hips wider than shoulders. In certain endocrine disorders, alterations in secondary sex character- istics occur, and the general habitus of an individual may resemble the opposite sex. Wide variations occur, for instance, the rugged "he-man" versus the effeminate type, or the mannish woman versus the ultrafeminine type.

In summary, a statement regarding general appearance is the end product of evaluation, interpretation, and integration of all the information gathered almost in a "blink of the eye." The amount and validity of the data and the conclusions drawn from them depend on the astuteness of the observer.

SKIN

The skin can be thought of as a mirror which often reflects a person's general health and well-being. The skin may sparkle and glow with vitality, or it may be dull and lifeless. Like the eye, it is important as a point of contact between the person's inner and outer worlds. It helps to regulate body temperature, transmit sensations, combat infections, and express emotions. Though this frontier of the human body is tough and resists the irritants and abrasions of daily living, the cliché "He is thin-skinned," with its numerous connotations, emphasizes the importance of skin reactions in revealing a person's true functional abilities (i.e., physical, social, and emotional). Accurate assessment of skin condition is dependent on the development of one's physical appraisal skills and an underlying knowledge of skin physiology. Specifically, the two tools most often needed and utilized in assessing this vital mirror of function are inspection and palpation.

Skin Composition and Function

Before the technique and principles of physical appraisal of the skin are discussed, its anatomy and physiology will be reviewed. When assessing the skin, one needs to know its basic structural components and understand their function. The skin is the largest body organ, comprising approximately 16 percent of the total body weight. It consists of three layers: the epidermis (outer layer), the dermis, or cutis (middle layer), and the subcutaneous tissue, or sub-cutis (inner layer) (see Fig. 6-2). The epidermis is covered with a fine layer of horny protein called keratin, which forms the strateum corneum, or protective layer. Melanocytes, which produce melanin for shielding the body against the sun's rays, are present in the basal layer of the epidermis. From the epidermis the accessory appendages (hair, nails, sebaceous glands, apocrine glands, and eccrine glands) extend into the dermis. The dermal layer is composed of bundles of collagen fibers, which act as a supporting framework for the epidermis, and it contains blood vessels, nerves, and lymphatic vessels. The sub-cutaneous, or fatty, layer is innermost and is the principal area of fat storage. In brief, the functions of these three layers are protection, heat regulation, sensory control, synthesis of vitamin D and antibodies, and excretory control (see Table 6-1).

Interview

The part of the nursing interview relating to the skin complements the general history. Questions are asked that elicit data on skin behavior and emphasize the following points:

1. *Family history.* Some skin diseases are familial or hereditary. When this is ascertained, one may have the opportunity both to correct misconceptions and allay fears about the presence or absence or prognosis of disease. What are the current familial dermatologic diseases?
2. *Personal history.* Age at onset of problem? How has the patient adjusted to the problem? By social withdrawal? Cosmetic cover-up? Withdrawal from school athletic activities that

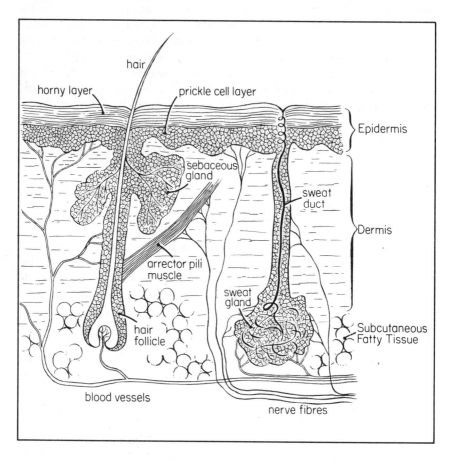

FIGURE 6-2. Structure of the skin.

require showers (e.g., football, tennis)? Does the problem threaten patient's self-image of masculinity or femininity? What is race or ethnic origin? (Some skin diseases are more common in certain ethnic groups.)

3. *Geographic origin and present abode.* Length of time spent in each area? (Some skin diseases are indigenous.) This may be important because of increased exposure. Occasionally, a contact of only five minutes is all that is necessary for acquisition of a disease.

4. *Season.* Seasonal occurrence of problem? Pollen? Sunlight?

5. *Occupation.* Type of work? Skin contact material, e.g., chemicals, dusts, gases; excessive heat and abnormal lighting; unhygienic surroundings; possible infected insects; other family members' occupational exposures?

6. *Leisure activities.* Does the problem occur only on weekends? After yard activities? Painting? Woodwork? Camping? Fishing? Hiking? Associated with children's play habits?

7. *Accompanying diseases.* Collagen disease? Drug therapy for collagen disease? Other diseases and their drug therapy?

Table 6-1.   Structure, Composition, and Function of Skin

Structure and Composition	Function
Epidermis	
Keratinocytes	Protection from bacterial and foreign-matter invasion
	Prevention of water and electrolyte loss
	Heat regulation
	Thickens with continual pressure or friction
Melanocytes	Pigmentation — protection from ultraviolet radiation
Epidermal or accessory organs	
Eccrine sweat glands	Heat regulation — evaporation
	Slight excretory function
Hair	Ornamentation
	Protection from dust and particulate matter
	Reduces surface area for heat conservation
Nails	Semivestigial
Sebaceous glands	Sebum for lubrication of strateum corneum and hair
	Limits absorption and evaporation
Apocrine glands	Semivestigial
	Additional function of epidermis: Vitamin D synthesis
Dermis (cutis)	
Collagen tissue	Supporting framework
Vasculature	Heat regulation
Lymphatics	Filters out antigens
Nerve endings	Sensory perception: heat, pain, touch, cold
Reticuloendothelial system	Antibody formation
Elastic fibers	Flexibility, elasticity, strength
	Additional functions of dermis: Protection from gross physical trauma Storage of water and electrolytes
Subcutaneous (subcutis)	
Subcutaneous fatty layer	Fat storage; heat regulation

8. *Previous treatments.* Self-treatment? Other drugs prescribed?
9. *Special history.* Onset of skin lesion (abnormality)? Exacerbations or recurrences? Site of onset? Character of lesions? Original character and subsequent changes? Course or extension? Symptoms? Itching? Ability to perform duties? Topical therapy? Self-treatment? Psychological factors? What does the patient associate with exacerbations of the problem (e.g., stress of a family argument, tax time, report time)?

Physical Appraisal Guidelines

Assessment of skin begins with inspection, the most important aspect of the physical appraisal process. Palpation is used to verify and support the findings of inspection. Frequently, these two processes are interrelated and are performed simultaneously. Several basic principles valuable in assessment of the skin should be kept in mind. These principles, as modified from Judge and Zuidema [1], are:

1.   Provide the patient with a comfortable environment and adequate room illumination. Nonglare (indirect) daylight is optimal. Flashlights and the usually dim lights over the bed are not adequate. Some of the newer lights that simulate daylight are acceptable. Observations made at night should be confirmed by the same person or another person in daylight.

2.   Use metric measurements when possible. (A number of helpful aids are available from pharmaceutical companies for use in assessing the size of skin lesions.)

3.   Compare each symmetrical or functional area with its opposite: for example, one side of the body against the other, or a sun-exposed area with an area not exposed to the sun.

4.   Learn and use precise terminology and nomenclature when describing skin (see Glossary and Fig. 6-3).

5.   Record the findings in the patient's record, and use this information as baseline data for determination of change. With each change in patient status, record progress notes.

6. Begin the examination by a brief careful survey of the entire skin, including the mucous membranes when possible. Start with the scalp and proceed to the toes. It is important to examine the entire skin, even though patients frequently deny the existence of skin changes. The expert nurse practitioner can usually list numerous examples of patients who denied any skin abnormalities but in whom major alterations were uncovered on direct visualization. One such nurse discovered a thumbtack implanted in the sole of the patient's foot, to the patient's dismay. The patient had diabetes mellitus with peripheral neuropathy and was unable to feel any abnormalities or to perform daily foot inspection to detect deviations. Often, patients are unwilling or hesitant to undress, which can be a hindrance to physical examination if the patient is not enlightened as to the importance of examining the whole integument even when he is "sure" there are no possible problems.

7.   Proceed systematically, examining the smooth skin (back, chest, abdomen, and extremities); intertriginous areas (deep folds where skin surfaces are opposed); hair (scalp, facial, chest, axillary, and pubic); mucous membranes (buccal cavity and sclera); and nails.

8.   When specific skin lesions (see Fig. 6-3) are noted, look first at their general distribution and then more closely at specific affected areas. Primary lesions appear first as a direct result of a causative factor (e.g., erythema following trauma such as a blow with a baseball). Secondary lesions are modifications of, or changes appearing after, the primary lesion (e.g., ecchymosis following the erythema of trauma). Later, the secondary lesion may undergo a series of characteristic changes until resolution of the lesion occurs (e.g., ecchymosis may change from its characteristic black-and-blue color to yellow and brown and then fade and disappear).

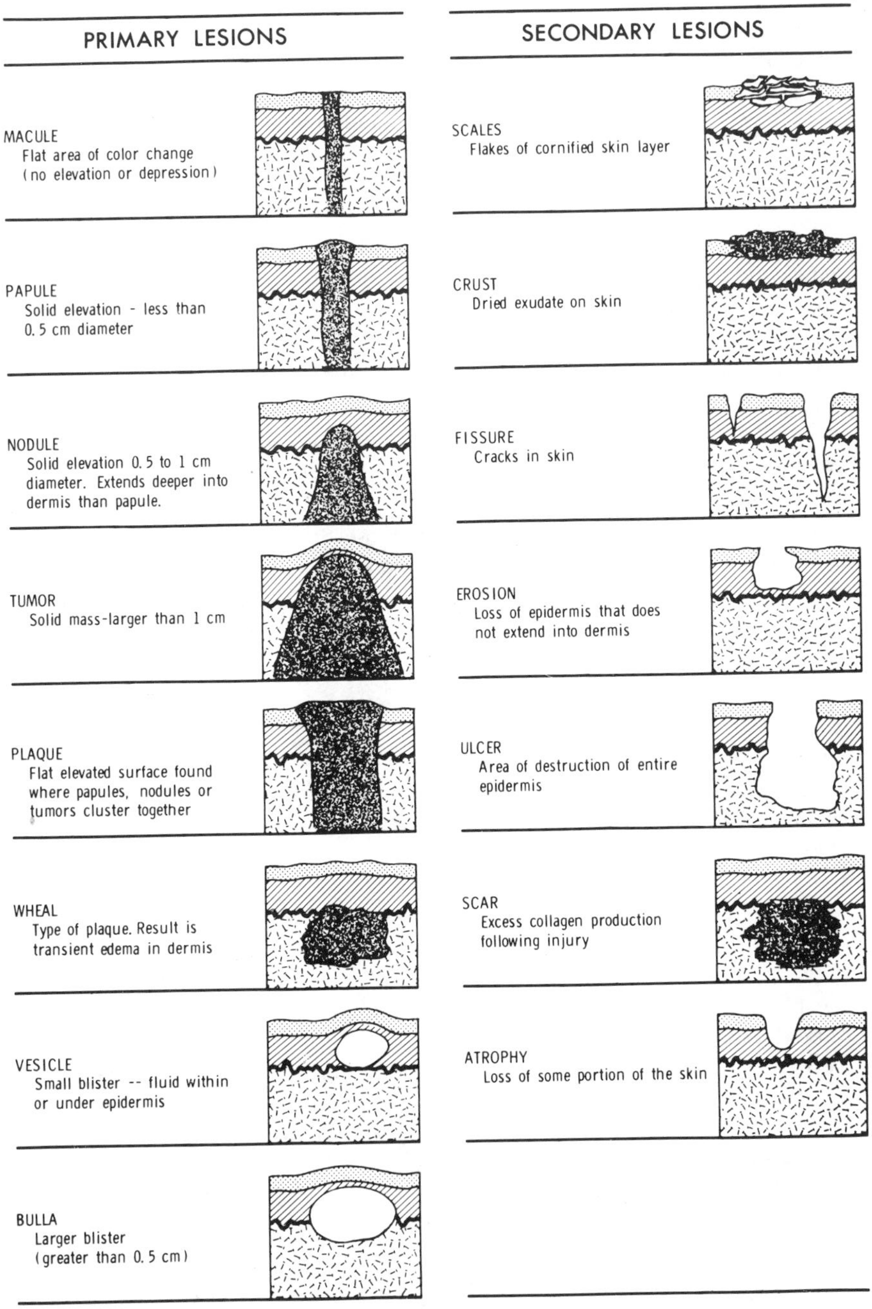

PRIMARY LESIONS

MACULE
Flat area of color change
(no elevation or depression)

PAPULE
Solid elevation - less than
0.5 cm diameter

NODULE
Solid elevation 0.5 to 1 cm
diameter. Extends deeper into
dermis than papule.

TUMOR
Solid mass-larger than 1 cm

PLAQUE
Flat elevated surface found
where papules, nodules or
tumors cluster together

WHEAL
Type of plaque. Result is
transient edema in dermis

VESICLE
Small blister -- fluid within
or under epidermis

BULLA
Larger blister
(greater than 0.5 cm)

SECONDARY LESIONS

SCALES
Flakes of cornified skin layer

CRUST
Dried exudate on skin

FISSURE
Cracks in skin

EROSION
Loss of epidermis that does
not extend into dermis

ULCER
Area of destruction of entire
epidermis

SCAR
Excess collagen production
following injury

ATROPHY
Loss of some portion of the skin

FIGURE 6-3. Characteristics of common skin lesions.

Appraisal and Interpretation of Skin Findings

An important but difficult element of skin inspection is assessment of color. There is great variability in skin color from person to person and in the same person. Heavily pigmented skin poses additional difficulties for the inexperienced eye, but with practice there are few skins that cannot be accurately evaluated.

The color of normal skin depends primarily on its content of melanin, carotene, oxyhemoglobin, or reduced hemoglobin. The melanin content of the keratinocytes and melanocytes determines the skin pigmentation. Contrary to popular belief, skin in all races has the same proportion of melanocytes. The variations in color are due to genetically determined and acquired differences in production of melanin and its transfer to the keratinocytes.

Both skin color (e.g., yellow, brown, white) and intensity (light or dark) are assessed. Areas of least pigmentation are best for assessing color (e.g., the sclera, conjunctiva, nail beds, lips, buccal mucosa, tongue, palms, and soles). Heavily calloused areas on the hands and feet will usually have an opaque yellow color.

Skin color may be affected by position or gravity. For example, a person with a peripheral vascular disorder will have marked color changes of an extremity depending on whether it is elevated, level with the heart, or in a dependent position. A useful method for evaluating color of an extremity is to position it at all three levels: heart level, elevated at 15° for at least five minutes, and finally lowered 30° to 90° for at least five minutes [3].

Convolutions of the skin often distort the true coloration by intensifying the color. These areas, such as knees, elbows, nipple and areola of the female breast, and fat folds, should be smoothed or spread out when being assessed. Similarly, edema reduces skin color intensity by increasing the distance between the pigmented surface and its vasculature. These factors may lead to inaccurate appraisals if their significance is not considered.

The patient's activities immediately prior to assessment can influence skin color. Emotional factors such as anger and fright or embarrassment and self-consciousness may contribute to generalized pallor in the former two or superficial vasodilatation (blush) in the latter two. Since cigarette smoking causes vasoconstriction, it may affect correct assessment of nail bed color. Application of warm soaks, use of hypothermia, and other such treatment modalities can also alter color. Distortion of skin color may be externally induced by other agents such as lipstick, powders, tanning agents, and tattooing. Comprehensive history-taking will help prevent observational mistakes. Recognition of these distorting factors and their influence on skin color is important.

Normal color distribution patterns vary from person to person and race to race. For example, dark-skinned people like those of Mediterranean origin may have very blue lips, contributing to a mistaken judgment of cyanosis. Blotchy bluish pigmentation of the gums and brown melanin deposits in the scleras, nail beds, or both are often normal findings in blacks who are very dark-skinned. In the dark-skinned person, the areas of lighter melanization (abdomen, buttocks, and volar surface of the forearm) allow for more accurate evaluation of pigmentation. Some types of skin abnormalities such as erythema are often visible in lighter-skinned persons but not in those whose skin is dark; however, the affected part may become an even deeper shade of brown. When inflammation is suspected in the dark-skinned person, other parameters are assessed by palpation — increased skin temperature, tight skin suggestive of edema, induration of deep tissue or blood vessels, and tenderness. Since the dorsal skin surface of the fingers is more sensitive to subtle skin temperature differences than the palmar surface, use the dorsal portion of the fingers to move from one skin area to another for comparison. The patient's family and friends are also helpful in validating color change, particularly when it has occurred gradually.

The nail beds, lips, and conjunctivas are observed primarily for assessing the patient for pallor. When observing the inferior palpebral conjunctiva (lower eyelid) for pallor, the lid should be lowered sufficiently to see the conjunctiva near the temporal (outer) canthus in addition to the inner canthus, since the coloration of the former is often darker. When assessing the darkly pigmented individual for pallor, greater perception is necessary because the changes are subtle. There may be an absence of red tones; the brown-skinned person may appear more yellowish-brown; and the black-skinned person may appear ashen gray. This supports the need for accurate baseline data for comparison.

Jaundice and cyanosis are observed in the usual sites (e.g., mucous membranes, nail beds). Since many factors can alter these findings, one single positive finding should not be held as conclusive. Other parameters, such as environmental temperature, drugs, smoking, amount of hemoglobin, color of urine, stools, or both, can support a description of cyanosis or jaundice. Both in the dark-skinned and light-skinned person, yellow scleras may indicate jaundice, but other factors can cause yellow scleral pigmentation; fatty deposits that contain carotene are a common finding in dark-skinned people. To determine if the yellow scleras signify jaundice, observe the hard palate in bright daylight. Jaundice can be detected there quite early, i.e., when serum bilirubin is 2 to 4 mg per 100 ml, if the palate does not have heavy melanin pigmentation [3]. If the hard palate does not show jaundice when the scleras are yellow, the pigmentation is due to some other factor, such as carotene accumulation. All these factors support the importance of repeated observations and accurate descriptions of what is seen. As often as possible the same person should perform the entire examination and should confirm specific findings in one area with additional data from other areas.

Palpation is used to validate further the data that are gathered from inspection and to ascertain other qualities such as texture, temperature, hydration, and turgor. The character of the skin's surface (i.e., fineness, coarseness) and the feel of deeper portions are its *texture*. The presence or absence of such textures as rough, dry, smooth, or velvety is best ascertained by stroking the volar surface of the forearm with the dorsal side of the fingers. Feeling the deeper portions of the skin may reveal areas of induration such as those resulting from multiple intramuscular or subcutaneous administrations of medication. These lipodystrophies may consist of smooth, large depressions in the skin that indicate atrophy of the subcutaneous fat layer or marked hypertrophy of the subcutaneous fat layer, which is of a spongy consistency. Both of these conditions are often seen at sites of repeated insulin injections.

Another skin quality is its *surface temperature*. Although skin temperature is an inadequate measure of the body's internal temperature, it gives valuable data about the patient's functional status. If a febrile patient is warm and dry, the temperature is probably rising, since the thermoregulatory mechanism of sweating is not functioning. Likewise, if the skin is warm and wet, the temperature can be expected to fall, due to the cooling mechanism of sweating. Since the skin temperature is dependent on the amount of blood circulating through the dermis, decreased localized blood flow such as to the feet may indicate a peripheral vascular dysfunction. Generalized skin coolness may indicate decreased metabolism such as that occurring after general anesthesia. If the temperature is very low, signs of shock may be evident. An increase in skin temperature may indicate a hypermetabolic state such as that occurring in hyperthyroidism and after sun exposure or sunburn.

Of the total body heat produced, 85 percent is lost through the skin by conduction, convection, radiation, and evaporation. Cooling of the body by evaporation, through sweating, is of various types and has many etiologies. Identification of the type of sweating often helps in differentiating normal from abnormal body functioning. The exocrine sweat glands, which are found over the entire body, respond principally to thermal and emotional stimuli. Maximal sweating due to emotion occurs on the palms, soles, and axillae, while maximal thermal sweating is seen on the fingers, arms, forehead, and axillae. When evaluating thermal causes of sweating, factors which may raise body temperature and induce sweating must be looked for. Has the patient been active, walking up and down stairs, for example, or has he been confined to bed? Is his room environment exceptionally warm? Has he just had a hot bath or shower? Is he receiving any medications that may induce sweating? Has he just eaten? After eating highly spiced foods, some people may exhibit gustatory sweating, indicated by sweat on the forehead, upper lip, scalp, and back of the neck. Sweating primarily of the palms and soles leads one to look for other evidence of fear or anxiety.

Sweating can also occur when there is a rapid fall in blood glucose, with resultant rise in the blood epinephrine level. This cause of sweating can usually be distinguished from the others because of the additional symptoms of weakness, tachycardia, hunger, headache, and "inward nervousness," or mental irritability or confusion, or both.

The apocrine sweat glands are less numerous than the exocrine and are found in hair-bearing areas. They do not play a role in thermoregulation and respond only to emotional and sensory stimuli. These glands are responsible mainly for the sweat which produces "body odor," particularly in the axillae.

Other skin qualities useful to the nurse in patient assessment are *hydration* and *turgor.* The state of hydration of skin and mucous membranes helps to indicate body fluid disturbances. A dry, leathery appearance of the tongue may not be a reliable indicator of negative water balance since mouth breathing frequently makes the tongue look dehydrated. A more reliable method of assessing hydration of the oral cavity is to palpate the mucous membranes along the area of the gum and cheek where the membranes approximate. If the membranes are dry and the finger does not slide easily, the patient may be water-deficient.

Skin turgor can be assessed by picking up and releasing the skin, particularly on the dorsa of the hands or forearms. Normal skin will usually snap back immediately into its resting position. If the skin is loose and wrinkled or lacks tone, or both, the patient may be dehydrated. Remember, though, that with aging there is normally a loss of elasticity in subcutaneous tissue. If the skin over the hands, feet, ankles, and sacrum is firm and indents easily (pitting edema) on moderate pressure from the examiner's fingertips, fluid excess is present.

The Dermal Appendages

Hair. All hair has phases of both activity and rest. Each individual scalp hair grows from about 0.3 to 0.4 mm per day during the growing phase [1]. The resting phase occurs every few months to a few years. The rate of growth varies with general health and age.

The distribution of hair over the body warrants careful observation. The scalp hair, eyebrows, eyelashes, and downy hair of the body are present in both sexes. After puberty coarse body hair evolves in distinct male and female patterns of the axillary and genital areas. Disturbances in body function are often reflected by changes in amount, texture, color, and growth pattern of the hair.

Alterations in amount of body hair can be extremely anxiety-provoking for both males and females. In the female with hirsutism, hair growth is intensified on the upper lip, chin, cheeks, chest, and from the pubic crest to the umbilicus (along the linea alba); and the downy hair on the arms, legs, and back becomes coarse. The pubic hair often takes on the upright triangular distribution typical of the male as opposed to the female's usual inverted triangle. An endocrine malfunction such as excess androgen production may sometimes be associated with hirsutism, but ethnic background (Mediterranean groups predominantly) may also be responsible for the excessive hair growth. This is especially true of the hair on the arms, legs, back, and face. Other ethnic group members such as the full-blooded black female and the male Indian rarely have facial hair or a beard. Distribution of the hair in family members and consideration of ethnic background are important in ascertaining the normalcy of hair growth.

Common disturbances of scalp hair involve its thickness. Baldness (alopecia) or thinning of the hair that is generalized or creates a receding hairline often is genetically determined. Some rare genetic defects in the hair shaft itself may produce breaking of the hairs and be mistakenly diagnosed as alopecia. General and localized baldness may result from treatment modalities such as radiation or chemotherapy. In addition, various types of scalp diseases (e.g., fungal, lupus) and telogen effluvium (transient hair loss occurring two to three months after general anesthesia, febrile illness, or giving birth) can cause hair loss. Other traumatic types of hair loss may occur from pulling of the hair because of a nervous habit; hairstyles such as braiding or ponytails; or constrictive wearing apparel such as a hat. The normal scalp sheds about 20 to 100 hairs per day, so one needs to determine if hair loss is in excess of this amount [4]. Frequently, an estimate of daily hair loss can be ascertained by asking the patient how much hair is left in his hairbrush or comb after each use and if this amount of hair has changed.

Since hair is essentially an adornment for many men and women, its loss or excess often provokes embarrassment and anxiety and conflict with the patient's self-image of masculinity or femininity. Awareness and sensitivity to the patient's need for personal expression of concerns and privacy is important in planning the care program.

Another pertinent feature relating to the hair is its amount of lubrication. Sebum from sebaceous glands anoints the hair and keeps it from drying and becoming brittle by limiting the amount of absorption and evaporation of water from the surface. The sebaceous glands are most numerous over the face and scalp. Assessing these areas gives one the best indication regarding the amount of skin oiliness. Hyperfunction of these glands is associated with androgen stimulation such as occurs with the excessive scalp oiliness and facial acne in adolescence. Dry, brittle hair is commonly the result of excessive washing or the application of chemical agents (coloring, bleach, or detergents) to the hair. In addition to the direct observation of the scalp and face, correlation of the findings with the data from the interview helps to determine dysfunctional states.

The Nails. The fingernails and toenails grow at a fairly constant rate, except when altered by generalized disease or injury. This makes them useful as an indicator of the person's general health. The visible nail plate is a dead sheet of hard keratin, and changes seen in the nails reflect damage that occurred earlier. Fingernails normally grow at the rate of 0.1 mm per day. By measuring the distance between abnormalities (pits, grooves, and lines) and the proximal nail border, one may estimate the time of initial illness.

Normal nails are transparent, with pink nail beds and translucent white tips at the point of separation of the nail from the nail bed. Surface longitudinal ridges and flecks of white spots in the nail are within normal limits. Transverse furrows (Beau's lines) in the nail indicate that nail growth has been disturbed. This can result from infection, systemic disease, or injury.

The nurse most often uses nail color as an indication of the amount of blood oxygenation. Bluish or purplish discoloration of the nail beds occurs with cyanosis, while pallor often indicates anemia. To compare color of the nail beds, apply slight pressure on the free edge of the second or third fingernail. The blanching which results is then compared to the normal color of the nail. The rate of color return also indicates the quality of peripheral vasomotor function.

Oral Mucous Membrane Examination. As with the skin, the mouth itself may reveal not only local but systemic disease and should be thoroughly examined. The recognition of poor oral hygiene early in hospitalization opens the path to immediate intervention, with the possibility of preventive nursing care. The purpose of a program of care is prophylaxis, or at least a lessening of the invasion of the oral mucosa by opportunistic organisms.

Repeated examination of the mouth provides a clinical knowledge base from which to recognize beginning and ongoing problems and to evaluate the effectiveness of prescribed care. The techniques used are inspection and palpation. The instruments needed are a tongue blade, bright mobile light source, and glove or finger cots. The patient may be sitting or recumbent. If both the examiner and patient are sitting, the examiner should face the patient at the same level.

The oral mucosal surface has a rich vascular supply. Normally the color of this surface is pale coral pink and is kept moist by numerous submucosal accessory salivary glands augmenting the major salivary gland secretion. Bright red surfaces usually indicate inflammation, while pallor indicates localized ischemia or generalized anemia. Cyanosis suggests hypoxemia, which may indicate local congestion or a systemic disease. The oral buccal cavity is pigmented with generalized and local melanin in accordance with racial background. Normally, the gums of pure blacks may be a bluish color, occurring either diffusely or in splotches; in other blacks, brown pigment is present in the gingival mucosa. On the tongue, brown pigmented dots, single or in groups, especially at the borders of the tongue, are not uncommon in blacks. Pigment changes in the oral mucous membrane may indicate many systemic conditions.

Begin the oral examination by explaining to the patient what is to occur. Observe the symmetry in form and function of the lips as the patient attempts to whistle. Observe the function and fit of dentures and then ask the patient to remove them. Always use direct lighting for the examination. Inspect the inner lip, cheek surfaces, and all the recesses of the gingivobuccal folds and gums by retracting the lips and cheeks with a tongue blade. Next ask the patient to open his mouth wide. Inspect the hard (anterior) and soft (posterior) palates. Depress the tongue with a tongue blade (being careful that the tongue is within the teeth) and request the "ah" phonation to observe midline uvula elevation and pharynx constriction (see Fig. 6-4a). Have the patient protrude his tongue. Assess its size, symmetry, involuntary movements, and restricted protrusion, in addition to the dorsal surface characteristics. Finally, retract the patient's tongue laterally, and view the posterior surface of the floor of the mouth (see Fig. 6-4c). Ask the patient to raise the tip of his tongue to the roof of his mouth while he keeps his mouth open. Inspect the ventral surface of the tongue and the anterior

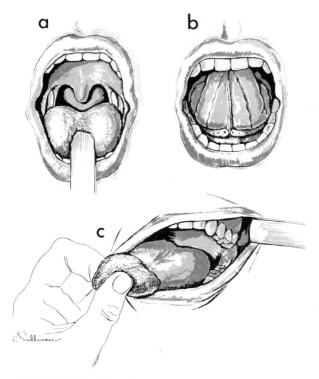

FIGURE 6-4. Positions for mouth examination. a. View of dorsum, palate, and pharynx. b. Inspection of ventral surface and floor of the mouth. c. Inspection and palpation of posterior surface of floor of mouth. (Reprinted from Judge and Zuidema [1].)

floor of the mouth (see Fig. 6-4b).

With the patient maintaining the open-mouth position, inspect the teeth for their form and support in the mouth. Using a probe, tap each tooth lightly for tenderness. Observe the movements of the mandible and occlusion of the teeth to evaluate their effectiveness during mastication.

Before proceeding with palpation of the oral mucosa, stop and explain the procedure to the patient. Ask the patient to protrude his tongue. The tongue can be controlled by grasping it between layers of gauze. The mucosa can now be adequately palpated. Using the index finger covered with a glove, gently palpate the soft, smooth surfaces. Release the tongue and continue palpation to the floor of the mouth. Palpate this oral mucosa with the opposite hand, supporting external tissues. Continue this bimanual palpation in the cheek and lip region. Conclude by palpating the hard and soft palate areas. Note the flow and quality of secretions from the orifices of the submaxillary and parotid ducts [1, pp. 101–103].

Guidelines for examination of the mouth are presented in Table 6-2, p. 100.

LYMPH NODE EXAMINATION

When inspecting and palpating the skin, also examine the lymph nodes. The groups of nodes that are generally examined are the cervicofacial, supraclavicular, axillary, epitrochlear, inguinal, and femoral. The tools that are required for assessment of the lymph nodes are inspection and palpation. The description of each node should include:

1. Exact location.
2. Extent of enlargement (usually the diameter is expressed in centimeters or in some familiar size, e.g., split pea, bean, almond).
3. Presence or absence of tenderness.
4. Presence or absence of visible or palpable surrounding inflammation.
5. Whether they are freely movable, adherent to the deeper structures, or matted together as a result of extensive inflammatory changes.
6. Texture (hard, soft, firm).

Inspect both sides and compare. Use the middle three fingers for palpation and notation of any visible lymphadenopathy. Movements should be slow and gentle; the fingers should move up and down, back and forth, and in a rotary motion. Palpation should be light or small nodes will be missed.

Cervicofacial and Supraclavicular Nodes

Proceed in an orderly fashion with the examination. Begin by examining the superior and posterior lymph nodes, proceeding downward as follows (see Fig. 6-5A): (a) occipital and postauricular; (b) submaxillary and submental; (c) anterior angle (upper end of deep cervical chain); (d) downward along the sternocleidomastoid muscle (superficial cervical nodes); (e) posterior triangle (lower end of deep cervical chain); (f) supraclavicular. The two approaches to examination of the nodes are shown in Figures 6-5B and C.

Axillary and Epitrochlear Nodes

For examination of the axillary and epitrochlear nodes the patient may be either sitting or supine. The axilla can be thoroughly assessed with one hand while the examiner's opposite hand holds the ipsilateral arm of the patient. The axilla should be thought of as having an apex and three walls: anterior or pectoral group, central group, and posterior group. Each of these areas should be palpated with the patient's arm at the side and again while the arm is moved through a full range of motion. This is done to uncover any lesions hidden under a muscle or in a fatty layer. Be aware of the patient's comfort and move the arm gently. Proceed by cupping the hand slightly and reach high into the apex of the axilla. Pull down, exerting gentle pressure with the fingertips against the thorax (see Fig. 6-6A).

Repeat this procedure, checking each group of nodes respectively.

Table 6-2. Regional Observations of the Mouth

Regions	Functions	Normal Characteristics	Assessment Guidelines
Lips	Speech Oral intake Control of secretions Contribute to facial expression	Pink, smooth, soft Exposed portion: dry, vermilion, usually marked by slight superficial vertical wrinkling Inside lips: grayish red	Color, form, position, function, texture, asym- metry, chapping, cracking of the mucosa, irritations at the corners or angles of the mouth, congenital or acquired defects
Teeth	Mastication	White enamel surface; no debris, film, or hard deposits Number: 32 (full adult dentition) Number: 20 (deciduous)	Color, number, caries, size, discoloration, occlusion, notched or peglike, bridges, alveolar swelling
Gums	Supporting structure Mastication	Pale, coral-pink, firm, slightly stippled surface (like an orange), attached to teeth and projecting to fill interdental space as papillae	Color, form, density, retrac- tion of gingival margin, pus in margins, inflammation, spongy or bleeding gums, localized gingival swelling
Tongue	Speech Mastication Taste Swallowing	*Dorsal:* moist, glistening coating, muscular; four types of papillae include: filiform (most important and numerous), fungi- form (grayish-red), foliate (located along the lateral portion of the posterior of the tongue), vallate papil- lae (form a V near the back of the tongue) *Ventral:* pink, smooth, shows large veins	Color, size, texture, papillae cleanliness, moisture, voluntary or involuntary movements, deviation from midline, restricted protrusion, tenderness, position Varicose veins
Buccal mucosa (cheeks)	Mastication Houses paro- tid gland	Grayish-red color; may be crossed by fine grayish ridges where it settles between rows of teeth when the mouth is closed; the parotid gland emits a clear secretion	Color, texture, parotid gland, ulcer, melanin deposits, vesicles, neoplasms, cysts or swelling of parotid gland, ductal orifice
Hard palate	Mastication Houses mucous glands	Pale pink, immovable, moist underlying bony process of the maxilla; no debris; irregular; rugae running trans- versely; orifices of ducts of mucous glands in the posterior part of hard palate; midline, hard swelling is a common variation	Color, texture, glands, ductal orifices; ducts may look like red dots in heavy smokers (nicotine stoma- titis); swelling; rugae
Soft palate	Swallowing Speech Houses mucous glands	Pink, muscular; has abundant submucosal accessory salivary glands; shows fine vessels under the mucosa	Color, texture, glands, ulcers, fungal infections, inflamma- tion

Table 6-2.   (Continued)

Regions	Functions	Normal Characteristics	Assessment Guidelines
Breath odors	Manifestation of condition of mouth, oral intake, systemic disease, lung disease	Absent or sweet	*Fetid:* infections of oral cavity, poor oral hygiene, putrefactive disease of the lung *Acetone:* diabetic acidosis *Ammonia:* renal failure *Musty:* liver disease
Floor of the mouth	Supporting Structures Houses submaxillary gland, sublingual gland, lymph nodes	Pale, coral pink, loose tissue Submaxillary glands emit a clear mucous secretion Submental and submaxillary lymph nodes	Neoplasms here are sometimes detectable only by palpation; cysts of sublingual glands; sublingual and submaxillary ductal orifices; lymph nodes are palpated for swelling

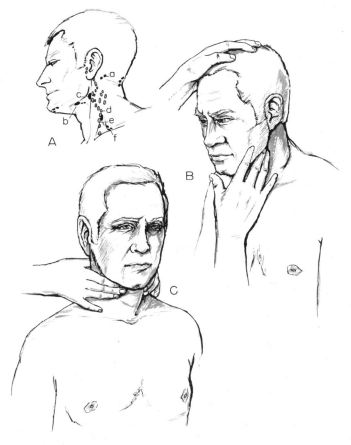

FIGURE 6-5.   Technique of examination of cervicofacial lymph nodes. A. Location of major groups of nodes. B. Anterior approach. C. Posterior approach. (Modified from Judge and Zuidema [1].)

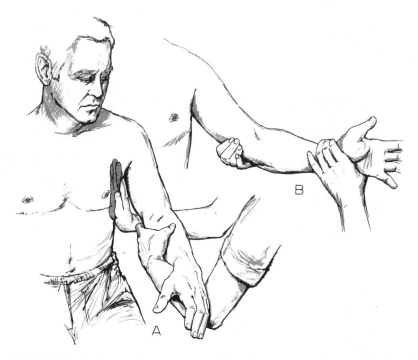

FIGURE 6-6.   Technique of examination of (A) axillary lymph nodes and (B) epitrochlear lymph nodes. (Reprinted from Judge and Zuidema [1].)

The epitrochlear nodes are palpated as shown in Figure 6-6B. The nodes are located in the fossa above and behind the medial condyle of the humerus.

Inguinal Nodes

The superficial inguinal and femoral nodes are palpated using the rotary motion described in Chapter 11.

Normal Findings

Lymph nodes are not normally palpable but are frequently noted because of prior inflammation. Cervical nodes are almost always felt in children up to 12 years of age. These nodes are referred to as "shotty," which is generally interpreted as firm, freely movable, and nontender, and indicates a chronic inflammatory process. Palpable inguinal lymph nodes in the adolescent and the adult are a common finding [1, pp. 264—269]. Rarely, enlarged lymph nodes may interfere with body function (e.g., movement of the head, swallowing, adduction and abduction of the arm). Identification of these alterations in function requires that they be considered in the nursing care plan.

REFERENCES

1. Judge, R. D., and Zuidema, G. D. (Eds.). *Methods of Clinical Examination: A Physiologic Approach* (3rd ed.). Boston: Little, Brown, 1974.
2. Marples, M. J. Life on the human skin. *Sci. Am.* 220:108, 1969.
3. Roach, L.B. Color changes in dark skins. *Nursing '72* 2:19, 1972.
4. Sneedon, I. B., and Church, R. E. *Nursing Skin Disease.* London: Arnold, 1968.

SUGGESTED READINGS

Brown, M. S., and Alexander, M. Physical examination. *Nursing '73* 3:39, 1973.

Prior, J. A., and Silberstein, J. S. *Physical Diagnosis* (4th ed.). St. Louis: Mosby, 1973.

Rook, A., Wilkinson, D. S., and Ebling, F. J. S. *Textbook of Dermatology* (vol. 1). Oxford, England: Blackwell, 1968.

Stewart, W. D., Danto, J. L., and Madden, S. *Synopsis of Dermatology* (2nd ed.). St. Louis: Mosby, 1970.

Sulzberger, M. B., et al. *Dermatology: Diagnosis and Treatment* (2nd ed.). Chicago: Year Book, 1961.

Wilkinson D. S. *The Nursing and Management of Skin Diseases* (3rd ed.). London: Faber and Faber, 1969.

7

PHYSICAL APPRAISAL OF THE EYE AND VISION

Patricia Mitchell Butler

GLOSSARY

abduction   Outward rotation of the part away from axis of the body.

adduction   Movement of a part toward the midline of the body.

aqueous humor   Fluid produced in the ciliary body and occupying the anterior and posterior chambers.

arcus senilis   Opaque white ring around the corneal periphery from fatty degeneration, seen in older persons.

blepharospasm   Twitching or spasmodic contraction of the orbicularis oculi muscle.

diplopia   Double vision.

ectropion   Eversion of the lid border.

emmetropia   Normal condition of the eye in refraction; with eye at rest rays parallel to the optic axis are focused on the retina.

entropion   Inversion of the lid border.

epiphoria   Abnormal overflow of tears down the cheek.

extorsion   Tilting of the eye (superior pole of the cornea temporally) outward.

fundoscopy   Examination of the interior of the eyeball using an ophthalmoscope.

glaucoma   Disease of the eye characterized by increased intraocular pressure.

hyperopia   Eyeball is too short from front to back, and the retina lies in front of the posterior principal focus of the eye; farsightedness.

hyphema   Blood in the anterior chamber of the eye in front of the iris.

hypopyon   Presence of pus in the anterior chamber.

intorsion   Tilting of the eye (superior pole of the cornea nasally) inward.

limbus   Edge of the cornea where it joins the sclera.

myopia   Eyeball is so long from front to back that the posterior principal focus of the eye lies in front of the retina; nearsightedness.

nystagmus   Rapid involuntary eye movements.

O.D.   Oculus dexter; right eye.

optic disc   Area in retina for entrance of optic nerve and blood vessels.

O.S.   Oculus sinister; left eye.

O.U.   Oculi unitas (both eyes); oculus uterque (each eye).

palpebra   Eyelid.

papilledema   Swelling of the optic disc.

photophobia   Abnormal intolerance of light.

presbyopia   Decreased or weakened ability of the eye to accommodate, due to loss of elasticity of the crystalline lens with advancing age.

ptosis   Drooping of the upper lid.

The role of the nurse in assessing eye function will vary, depending on the patient's age and health, but will include an appraisal of the functional status of the eyes, referral to ophthalmologist, orthoptists, and other specialist services, and counseling the individual for optimal visual functioning in his everyday life situation.

Appraisal of the eye and vision includes both a history and physical examination. The examination encompasses measurement of visual acuity, testing ocular movements, evaluation of visual fields, inspection of external eye structures, testing nerve reflexes, and fundoscopic examination as well as gross determination of intraocular pressure. Equipment needed for the ophthalmologic examination includes:

1. Snellen chart
2. Jaeger chart
3. Penlight
4. Cotton-tipped applicator
5. Cotton ball
6. Ophthalmoscope
7. Eye cover or shield

HISTORY AND EXAMINATION

History

The assessment of the eye is begun with a careful and detailed history. Throughout the history-taking and physical examination, observation is made of the physical appearance of the eye. Eye and head movements and facial expressions should be noted. These can provide clues both to systemic functional alterations of body systems and to alterations of the eye. Physical examination of the eye may also give clues to systemic disease, as many diseases manifest eye changes [1, 3].

A familial history is necessary, as many eye disorders are hereditary. A past history of eye disorders must be elicited, including previous diagnoses, treatments, and results. When taking a child's history, determine what the parents or guardians perceive the child to be able to see. Also, determine if the infant or child looks at objects or reaches for people or large and small objects and whether or not any change in this pattern has been noticed.

The history should provide answers to the following:

1. Have any changes occurred in vision?
2. Are there any signs or symptoms of pain, light sensitivity, itching, tearing, redness, blurring or veiling of vision, or are spider-web—type lines or spots seen?
3. Are specific activities associated with these symptoms?
4. When do the symptoms occur, what is their duration, and how does the person obtain relief from them?

Measurement of Visual Acuity

The examination should be done in a specific order according to an established system, so that no part will be omitted. Visual acuity measurement can be done first and may serve, especially with children, as a means of establishing a relationship. The Snellen chart is the most readily available and easiest method to use for testing distant vision. There are many variations of this chart, but the most versatile is the block E chart, which can be used with children, illiterate persons, or those who do not read English. Cut-out block Es are available to familiarize the child with the "three-legged table." Children and other persons using this chart are asked to indicate the direction of the "legs" of the table, and the nurse must make certain that they clearly understand what they are to indicate. Children 2 years of age and older can be tested with this chart after some time is spent in teaching and game playing.

The Snellen chart uses standardized sizes and forms of letters or objects to test visual acuity. The distance and size of the letters determine the size of the retinal image. A person's visual acuity is indicative of the functioning of the fovea, the most sensitive area of the retina. The numbers at the ends of the row are the visual acuity measurement recorded for the patient. Figure 7-1 indicates the distance (in feet and meters) of the patient from the Snellen chart. The angles of arc (5 minutes) are also indicated i.e., 5 minutes of arc at 20 ft (6 M), 100 ft (30 M), and 200 ft (60 M).* Visual acuity numbers, e.g., 20/30 are not fractions. The upper figure always indicates the distance the person being tested is from the chart. The lower figure indicates the distance at which the normal eye would see the letter; 20/30 vision means that the person tested was seated 20 ft. (6 M) from the chart and could read the line that those with normal vision can read at 30 ft (9 M) but could not read beyond this line.

Testing is begun with the person comfortably seated 20 feet (6 M) from the chart. One eye should be tested at a time. The patient's hand should not be used to cover his other eye. A tongue blade with a round piece of construction paper secured to it will do well as an eye shield. The nurse must make certain periodically that the person is unable to see with the covered eye, particularly when testing a child. Adults should be asked to read the line most comfortably read and should identify all the letters correctly. When testing the child, it is well to start at the top of the chart. Encourage the reading of as many letters as possible. If the person reads with the right eye the 20/30 line "missing" two letters, 20/30-2 O.D. is recorded. How the line was read is described also, i.e., "quickly and rhythmically," or "hesitantly, with great effort." A different set of letters or E chart should be used for each eye, however; if this is not possible, then the known or suspected "poorer" eye should be tested first and the uncorrected vision tested before the corrected.

---

*The metric system is being used by many ophthalmologists. To convert from feet to meters, divide roughly by 3.3 or multiply by 0.3048. To convert meters to feet multiply by 3.281.

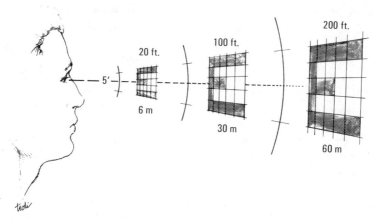

FIGURE 7-1. Visual acuity test using Snellen chart (20 ft = 6 M; 100 ft = 30 M; 200 ft = 60 M). (Reprinted from Judge and Zuidema [6].)

The person who cannot read the chart at 20/200 (top letter) is moved closer to the chart until able to read this top large letter. The distance and letter are recorded, e.g., 3/200. If no chart letters can be read, a finger test is done. The nurse holds her hand in front of the patient to determine if variable numbers of fingers held up can be seen and accurately counted. If the finger count cannot be done, the nurse will then determine if hand movements (HM) can be identified or, last, if the patient has light perception (LP). When an eye cannot perceive light, it is termed "blind" by the physician. Legal blindness is defined as less than 20/200 (big E) vision in the best eye with full correction, or less than 20 degrees field of vision [4]. Legal blindness should be established by a physician, as the patient is then entitled to tax and other benefits.

The importance of testing visual acuity, particularly in children, cannot be stressed enough. Many children have defects in eyesight which may or may not be refractive errors. With one eye patched, children under 2 years of age can play games in which objects of varying sizes are picked up, permitting the nurse to make a gross estimate of visual acuity and functioning of each eye.

Amblyopia is defined as reduction in visual acuity with proper correction in place in an eye that appears normal by ophthalmoscope. Approximately 1.5 to 2 percent of the young adult population in the United States has some form of amblyopia [8]. Although there are several types, the most frequently encountered is strabismic amblyopia (amblyopia resulting from constant macular suppression to prevent double vision resulting from the strabismus). Careful examination of visual acuity using the Snellen chart can usually detect amblyopia. If the visual acuity in each eye differs by two or more lines on the Snellen chart, the child should be referred to an ophthalmologist for further study.

The Jaeger chart can be used for testing near vision. Newsprint can also be used. The Jaeger card contains varying size print with scores beside each size. This card should be held 14 in. (35 cm) from the eye, and the person is asked to read as many lines as possible. The revised Jaeger card has the score in Snellen, metric, and percentage figures. This test is particularly useful for persons over 40 years of age who are beginning to experience presbyopia. Patients with hyperopia, astigmatism (defective refraction), accommodative curvature of cornea and lens (IIIrd cranial nerve) impairment, or other pathological condition may have poor near vision, and this test should be done routinely. Testing games for children are available and recommended for the nurse who has many preschool children for visual screening. (The E Testing Game and Titmus Stereotests can be obtained from the Benson Optical Co., 1812 Park Avenue, Box 679, Minneapolis, Minn. 55440.) Any person with vision less than 20/30 O.D. or O.S. should be referred to an ophthalmologist for further testing and treatment.

Testing for Ocular Movements

Ocular muscles should be tested routinely from infancy through old age. In infants, the nurse observes particularly for muscle weakness which may be too subtle to be detected easily. The nurse also observes for nerve impairment to the muscle. "The maintenance of parallel eyes (and therefore of corneal light reflexes which are equally centered) occurs in most persons because of the fusion reflex which makes binocular vision possible [5]." Man has learned to adapt to a certain degree of muscle weakness so that, despite it, he still achieves fusion and binocular vision. This is often to the detriment of one eye. When one eye is covered, this fusion is not possible, and one eye will realign to its visual axis to fixate the target on the fovea, i.e., it will move so that the object looked at is centered on the fovea.

The patient should be seated, looking directly at the nurse examiner, and asked to look straight ahead. As the nurse shines a penlight on the cornea, the corneal light reflex appears on the cornea's shiny surface. The location of the corneal light reflex should be parallel to the pupils of both eyes [5, 7, 8].

To perform the cover test the patient is asked to fix his vision on a target. If testing a child, the target may be a toy with blinking eyes or a bright picture. The right eye is first covered while the nurse observes the left eye for movement; if none is noted, the eye was probably centering the object on the fovea. The cover is then removed from the right eye and placed on the left eye after several seconds. The test is then performed on the right eye (the reflection of light from the corneas of each eye, normally, should be in exactly the same position on each pupil).

In the alternating cover test, the patient continues to watch the fixation target. The nurse alternately covers the right and then the left eye. This alternating back-and-forth movement prevents the use of both eyes together (fusion). The eye alternately uncovered is observed for movement. If movement of the eye occurs, it is an indication of muscle imbalance; that is, the eyes are not aligned when fusion is interrupted [9]. The test should be performed for both near (1 ft, or 0.3 M) and distant (20 ft, or 6 M) fixation.

Muscle balance testing can be done in the eight diagnostic positions of gaze as well as in the primary (straight ahead) position of gaze. The eight diagnostic positions of gaze are: (1) right gaze (dextroversion), (2) left gaze (levoversion), (3) straight-up gaze (supraversion), (4) straight-down gaze (infraversion), (5) up and right gaze, (6) down and right gaze, (7) up and left gaze, (8) down and left gaze.

The 12 extraocular eye muscles that control eye movement are evaluated for the specific direction of their maximum action. The functions of these muscles are listed in Table 7-1.

The muscles of the same eye that act together to rotate the globe are termed *agonist*, e.g., right superior rectus (RSR) and the right inferior oblique (RIO) are agonist in elevating the right globe. The muscles of the same eye that act in opposite directions and therefore require reciprocal inhibition of one while the

Table 7-1. Muscles Controlling Eye Movement and Their Action and Innervation

Muscle	Movement Controlled	Innervation (Cranial Nerve)
Medial rectus		Oculomotor (IIIrd)
Right	Eye to left	
Left	Eye to right	
Lateral rectus		Abducens (VIth)
Right	Eye to right	
Left	Eye to left	
Superior rectus		Oculomotor (IIIrd)
(right and left)	Elevates eye	
	Rotates eye upward and inward	
Inferior rectus		Oculomotor (IIIrd)
(right and left)	Depresses eyes	
	Rotates eye downward and inward	
Superior oblique		Trochlear (IVth)
(right and left)	Depression	
	Intorsion	
	Abduction	
	Rotates eye downward and outward	
Inferior oblique		Oculomotor (IIIrd)
(right and left)	Elevation	
	Extorsion	
	Abduction	
	Rotates eye upward and outward	

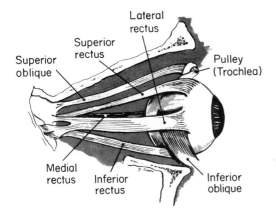

FIGURE 7-2. Extraocular muscles controlling eye movements (right eye).

other is contracting are termed *antagonists.* For example, when the left lateral
rectus (LLR) is contracting to move the left eye to the left, its antagonist, the
left medial rectus (LMR) is being inhibited [8]. "Two antagonistic muscles may
contract at the same time but in one it may be with increasing intensity whereas
in the other with decreasing intensity. This phenomenon allows a finely graded
response and steady movement [8]."

The *yoke muscles* are the muscles in the opposite eye that work together to
move the eyes to a given position of gaze; i.e., the right lateral rectus (RLR) and
the left medial rectus (LMR) are yoke muscles in that they are the leading
muscles in moving the gaze to the right [5].

Only with knowledge of the agonist, antagonist, and yoke muscles and their
innervation and positions of gaze can the nurse effectively examine the patient's
ocular movements.

Using a penlight as a target, the nurse has the patient fix his gaze on the light
while she moves it from the primary position through the other eight positions.
The nurse watches closely the parallel position of the corneal light reflexes in all
positions of gaze. Deviation of light reflexes is abnormal and requires further
testing by an ophthalmologist.

Any vertical shifting (or movement) in the cover test is abnormal, as is
diplopia. A slight horizontal shift of the visual axis may be seen with the
alternating cover test. At the extreme of gaze, physiologic or end-point
nystagmus may occur and is considered normal; any other nystagmus is
considered abnormal. The nerve innervation for the ocular muscles listed in
Table 7-1 will be helpful in the neurologic examination as well as in vision
testing. Any abnormalities noted call for additional testing and referral to an
ophthalmologist. Follow-up by the nurse is necessary to determine whether or
not the patient or family has proceeded as directed.

Testing Visual Fields

The visual field and perimetry testing is done next. The visual field is that portion of the external world that the eye can encompass. The images formed on the retina are inverted and reversed representations of objects in the real world, but are subsequently inverted and reversed again by higher brain centers, so that we ultimately see objects as they really are.

Lesions or defects in the retina, optic pathways, and brain are described in terms of the field of vision they affect rather than the part of the retina affected by them. Severing of, or severe damage to, the optic nerve or retina of one eye will obliterate the visual fields, both nasal and temporal, of that eye.

When lesions occur in the optic chiasm,* optic tract, or brain they usually affect the visual fields of both eyes because of the crossing of fibers. Therefore when there is a lesion at the optic chiasm there is a loss of visual impulses from the nasal halves of each retina (right retina of left eye, left retina of right eye). This results in the loss of the temporal visual field of both eyes and is called heteronomous hemianopia. Lesions of the right side of the brain or right optic tract result in visual field defects of the left nasal field and right temporal field (right side of left eye or left side of right eye are affected). Conversely, lesions of the left optic tract and brain affect the nasal side of the left eye, left temporal field defect, and the right side of the right retina, right nasal field defect. This condition is called homonymous hemianopia [2, 4]. Interestingly, macular vision is commonly spared in homonymous hemianopias [2, 8].

There is considerable separation of nerve pathways in the brain, and lesions in many areas of the central nervous system, the retina, or the optic tract may result in various patterns of visual field defects.

Glaucoma, elevated intraocular pressure, decreases peripheral vision because the increased intraocular pressure damages the optic nerve at its head or optic disc. Central vision, that vision in the central part of the retina, macula, and fovea, is unaffected until the disease has progressed.

The confrontation test is a rough measurement of the visual fields, and peripheral vision should be performed on all persons examined. Both the nurse and the patient are seated about 3 ft (1 M) apart. One eye of the patient is patched and one eye of the examiner is closed. The nurse should have a dull surface behind her, with illumination preferably coming from behind the patient [8]. This test presumes a previously established normal field for the nurse examiner. The nurse and patient fix their open eye on the other's uncovered eye.

For children, a small light or toy is used; for adults, a moving (wiggling) or cotton-tipped finger, small ball, or light. The objects are moved inward from outside the visual field until seen by the person being tested. If the fields are

---

*The point at which fibers from the left side (nasal) of the retina of the right eye cross to the left side of the brain, forming the left optic tract with fibers from the right (temporal) side of the right eye; and fibers from the right (nasal) side of the retina of the left eye cross to the right side of the brain to join the fibers from the left (temporal) side of the left eye to form the left optic tract.

normal, the nurse and patient should detect the object at the same time. With cooperative patient and astute examiner, it is possible to detect the blind spot but the test is not refined enough to detect its enlargement.

For small children, one can use a target for fixation that moves and can be placed on the examiner's headpiece or on her glasses. Then the use of a figure on a wand instead of the usual finger will attract the child's attention when brought into his field of vision. Patients with any abnormalities in the visual fields should be seen by an ophthalmologist or a neurologist.

The confrontation test is an imprecise test; many precision instruments must be used for accurate perimeter examinations. If the person has symptoms that indicate the possibility of visual field defects, he should be referred for precise testing.

External Ocular Structures

Eyebrows are examined for hair, loss of hair, scaling, and movement. Loss of movement of both brows would indicate central impairment of the facial nerve, while unilateral loss indicates a peripheral impairment [2, 7].

The appearance of the eyelids should be noted. The eyelid is subject to all the dermatologic conditions manifested by the other skin surfaces of the body. The color, texture, mobility, and position of the lids should be observed and the palpebral fissures examined. Differences other than normal racial differences in the upper lid folds should be described. Localized swelling, inflammation, generalized periorbital edema, and scars from previous ocular injuries should be recorded.

The size of the palpebral fissures is altered by the position of the lids. The margins of the lid in normal position expose no sclera and overlay the cornea above and below. Frequent involuntary lid-blinking should be present. The lids should close easily by voluntary movement. Equal elevation and movement of the lids with the globe should occur in all positions of gaze. Motor innervation of the levator palpebrae superioris muscle, which raises the lid, is via the facial nerve (see Table 7-2). The lids should be in close approximation to the eyeball. Inverted (entropion) or everted (ectropion) lids are abnormal. Protrusion of the eyeball is difficult to determine, but if it is suspected, the patient should be sent to an ophthalmologist for instrument measurement [2, 7, 8].

The *conjunctiva* is the smooth transparent muscosal layer which unites the lids and globes. The *palpebral conjunctiva* lines the eyelids; the *bulbar conjunctiva* covers the exposed surface of the eyeball. The conjunctiva is an indicator of both systemic and local disease. The sclera should be seen through this transparent membrane and should be the color of white porcelain. There may be slight yellow pigmentation at the circumferential edge of the limbus. Normal conjuctiva contains a few large and tortuous visible episcleral vessels. Congestion of the conjunctiva may be superficial or deep. The superficial congestion may involve the whole conjunctiva. The vessels of the conjunctiva both large and small, especially in the peripheral area, are engorged. Deep congestion involves the cornea and deeper structures within the eye. This congestion is found immediately around the limbus, producing a diffuse, deep flush. The flush or vessels do not move when the conjunctiva is manipulated [8].

The bulbar and palpebral conjunctiva and the conjunctiva cul-de-sac (fold at junction of the two) should be inspected for edema and pallor. The lower lid is everted by pulling downward with the index finger at the midpoint of the lid above the bone of the lower orbital rim. Have the patient look up. The upper lid is everted to expose the upper palpebral conjunctiva and the conjunctival cul-de-sac. Visualization of this conjunctiva and underlying sclera is an important part of appraisal, as this is an area where melanomas and lymphomas may go undetected by both patient and examiner. To perform eversion of the upper eyelid, have the patient look downward with the eye open, grasp the lashes of the upper lid, pulling the lid downward and away from the globe. A cotton-tipped applicator is pressed against the upper edge of the lid while pulling upward on the lashes [8]. As long as the patient continues to look down the eyelid will remain in eversion. The upper lid is returned to its normal position by directing the patient to look up.

The *lacrimal gland,* which secretes the tears that flow across the eye and moisten the conjunctiva and cornea, is in the upper outer wall of the anterior portion of the orbit. There is a small palpebral portion located in the upper lid [8]. The lacrimal tissue sometimes can be seen when the upper lid is everted, particularly in the elderly. The lacrimal glands develop malignancies, and mixed cell tumors not uncommonly. The area should be examined for swelling,

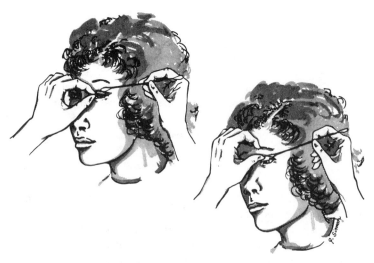

FIGURE 7-3. Eversion of lid for examining the conjunctiva of upper lid and under the upper lid. (Modified from Judge and Zuidema [6].)

tenderness, redness, and pain. Infections and abscesses of the lacrimal gland occur but are uncommon [7].

Tears flow to the inner canthus, where they drain through the lacrimal puncta into the lacrimal sac, lacrimal duct, and nose. The lacrimal puncta are visible on slight eversion of the lower lid near the inner canthus. Exert pressure on the lacrimal sac. Regurgitation from the puncta indicates blockage of the lacrimal duct. Infection of the sac is indicated when the material regurgitated is purulent. The patient should be asked whether tears overflow the lower lid onto the cheek (epiphora) when not crying or tearing due to irritation [7].

Corneal Reflexes

The cornea is observed and examined for smoothness, clearness, and its reflective properties. Dullness in any area or irregularities are abnormal. The size and shape of one cornea is compared with that of the other. A penlight can be used for examination and reflection. Since a detailed examination of the cornea requires fluorescein staining and a corneal microscope, it is not usually done in the nurse's general assessment situation. Any patient who has photophobia, dullness, irregularities of the cornea, opacity, blurring of vision, or blepharospasm should be referred to an ophthalmologist for diagnosis and treatment.

The corneal reflex tests the sensitivity of the cornea to pain, touch, and pressure and is done as a part of the appraisal. This is a test of an afferent sensory branch of the trigeminal (Vth cranial) nerve. The motor response is via the facial nerve and consists in activation of the orbicularis oculi muscle, which, among other functions, closes the eyelids [2]. In the reflex both eyes are closed, due to connecting fibers to the facial nuclei [2]. The response of the stimulated eye is called the *direct corneal reflex;* the response of the other eye is the *consensual corneal reflex* [5]. Both consensual and direct responses are obliterated by interruption of the trigeminal nerve pathways.

To test for the corneal reflex, the patient is informed of what to expect and seated opposite the nurse examiner. The patient is asked to look to the right. A twisted wisp of cotton is lightly touched to the corneal surface. An attempt should be made to approach the eye with the cotton from the side to prevent an avoidance response. The normal response should be (1) closing, and blinking of both eyes, that is, the direct and consensual corneal reflex, (2) increased lacrimation, and (3) a report of slight discomfort [6]. A consensual reflex but no direct reflex is obtained if the facial nerve on the same side is destroyed. There will, however, still be increased lacrimation [2].

The *arcus senilis* is seen around the limbus but separated from it by a clear zone in most persons over the age of 50 [5].

Anterior Chamber

The anterior chamber is viewed for a general impression of depth and for clearness of the aqueous humor. Cloudiness of the aqueous, hyphema, or accumulation of any exudate is abnormal. A general impression of the depth of the chamber is achieved by directing a penlight beam across the iris from the temporal side. If the chamber is shallow, only the temporal side of the iris will be illuminated, because the iris is bowed forward and the nasal half will be shadowed [7]. Any bulging forward of the iris, or a shadow on the nasal half of the iris, would indicate narrow-angle anatomy, predisposing to glaucoma, and the patient should be referred to an ophthalmologist for gonioscopic and tonometric examination [6].

Iris, Pupillary Reflexes, and Lens

Examination of the iris should include observation of color, texture, and pattern. Any unusual markings or growths should be noted. Compare and contrast pupil size, recognizing, however, that 25 percent of normal persons have unequal pupils [9]. Contraction and dilatation of the pupil can be demonstrated by shining a penlight into the eye in a semidarkened room. The pupillary light reflex is tested by shining a penlight into one eye and then the other eye. The constricting response of the illuminated eye is the direct light reflex. Abnormalities of the pupillary response may be due to any of a number of neurologic lesions as well as demonstrating the effect of drugs on the iris muscles. See Keeney [7] for more extensive discussion of the neurologic implications.

The near-point pupillary reflex is tested by having the patient look into the distance and then at an object 6 in. (15 cm) from his nose at the nose level. Illumination should remain constant. The response evokes three reflexes: (1) convergence, (2) accommodation, and (3) pupillary constriction [2, 8]. Equality of response in both eyes is normal and is the important factor. Rapidity of response will vary and tends to slow with age, particularly when accommodating for near point reflex.

Table 7-2. Muscles of the Eyelid and Iris and Their Action and Innervation

Muscles	Action	Innervation
Levator palpebrae superioris	Raises upper lid	Oculomotor (IIIrd)
Orbicularis oculi	Closes eyelids, acts as a sphincter (activates corneal reflex), wrinkles forehead, compresses lacrimal sac	Facial (VIIth)
Sphincter pupillae	Contracts pupil (miosis)	Oculomotor (IIIrd)
Dilator pupillae	Dilates pupil (mydriasis)	Sympathetic fibers

The lens of the eye is viewed and examined through the pupillary aperture. The lens normally is clear and transparent. Oblique illumination will reveal opacities. The transparency of the lens decreases with age, and it may appear gray in elderly persons.

Fundoscopic Examination

Currently, the nurse's use of the ophthalmoscope is somewhat limited. Ophthalmoscopic examination is a necessary part of the eye examination, and as nurses gain the knowledge and skill in this area of appraisal, it will become more and more a part of general nursing practice.

For basic ophthalmoscopy the direct ophthalmoscope is used. The nurse should become familiar with the instrument before using it on the patient. Position the ophthalmoscope next to the right eye, with the right forefinger on the lens disc. Bring the left palm within 2 in. (5 cm) of the ophthalmoscope and practice focusing on the lines of the palm until the best image possible is achieved. Vary the distance between the instrument and the palm and change the lens disc setting for the best image. The newest instruments have two discs. The larger is the lens disc and changes the refractive power of the lens (measured in diopters). The other disc changes the image of light (i.e., slit, red-filter, grid). Use of the medium round light is advised. The ophthalmoscope has both concave (minus) lenses, indicated by red numbers, and convex (plus) lenses, indicated by black numbers. "A more deeply curved convex lens focuses the rays of light closer to the lens than one with a lesser degree of curvature [8]." The hyperopic eye affords a larger area of visualization under less magnification; the myopic eye provides a smaller area of visualization with more magnification.

The nurse examiner should wear her normal corrective lenses if she has any. Patients who have severe astigmatism should wear their contact lenses or glasses for the examination, as the distortion which occurs without them cannot be corrected by the lens of the ophthalmoscope. However, hyperopic and myopic conditions in the examiner and patient are neutralized by the lenses of the ophthalmoscope. With hyperopia of the patient the nurse would use the convex lens, with myopia, the concave lens. However, the combination of the examiner's eye and the patient's eye will determine the actual diopter setting.

The fundoscopic examination is done in a room with subdued light and minimum activity to eliminate reflections and distractions. The patient and examiner should both be in comfortable body alignment, with the eyes at the same height. The ophthalmoscope is held in the examiner's right hand as the right eye is examined, and in the examiner's left hand as the left eye is being examined. The index finger is positioned on the lens disc (the thumb does not allow the rapidity of rotation allowed by the forefinger). The nurse examiner positions herself to the right of the patient's right eye. The patient is asked to fixate straight ahead on a mark on the wall over the examiner's shoulder.

The ophthalmoscope is positioned immediately in front of the examiner's eye and approximately 6 to 8 in. (15 to 20 cm) from the patient's eye. The lens is set at zero, and the cornea and lens are studied for opacities; these appear as black areas against the reddish-orange background of the retina. The normal fundus is seen as a red reflex (circular-reddish orange retinal reflection) also called the *fundus reflex.* The opacities appear black on the red reflex because they prevent the reflected light from reaching the observer's eye. The ophthalmoscope is moved to 1-½ to 2 in. (3.8 to 5 cm) from the patient's eye. The lens is set at +8 to +10 diopters for studying the cornea for opacities. The lens setting is then changed to a lower power (+2 to +4 diopters) to focus back toward the retina. The lens disc is rotated until a vessel is located on the retina and focused on. The vessel is followed as it grows progressively larger until the optic disc is located.

The *optic disc,* which is the site of entrance of the optic nerve and retinal blood vessels, may be oval or circular and is lighter than the retina in color, often described as reddish or pink (see Fig. 7-4). The *physiologic cup* of the disc is a pale area of depression with a rim between the cup and the disc border. The border may be a clear-cut edge, may be demarcated by a white ring, or may merge gradually into the retina [8]. A black ring or crescent may be seen occasionally as a result of thickened pigmented retinal epithelium. Myopic eyes tend to have a larger disc than hyperopic eyes. In glaucoma, the rim and border are sharp, the physiologic cup is deep, and the disc is paler. A pale disc may indicate optic atrophy. When papilledema or papillitis is present, the disc borders may be blurry and the disc congested [8]. Elevation of the nerve head may also be present and is abnormal.

The central retinal artery enters at the optic disc and immediately bifurcates into the superior and inferior papillary arteries. After the second bifurcation the vessels are arterioles (venules before the second major junction). The veins are larger and the column of blood is darker than in the arteries (Fig. 7-4). A 3:2 vein-to-artery ratio is seen in normal persons [7]. Some sources give a ratio of 5:4 [8]. With arteriosclerotic and hypertensive changes, the arteries narrow (3:1 ratio), change color, become more opaque, show a copper-wire effect, and show changes at the arteriovenous crossings [8]. Indentation of the vein where the artery crosses, enlargement of the vein distal to the arterial crossing, and disappearance of the vein on either side of the artery indicate thickening of the arteriolar wall [5]. The entire fundus is examined by having the patient rotate the globe so that different areas can be examined. Avoid the center of the fundus *(macula)* until all the periphery has been examined.

The macula is approximately 2 disc diameters temporally from the optic disc and is normally darker than the surrounding fundus. The darkness of the macula varies with complexion. In blondes the macula may not be differentiated by color, and location may be determined by relation to the optic disc and retinal vessels. Brunettes have a dark macular area. The area of darker red in the center of the macula is the *fovea centralis.* In the center of the fovea is seen a tiny light reflex, which is a reflection of the light of the ophthalmoscope on the concave

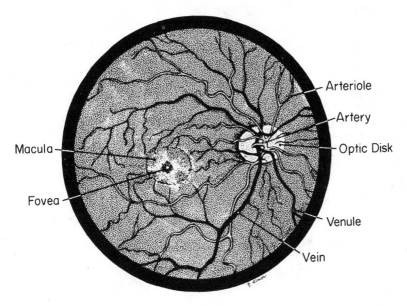

FIGURE 7-4. Structures seen in examination of the fundus by ophthalmoscope.

surface of the fovea. The macula and the fovea are the last areas of the fundus examined, as the patient will become light-dazzled, and his eyes will tear during this part of the examination. The variations of normal are great and it will take considerable skill, knowledge, and practice to be able to identify more than the grossly abnormal.

Intraocular Pressure

A rough estimation of intraocular pressure is done by using the finger tension test. The patient is asked to close his eyes and look down while the nurse places two forefingers on the upper lid over the sclera of the eyeball. Pressure is exerted by alternating the forefingers in a back-and-forward movement. The globe should indent slightly with the pressure. The examiner must first learn what the "feel" of normal globe pressure is. Normal intraocular pressure is 12 to 22 mm Hg [5]. A comparison is also made between the two eyes. This estimation is made on all patients and is of particular importance for those over 40 years of age. Any suspected increased pressure or symptoms of glaucoma require the immediate referral of the patient to the ophthalmologist.

   Nurses can and do use the Schiötz tonometer, but this special test needs to be done in collaboration with the ophthalmologist since medication of the eye is involved. Other tests may be required for patients with suspected or confirmed eye abnormalities but are outside the scope of the general examination ordinarily done by nurses in most nonspecialized settings.

REFERENCES

1. Ganong, W. F.   *Review of Medical Physiology* (3rd ed.). Los Altos, Calif.: Lange Medical Publications, 1967.
2. Gatz, A. J.   *Manter's Essentials of Clinical Neuroanatomy and Neurophysiology* (4th ed.). Philadelphia: Davis, 1970.
3. Gordon, D. M.   Diseases of the Eye. *Clinical Symposia Reprint.* Ardsley, N.Y.: Ciba Corporation, 1962.
4. Havener, W. H., Saunders, W. H., and Bergersen, B. S.   *Nursing Care in Eye, Ear, Nose, and Throat Disorders* (2nd ed.). St. Louis: Mosby, 1964.
5. Henderson, J. W.   Eye. In R. D. Judge, and G. D. Zuidema (Eds.), *Methods of Clinical Examination: A Physiological Approach* (3rd ed.). Boston: Little, Brown, 1974.
6. Judge, R. D., and Zuidema, G. D. (Eds.).   *Methods of Clinical Examination: A Physiologic Approach* (3rd ed.). Boston: Little, Brown, 1974.
7. Keeney, A. H.   *Ocular Examination Basis and Technique.* St. Louis: Mosby, 1970.
8. Scheie, H. G., and Albert, D. M.   *Adler's Textbook of Ophthalmology* (8th ed.). Philadelphia: Saunders, 1969.
9. Taber, C. W.   *Taber's Cyclopedic Medical Dictionary* (10th ed.). Philadelphia: Davis, 1965.

PHYSICAL APPRAISAL OF THE EAR AND HEARING   8

Patricia Mitchell Butler

GLOSSARY

atresia   Pathological closure of a normal anatomic opening or congenital absence of the same, used here in relation to external auditory canal.

cerumen   Waxlike, soft, brown secretion found in the external canal of the ear.

cochlea   A winding cone-shaped tube forming a portion of the inner ear which contains the organ of Corti.

dizziness   Disturbed sense of relationship to space.

endolymph   Fluid in the membranous labyrinth of the inner ear.

frequency   Number of vibrations per second made by a sound wave (expressed in cycles per second) (cps).

injection   Prominence and dilatation of the normal vascular bed.

intensity   Pressure exerted by a sound (expressed in decibels) (db).

labyrinth   Intricate communicating canals in the inner ear.

nystagmus   (labyrinthine or central)   Slow movement of the eye in one direction followed by a rapid involuntary compensatory movement in the opposite direction (rhythmic).

ossicles   The three small bones of the middle ear: the malleus, incus, and stapes.

otalgia   Pain in the ear.

otitis   Inflammation of the ear.

pinna   Projecting part of the external ear; auricle.

recruitment   Abnormally rapid increase in loudness with increasing sound intensity, which occurs in deafness of neural origin.

tinnitus   Noise often of ringing, in the ears, originating within the body.

tragus   Cartilaginous tonguelike projection in front of the external auditory meatus.

tympanic membrane   Membrane serving as the lateral wall of the tympanic cavity and separating it from the external acoustic meatus.

umbo of the tympanic membrane   The point where the handle (manubrium of the malleolus) is attached to the inner surface of the tympanic membrane.

vertigo   Sensation of whirling motion of oneself or of external objects.

vestibule   The middle part of the inner ear, behind the cochlea and in front of the semicircular canals.

Appraisal of the ear includes both physical and historical data collection by the nurse. The major objective is to determine the functional status of the ear, and, if there is abnormality, make the appropriate referral of the patient to a specialist or an agency. The appraisal of the ear and hearing includes the history, both past and present, testing for hearing, the physical appraisal of the external ear, otoscopic examination of the external canal and tympanic membrane, and vestibular testing. Equipment needed for the otologic appraisal includes:

1. Tuning forks (512 to 1,024, and 2,000 cps frequency)
2. Otoscope with pneumatic bulb attachment
3. Masking device, i.e. paper
4. Barany noise box

HISTORY AND EXAMINATION

The history should begin with questions about hearing loss in family members, and, insofar as possible, a determination of the type of loss. Next, a history of ear diseases in childhood is obtained. Specific inquiry is made regarding episodes of otalgia, drainage, stuffiness, fever, and decreased hearing. Occurrence and frequency of infections, treatment instituted, and response to therapy are determined also. An attempt is made to determine event-related and other potential causative factors, e.g., drainage and pain occurring after swimming, in cold weather, or when no hat or protective ear covering is worn.

In assessing infants and children unable to communicate verbally, behavioral changes are cardinal signs. Mothers should be asked about behavior changes observed and instructed to note these changes in the future. Explicit data about symptoms should be sought as indicated in the following:

1. *Otalgia.* Does the patient have otalgia, and if so, when did it begin? Is it described as constant or intermittent? Is it associated with movement, activity, or noise, and is the pain sharp or dull? How has the individual attempted to relieve the pain, and has the pain been relieved?

2. *Chills and fever.* Has the patient had fever or chills? Did he take his temperature, and if so, what was it? Has he had a recent history of colds, influenza, or other systemic disease? Was medical treatment sought, and if so, what was the diagnosis and treatment? If medical treatment was not sought, what was the course of the fever? Was there self-treatment? What kind, and what results were obtained?

3. *Drainage.* Is there drainage from the ears now and has there been drainage previously? What is the color, consistency, amount, and odor of the discharge? When was the drainage first noticed? Is the cerumen normally soft or hard? How are the ears normally cleaned? Has the drainage been separate from or associated with other symptoms?

4. *Medication history.* A medication history should be elicited. Is the patient now taking ototoxic drugs? Has the patient taken such medications recently, e.g., aspirin, quinine, streptomycin, kanamycin, gentamicin, neomycin, nitrofurantoin? If ototoxic drugs have been taken, the extent to which the patient has used the drug needs to be determined.

5. *Tinnitus, vertigo, and dizziness.* It should be determined whether the patient has or has had tinnitus, vertigo, or dizziness associated with the use of medications or with other diseases or symptoms. Evaluations of equilibrium, dizziness, and vertigo are made to determine the gross function of the vestibular

portion of the VIIIth cranial nerve. Dizziness and vertigo can be symptoms of neurologic and systemic problems as well as of vestibular alterations. It is important to have patients describe the sensation they feel. Does the dizziness or vertigo occur only in one position (horizontal or vertical) or when bending over, standing, or changing position? Does the person feel he is moving, or does he feel that he is stationary and the room is moving?

6. *Environmental noise.* A brief history of exposure to environmental noise in the work, home and social settings should be taken. Determine if the patient is exposed to loud noise in the work setting and whether he utilizes protective devices provided. What is the extent of exposure?

Throughout the history-taking and physical examination the nurse can gain further information through nonverbal clues the patient may give. Is the patient's voice loud or soft? Is it proportional to the environmental noise? Does he need to have questions repeated, or just certain words? Is body or head posture changed as if to facilitate hearing?

TESTING HEARING ACUITY

On completing the history, the nurse can begin the physical examination by testing the hearing. The ear examination, including hearing acuity testing, is conducted with the patient comfortably seated. For most of the examination the nurse is also comfortably seated, except during otoscopic examination of the small child or infant.

Tests for Conversational Hearing

Hearing for normal conversational purposes can be checked by the use of whisper and spoken-voice testing [1] (see Table 8-1). The whisper and spoken voice should be several inches from the ear being tested. When testing is done by air conduction, the opposite ear from the one being tested must be masked. Masking is also important when testing bone conduction, particularly when the hearing difference between the two ears is greater than 30 db (the intensity level of the sounds normally heard in a quiet room). The greater the discrepancy in hearing between the ears, the greater the need for the better ear to be masked.

Further testing can be done by determining the intensity level at which the individual can understand speech, called *sensitivity hearing.* Magnetic phonographic and tape recordings are available for this test. The live voice can be used but has the disadvantage of not being standardized and thus can be used only for gross measurement of sensitivity. *Spondee words* are bisyllabic, easily understood, and equally stressed words such as *airplane, oatmeal, daybreak, pancake, mousetrap, mushroom, stairway, headlight.* These are spoken to the patient at normal conversational intensity and with increasing levels of intensity as needed. Recordings of these words can be ordered from the address given below.*

*Techsonic Studios, 1201 South Brentwood Blvd., St. Louis, Missouri.

Table 8-1. Voice Test Equivalent[*]

Voice Level and Decibel Equivalent	Clinical Equivalent
Inaudible whisper, 15—25 db	Normal hearing or very mild loss
Soft or just audible whisper, 25—35 db	Mild hearing loss (socially adequate for adults, inadequate for children)
Loud whisper, 35—45 db (mild masking, i.e., finger in opposite ear)	Moderate loss (borderline for conversational purposes)
Soft spoken voice, 45—55 db (mild masking, i.e., briskly moving finger in opposite ear)	Socially inadequate; needs some form of correction if best ear
Moderate spoken voice, 55—70 db (loud masking, i.e., rubbing paper, radio static or Barany noise box in opposite ear)	Always involves some sensorineural loss, with or without associated conductive loss
Loud spoken voice, 70—90 db (very loud masking, i.e., Barany noise box, white noise, or alarm from watch in opposite ear)	Severe loss with large sensorineural deficit, with or without associated conductive component

*Modified from Boles, R. [1]. By permission of the author and publisher.

The level (in db) at which the person can correctly repeat 50 percent of the words is called his *speech reception threshold* (SRT).

Speech discrimination testing is another method the nurse can use for evaluation of hearing. Phonetically balanced (P-B), one-syllable words, phonetically difficult to understand, are presented at an optimal intensity for the patient. The percentage of words such as *knees, yard, carve, tin, sin, day, toe, felt, hunt,* and *stone* which are repeated correctly is used to give the nurse an idea of the patient's discrimination ability. Both sensitivity and discrimination ability is decreased with sensorineural loss.

Hearing testing in children is difficult but is imperative for early detection of loss. The presence or absence of the startle reflex can be used to test infants under 6 months of age. Testing the ability to localize sounds is another way of assessing hearing in infants and children. Or one can use toys that make varying noises at different intensities to test hearing levels. However, if this proves too difficult, gross measurement is better than none at all. Word games and play techniques can be used by the nurse or by the family for testing hearing.

Tuning Fork Tests

Tuning fork tests for hearing acuity are an important part of the otologic examination. Tuning forks with the frequencies of 512 to 1,024 and 2,000 cps (within the speech frequency range) should be used. The Rinne test (air and bone conduction) is performed by alternately placing a vibrating tuning fork on the mastoid bone and then opposite the external auditory meatus. The opposite ear is masked during the test. The tuning fork is held on the mastoid bone and at the auditory meatus until the sound is no longer heard. The sound vibrations are conducted via bone to the cochlea, activating hair cells that are connected to the fibers of the auditory (VIIIth cranial) nerve. When the still vibrating tuning fork is placed outside the external auditory meatus, conduction occurs by the usual route. The normal ear hears the tuning fork twice as long by air conduction (AC) than by bone conduction (BC). When this occurs, the result is designated as a positive Rinne (AC > BC). This relationship is reversed in advanced conductive loss (negative Rinne) and is designated as a negative or equal Rinne (BC > or = AC). With sensorineural loss (see Types of Hearing Loss) the normal relationship is maintained (positive Rinne, AC > BC), but the length of time the fork is heard is reduced.

The Schwabach test (bone conduction only) is a comparison of the patient's and the examiner's bone conduction. The vibrating tuning fork is placed alternately on the patient's mastoid process and on the examiner's mastoid process. When either stops hearing the tone, the number of seconds that elapse before the tone can no longer be heard by the other person is recorded. The tone will not be heard as long by the person with sensorineural loss as it is heard by the [nurse] examiner. If the tone is heard longer by the patient, he has a conductive hearing loss (provided the examiner's hearing is normal), which masks the environmental noises so that he hears the tone longer than the examiner.

In the Weber test, a vibrating tuning fork is placed in the midline of the skull or, unless the patient has dentures, on the maxillary incisors. The person with conductive loss hears the sound in the impaired (poor) ear if the other ear has normal hearing because the impaired ear is essentially masked for room noise. If there is sensorineural loss in one ear with the other ear normal, the sound is heard louder in the normal ear. With normal hearing the sound is not lateralized (i.e., to the right or left ear) but is heard equally by both ears (as if in the midline). The nurse should indicate on the record the ear to which the sound is lateralized.

Types of Hearing Loss

Hearing loss may be of three types [4] :

1. *Conductive hearing loss* occurs when there is interruption or attenuation of sound waves as they are conducted from the external meatus to the cochlea. This may occur in the external ear at the tympanic membrane or in the middle ear or its ossicles. Persons with conductive hearing loss speak softly, often hear better in a noisy environment (others speak above the noise), and are able to hear well on the telephone.
2. *Sensorineural or perceptive hearing loss* is an interruption or attenuation of impulses transmitted or interpreted at the level of the cochlea, auditory nerve, or hearing center of the cerebral cortex. Persons with a sensorineural hearing loss speak loudly, may hear sound but are unable to understand it (poor discrimination), and hear better in a quiet environment. These persons may also experience recruitment.

3. *Mixed hearing loss* is a combination of conductive and sensorineural hearing loss.

EXAMINATION OF THE EXTERNAL EAR

The physical appraisal of the ear begins with the examination of the auricle. The size and shape are noted, and the auricle (pinna) is inspected and palpated for lesions or abnormal growths. Movement of the auricle is normally not painful if the nurse examiner moves it gently. Pain on movement of the auricle or tragus is usually associated with abnormality, particularly with external otitis (otitis externa).

Deformities of the auricle such as macrotia (abnormal enlargement) or lop ears (projecting auricle) may be referred to a plastic surgeon if the cosmetic aspect is creating a problem for the person and corrective surgery is desired. Gnarled, thickened cauliflower ears are indicative of repeated trauma. Persons with hematomas of the auricle and damage to the external structures should be referred to a physician. Sebaceous cysts, nodules, and nonhealing sores may be seen on the auricle.

The external auditory meatus should be examined for the size of the opening, swelling, redness, discharge, cerumen, or any visible lesions. The external auditory meatus may be completely occluded by tumor or, in external otitis, by swelling.

Loss of touch and pain sensation in the external auditory canal indicates functional alteration of the afferent glossopharyngeal (IXth) and vagus (Xth) cranial nerves [3].

The nurse's role in appraisal of the ear is to determine its functional status. If any abnormalities are identified, the patient must be referred to a physician, particularly to an otologist if one is available. The nurse should also refer persons with hearing losses to audiologists for further evaluation and as appropriate to centers and local agencies where classes in lipreading and correct use of hearing aids are offered.†

OTOSCOPIC EXAMINATION

The external auditory canal and tympanic membrane are examined with an otoscope. The use of a head mirror and an appropriately sized aural speculum provides a better view of the ear and allows the examiner a free hand for instrumentation. These instruments take time and practice to learn to use safely and effectively. The otoscope provides for excellent visualization and a pneumatic device, consisting of a bulb and tube, when attached to the otoscope,

---

†Information on these classes can be obtained from the National Association of Hearing and Speech Agencies, 919 185th Street, N.W., Washington D. C., 20006.

permits manipulation of the tympanic membrane. The largest size speculum the ear will accommodate comfortably should be used on the otoscope for best visualization and to create a seal with the external canal for the use of the pneumatic device. Slight pressure on the pneumatic bulb will cause the tympanic membrane to move, since the normal tympanic membrane is sensitive to slight changes of pressure. The use of the pneumatic bulb requires care and expertise and is described here, although it may not be within the general practice of the beginning nurse examiner.

As the otoscope is introduced into the external canal, the nurse must be very gentle, as the epithelial lining is extremely sensitive. Any pressure against the wall of the canal may be painful, and the tissue may be traumatized and bleed easily. The otoscope should be held upside down, so the hand holding it may be steadied against the patient's head. This prevents the nurse from creating a lever-type movement against the canal with the tip of the speculum. If the person moves his head the nurse's hand and otoscope moves with it, preventing trauma and discomfort. The patient should be instructed to indicate any discomfort to the nurse during the examination. In examination of adults, both patient and nurse should be seated comfortably.

The small child or infant should be placed prone on an examining table with the arms beside his body and with the head turned on one side and then the other for the otoscopic examination. The nurse can position her body over the child's and stabilize the head both with the left hand pulling the pinna (lower

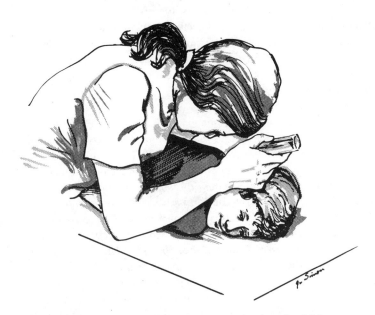

FIGURE 8-1.   Positioning for otoscopic examination of a child.

helix) back and with the right hand holding the otoscope or vice versa (see Fig. 8-1). The pneumatic bulb should be manipulated with the left hand while the nurse holds the pinna. The right ear is examined with the right hand holding the otoscope; the left ear, with the left hand holding the otoscope.

The external canal may need to be cleaned if cerumen is excessive or if drainage is obscuring a suspected lesion. Determination of the intactness of the tympanic membrane must be made before any solution is instilled and can be done in two ways: first, by asking the patient to create pressure to move the tympanic membrane by swallowing, or to equalize the pressure by yawning (the patient can feel the change of pressure as this is done); second, by placing the otoscope into the external ear and squeezing the pneumatic bulb to create the feeling of pressure on the tympanic membrane. Solution should not be instilled if a ruptured tympanic membrane is suspected; rather, the patient should be referred to an otologist without delay. If the tympanic membrane is intact, enough hydrogen peroxide (3%) warmed to body temperature is instilled to fill the canal. After instillation, the patient should lie on the opposite side for 5 to 10 minutes while the cerumen softens. The ear is then irrigated with tap water warmed to body temperature. Either an ear bulb or syringe can be used to irrigate. The force of the stream will not damage the tympanic membrane as long as water is allowed to escape via space around the syringe or bulb tip. The canal can then be dried with rolled tissue.

Once the canal is clean, the otoscope can be introduced slowly while the nurse examines the canal. The color of the epithelial lining is noted (e.g., is it pale, reddened, with vessels injected?). Any lesions, tumors, polyps, hematomas, exostoses, or chondromas (small, broad-based cartilaginous lumps) observed are to be described in the record. Foreign bodies or insects in the ear may be seen in children. Drops of mineral or olive oil should be instilled to immobilize the insects and facilitate their removal by irrigation. Any patient with a foreign body in the ear requiring manipulation or instrumentation for its removal needs the immediate attention of a physician.

To visualize the tympanic membrane, the pinna is pulled backward and upward (in the child, only backward) to straighten the canal. Landmarks to guide the nurse in her examination are seen in Figure 8-2. The normal eardrum appears translucent or pearly gray. The tympanic membrane is on an inclined plane, which creates the light reflex anteroinferiorly from the umbo. The umbo is visualized in the center of the membrane, behind which is the lower end of the malleus. Ascending from the umbo, first is the manubrium (long process or handle) of the malleus and then its short process, which stands out like a tiny knob. Directly upward and outward from the short process of the malleus are the anterior and posterior malleolar folds of the tympanic membrane.

The pars tensa is the area of the tympanic membrane which has a fibrous middle layer, while the pars flaccida, above the anterior and posterior fold, does not. Through some eardrums the long process of the incus and the chorda tympani nerve may be seen posterior superiorly behind the malleus and high

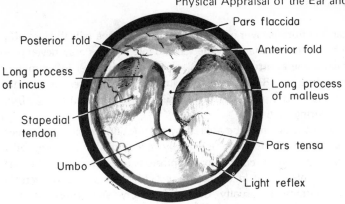

Pars flaccida

Posterior fold

Anterior fold

Long process
of incus

Long process
of malleus

Stapedial
tendon

Pars tensa

Umbo

Light reflex

FIGURE 8-2. Landmarks of the tympanic membrane, right ear. (See discussion in text.)

across the eardrum. The anulus is the thickened ring around the periphery of the tympanic membrane.

Vascularization of the eardrum varies significantly among individuals and is seen mainly along the manubrium, malleolar folds, and anulus. Injection of these vessels is abnormal. It may also be present after irrigation to cleanse the canal, or if daily self-cleansing measures are used by the patient. Intense injection is seen with external otitis.

After clear identification of the landmarks, the nurse should gently squeeze the pneumatic bulb to cause movement of the tympanic membrane. If there is a good seal between the otoscope and the ear, gentle repeated squeezing of the bulb should move the membrane. Membrane movement is frequently best seen by watching the light reflex. Inability to move the tympanic membrane (or the movement of air bubbles behind it) when the pneumatic bulb is used, along with evidence of retraction, or an amber color of the tympanic membrane, or both, may be signs of serous otitis media. Alterations of the color, position, and integrity of the tympanic membrane often reflect the presence of diseases of the middle ear. Patients with these alterations need referral to a physician.

The position of the eardrum may be altered in several ways. Retraction creates prominence of the landmarks. In a patient in a sitting position, a fluid level or movement of air bubble may be seen behind the eardrum. Bulging of the eardrum may occur from pressure within the middle ear. Then landmarks are faint or totally obscured. This is usually seen with purulent otitis media. With a cholesteatoma (extensive cystic mass associated with chronic middle ear infection) some bulging may occur, and the tympanic membrane may appear white.

The color and characteristics of the tympanic membrane vary with many disease processes. With acute external otitis it is injected and thickened and leathery [2]. Healed perforations may be present as flaccid areas that move more readily than the normal tympanic membrane on pneumatic stimulation.

This results when the fibrous layer of the tympanic membrane fails to close after perforation. Dead white or ashen gray flecks or dense plaques may develop on the tympanic membrane as a result of cartilaginous deposits after inflammatory disease or after perforation. Blueness of the eardrum indicates bleeding into the tympanic membrane (ecchymosis) and may result from barotrauma (e.g., from too rapid descent during air travel).

Integrity of the eardrum may be altered by perforation, tearing, or surgical incision (myringotomy). Perforation is usually the result of purulent otitis media. Tears may result from concussion (explosions or hard slap on the ear), skull fracture, or the placement in the ear of any object which cuts or tears the membrane. Myringotomy is usually done posteriorly and inferiorly as a therapeutic measure to facilitate drainage of the middle ear.

The epithelial cells on the surface of the tympanic membrane move outward toward the anulus and into the auditory canal (epithelial migration) as opposed to the usual flaking off of dead epithelial tissue. This process takes approximately 30 days or more. Markings on the tympanic membrane thus appear to move outward and remain on the membrane or epithelial lining of the canal for at least 30 days. Because of this movement, the nurse working with a patient who has had a previous pathological condition of the tympanic membrane should draw a sketch of any markings on the eardrum for later reference. The lesions may appear not to have healed or to be just remaining there. With a diagram the nurse can see the progression of the healed or scabbed area.

There are many probable causes of tinnitus which can be termed as subjective (patient experienced) or objective (heard by the examiner as well as the patient) [2]. As all tinnitus requires further testing, patients with this condition should be referred to a physician.

VESTIBULAR TESTING

In examination of the ear, vestibular function must also be tested. The vestibular portion of the auditory (VIIIth) nerve furnishes afferent fibers ultimately influencing the coordination of the neck, eyes, and body necessary for maintaining equilibrium in relation to movement of the head and posture [2]. The patient usually experiences symptoms of dizziness or vertigo when there is an abnormality in this system. The nurse can assess the functioning of the labyrinth system using several simple tests.

One test is for nystagmus. Vestibular nystagmus is produced by disturbances of the labyrinth and sometimes by disturbances of the central nervous system. It should be distinguished from normal eye movements and from ocular nystagmus (in both of which both excursions of the eye are of equal amplitude) [2]. Vestibular nystagmus is a slow movement of the eyes in one direction until they reach a limit, followed by a rapid compensatory movement in the opposite direction. The movements are rhythmic. Vestibular nystagmus indicates a disease process except when it occurs on extreme lateral gaze.

Nystagmus may be induced by use of the caloric test and the electronystagmogram. In the caloric test, either cold or hot water is used to douche the external auditory canal. Measurement of the resulting nystagmus gives important information on the location of the disease process. The electronystagmogram (ENG) is a refinement of the caloric test. Leads are placed around the eyes to record graphically the movements of the eye. These tests are usually done by nurses in the otologist's office or clinic.

Past pointing and falling is another measurement of labyrinth function. Past pointing and falling occur in the direction of the flow of the endolymphatic fluid in the labyrinth. The patient should sit with eyes closed and two index fingers and arms extended in front of him. The nurse sits opposite the patient and places her fingers on his. The patient is told to raise both hands and arms and then lower them to the nurse's fingers. The person with normal labyrinth function can do this, while the fingers of a person with abnormal labyrinth function will deviate to the right or left of the nurse's fingers.

To test the falling reaction the patient stands with feet together and eyes closed. The person with abnormal labyrinth function will tend to fall to the left or right. (For further discussion of labyrinth function, see DeWeese and Saunders [2].) Patients with detected vestibular alterations must be referred to an otologist.

The facial (VIIth cranial) nerve passes through the posterior part of the middle ear and is enclosed in a bony canal (facial, or fallopian, canal). Chronic mastoiditis, skull fracture with damage to the middle ear, and trauma during middle ear surgery may result in temporary or permanent facial paralysis. The chorda tympani nerve (branch of the facial) passes immediately behind the tympanic membrane and is distributed to the taste receptors (sweet, salt, and sour), in the anterior two-thirds of the tongue. Chronic infection of the mastoid or middle ear surgery may cause temporary or permanent loss or decreased taste.

Nurses today are often called on to appraise the patient's hearing and determine the presence or absence of many common ear problems. The data obtained from the examination will guide the nurse in making responsible decisions regarding the care and counsel she can provide the patient or the need for referral for medical evaluation and therapy.

REFERENCES

1. Boles, R. Hearing test without an audiometer. *Univ. Mich. Med. Cent. J.* 37:156, 1971.
2. DeWeese, D. D., and Saunders, W. H. *Textbook of Otolaryngology* (3rd ed.). St. Louis: Mosby, 1968.
3. Gatz, A. J. *Manter's Essentials of Clinical Neuroanatomy and Neurophysiology* (4th ed.). Philadelphia: Davis, 1970.
4. Montgomery, W. W. Ears, Nose, and Throat. In R. D. Judge and G. D. Zuidema (Eds.), *Methods of Clinical Examination: A Physiologic Approach* (3rd ed.). Boston: Little, Brown, 1974.

SUGGESTED READINGS

Ganong, W. F. *Review of Medical Physiology* (3rd ed.). Los Altos, Calif.: Lange Medical Publications, 1967.

Havener, W. H., Saunders, W. H., and Bergesen, B. S. *Nursing Care in Eye, Ear, Nose and Throat Disorders.* St. Louis: Mosby, 1964.

Naunton, R. F. *An Introduction to Audiometry.* Minneapolis: Maico Hearing Instruments, 1968.

PHYSICAL APPRAISAL OF RESPIRATORY SYSTEM FUNCTION

9

Susan Mengel Pinney

GLOSSARY

atelectasis Incomplete expansion of the lung; a nonspecific term referring to partial or complete airlessness or reduction in lung volume, or both, with or without locally obstructed bronchi.

bronchiectasis Chronic disease marked by dilatation of the bronchi or bronchioles and chronic suppuration.

bronchitis Acute or chronic inflammation of bronchial tubes.

collapse Reduction in lung volume, acute or chronic, due to any cause.

compression Mechanical reduction in lung volume by pressure.

consolidation Diffuse replacement of a large zone of pulmonary parenchyma with liquid and solid products of inflammation.

crepitation Crackling; specifically, noise produced by pressure on subcutaneous tissue containing an abnormal amount of gas or air; *crepitant rale* Rale of crackling quality, usually moist.

cyanosis Bluish coloration of the skin and mucous membranes due to insufficient oxygenation of the arterial blood.

emphysema Abnormal presence of or increase in air content. Most commonly, a disease associated with chronic bronchitis characterized by diffuse bronchial obstruction and breathlessness. *subcutaneous e.* Air or other gas in subcutaneous tissues.

empyema Accumulation of pus in the pleural cavity.

epistaxis Hemorrhage from the nose.

fremitus Palpable vibration. *friction f.* Vibrations due to friction rubs. *rhonchal f.* Vibrations due to passage of air through bronchial tubes filled with secretions. *tactile f.* Voice sound vibrations felt when applying hand to thorax; also called *vocal f.*

hemoptysis Expectoration of blood by coughing.

oropharynx Part of pharynx directly behind the oral cavity, extending from the inferior border of the soft palate to the lingual surface of the epiglottis.

paroxysmal Recurring suddenly or with suddenly increasing intensity.

pleural effusion Presence of fluid in the pleural space; the term includes bloody fluid (hemothorax), purulent fluid (empyema), and chylous fluid (chylothorax), which require thoracentesis for specific identification.

pneumonia Inflammation of the lungs due to infection.

pneumonitis Condition of localized acute inflammation of the lung without gross toxemia.

pneumothorax Accumulation of air or gas in the pleural cavity.

rhinorrhea Nasal discharge.

stridor Harsh, high-pitched crowing sounds during respiration.

suppuration Formation of pus.

voice sounds Vibrations of the spoken voice transmitted through the lungs and appreciated by auscultation; also called *voice resonance* and, rarely, *vocal fremitus.*

133

During recent years nurses have had increasing responsibility for extensive physical examination of the respiratory system. Since the introduction of intensive care units, nurses functioning in these areas have needed specialized knowledge and sophisticated skills in caring for acutely ill patients. These nurses have demonstrated the ability to percuss and auscultate the thorax competently, to monitor respiratory system function closely, and to be sensitive and responsive to symptoms of approaching respiratory distress.

Expanded knowledge and skill is now essential for nurses functioning in other than intensive care settings. Nurses in the general medical-surgical area of the hospital, or in the clinic, the home, or other nonacute care settings care for patients with respiratory alterations of varying severity. These nurses encounter patients either with a primary respiratory alteration or with a nonrespiratory acute alteration accompanied by chronic respiratory disease. It is equally important that these nurses have physical appraisal skills to monitor respiratory system function, enabling them to detect the often rapid changes in status of patients with acute respiratory problems. These nurses can also use their skills to help maintain chronic respiratory alterations in the nonacute state so that they do not become complications of alterations in other body systems. In either case, the nurse will use the physical appraisal data she collects to aid in the detection of respiratory alterations, to create her care plans, and to carry out their subsequent evaluation and revision.

One needs only a penlight, tongue blade, stethoscope, and careful thought to perform the basic respiratory examination. Some nurses, especially those in intensive care settings, are already practicing physical appraisal of respiratory system function in greater depth than is presented here. The readings suggested at the end of the chapter will assist those who want more specialized knowledge.

GENERAL APPEARANCE

Posture provides many clues to respiratory system function. Patients with obstructive lung disease have an easily recognized posture, assumed in an effort to expand the thoracic cage and use all available thoracic space. Characteristically, the patient is sitting, leaning forward, and attempting to prop his clavicles by placing his hands on his knees, or his elbows on the arms of a chair. The sternocleidomastoid muscles, used as accessory muscles of respiration, are often prominent.

General color and facial expression are also indications of respiratory difficulty. A dusky or bluish coloration may be present, especially on the lips, and the cheeks may be ruddy. The facial expression is often drawn, because of exertion, and anxious, due to a feeling of air hunger. The patient may be able to say only a few sentences before having to stop to catch his breath. Noting the number of words the patient can say before having to gasp for breath is a useful measure for making future comparisons of the degree of respiratory distress.

Neurologic status is an important parameter to note and monitor, because changes in the alertness and personality of the patient may reflect cerebral sensitivity to changes in oxygen, carbon dioxide, and hydrogen ion levels. As pulmonary decompensation and hypoxia progress, the neurologic picture changes from anxiety and restlessness to irritability, to drowsiness, and finally to coma.

Specific Findings

Cyanosis. Cyanosis is due to an increased amount of blue, reduced hemoglobin in the superficial capillaries. Cyanosis is often hard to detect in persons with dark skin, because their pigmentation either masks or mimics the cyanosis; it is therefore best detected in the nail beds of a darkly pigmented person, or under the tongue or inside the cheek. Cyanosis is also difficult to detect in the person who is anemic, since there is less hemoglobin, either oxygenated or reduced, to impart color to the skin. For this reason a severely anemic person can die of hypoxia without becoming cyanotic. On the other hand, a patient with polycythemia may appear more cyanotic than one with a normal hematocrit, but with the same arterial oxygen tension. This is because of the polycythemic patient's inability to fully oxygenate the abnormally large mass of red blood cells, and usually does not represent inadequate oxygen delivery to the tissues. In this circumstance the presence of cyanosis cannot be given the same significance as cyanosis in a nonpolycythemic person.

Cyanosis is a nonspecific sign, resulting from a number of cardiac and pulmonary problems. In a patient with chronic obstructive pulmonary disease cyanosis is often of little help in assessing respiratory function because it appears so late — when the arterial PO_2 is 45 mm Hg or less (80 to 100 mm Hg is normal). However, any change — either the sudden onset of cyanosis or variance in its degree — is a sure indication of some important physiologic change.

Clubbing of Fingers. The condition of the fingers may be a more reliable indicator of chronic hypoxia than cyanosis. Clubbing of the fingers is caused by a chronic decrease in the oxygen saturation of the blood supplying this area. This results in a bulbous enlargement of the tip of the finger, with convex overhanging of the nail and loss of the obtuse angle at the nail bed (Fig. 10-10). A coarse vertical ridging in the fingernails may also reveal chronic pulmonary insufficiency.

Another sign the nurse may detect when observing the nails is their tendency to become periodically flushed and then return to their original color. This is evidence of excess blood supply, or hyperemia. As the carbon dioxide builds up in the capillaries, the arteries dilate, and the blood rushes through the area. When more oxygen has been supplied to the area, the arteries return to their normal size and blood flow becomes normal.

Cough.   The nurse needs to observe a patient's cough for frequency, production or nonproduction of sputum, time of day during which it occurs, and changes with body position. The character of the cough can be described as hacking (frequent coughing, though not severe), paroxysmal (a sudden prolonged episode of forceful coughing), explosive, or brassy (harsh, unproductive, with a strident quality). In addition, the nurse should observe what measures the patient uses to relieve the cough and their effectiveness.

Sputum Production.   The nurse may want to ask the patient to save his sputum to assist her in assessing it. Important characteristics of the sputum are its color, odor, consistency, and volume. Mucoid sputum, or sputum that is grayish-white, translucent, odorless, and slimy, is often seen with bronchitis. Purulent sputum may be green, yellow, or brown and often has a distinctive odor. Foul-smelling sputum is present with lung abscess, bronchiectasis, and other types of necrotizing infections, which also give the breath an offensive odor. The volume of sputum may range from a few teaspoons expectorated on arising to more than a pint daily. In acute pulmonary edema, the sputum is frothy and either white or pink.

Hemoptysis is often a serious sign which may occur in the course of pneumonia, tuberculosis, or cancer. Any description of hemoptysis must include the amount and color of the blood for the recording to be meaningful. The amount of blood may range from small streaks on the surface of the sputum to the red, frothy sputum seen with copious bleeding. The color should be described as bright or dark, since the brighter the blood, the fresher the bleeding. The presence of clots or pus should be noted. The nurse should try to estimate the amount of blood expectorated within a given period of time. Patients may or may not be helpful in providing this information because they are usually frightened and prone to overestimate the amount of blood. In this situation, it may be especially helpful to ask the patient to save *all* of the sputum.

NOSE AND PARANASAL SINUSES

Technique of Examination

Following the cephalocaudal approach to physical appraisal, a description of the respiratory system will begin with the nose and the paranasal sinuses.

First, inspect the contour of the external nose for asymmetry, and then palpate for any loss of structure or support. Test the patency of each nostril by occluding the other with digital compression while the patient inhales with his mouth closed.

Position the patient's head to examine the interior nose by placing the palm of one hand on his upper forehead and then gently lift the bulbous portion of the nose with the thumb, so that the interior can be seen. You may, in addition, want to ask the patient to attempt to flare his nostrils by raising his upper lip. Holding a penlight in your other hand, examine the condition of the skin and the mucosa on the interior of the nose and the adequacy of each airway (Fig. 9-1).

Observe the septum for deviation and then perforation by closing one naris with a penlight and viewing the transilluminated septum through the open naris. The septal surface of the nasal chamber is normally planar and smooth. The lateral wall of the chamber, however, is made irregular by three projections, the superior, middle, and inferior *turbinates.* In looking through the anterior chamber you will probably see the anterior two-thirds of the inferior turbinate and the anterior half of the middle turbinate; the superior turbinate is rarely visible.

The paranasal sinuses cannot be seen and therefore are indirectly examined by palpation. Palpate the frontal sinuses by pressing upward just below and

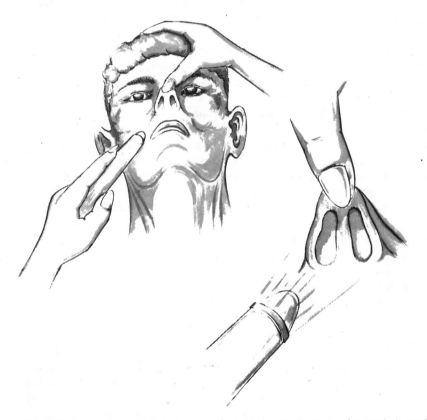

FIGURE 9-1.   Intranasal examination. One hand, placed on the forehead, is used to position and steady the head; the thumb is used to lift the bulbous portion of the nose. The penlight is held in the other hand.

behind the eyebrows. To detect tenderness of the maxillary sinuses, palpate along the ascending process of the maxilla and the canine fossa. Placing pressure simultaneously on both sides will often be more effective in demonstrating differences in tenderness.

Findings

The exterior nose may reveal chronic nasal obstruction and resultant mouth breathing, producing narrowing of the nose, described as *adenoid facies:* Tumors originating within the nose can cause marked deformity of its exterior. With increased respiratory effort, the nares may alternately dilate with inspiration and contract with expiration, and is called a *nasal flare.*

Unilateral nasal obstruction may be caused by a foreign body, deviated septum, or neoplasm. An S-shaped deviation of the nasal septum may cause bilateral obstruction. Obstruction of both nares is most commonly due to rhinitis but may also be due to the presence of nasal polyps.

The anterior chamber, or vestibule, of the naris is normally lined with skin, contains nasal hairs (vibrissae), and is the most common site for furuncles of the nose. The posterior vestibule is covered with nasal mucosa, which can be expected to be redder than oral mucosa. A blanket of mucus secretion covers the entire interior nasal cavity and functions to collect bacteria and debris from inspired air. A nasal allergy produces stuffiness, sneezing, and a watery nasal discharge. The common cold begins with a discharge of clear, watery mucus, indicating the viral etiology; later, the discharge may become thick and purulent, with superimposed bacterial infection. In acute and chronic infection of the paranasal sinuses the discharge is purulent, often viscid, and may tend to flow backward into the nasopharynx, causing a postnasal drip.

Epistaxis may result from trauma, but may also be a sign of serious local or generalized disease. A history of its repeated occurrence should always be reported to the physician. Bleeding commonly occurs from a vascular network in the anterior nasal septum, often caused by repeated nose-picking. Epistaxis may also be caused by hypertension or polycythemia, resulting from erosion of the small vessels. Often a neoplasm will produce a bloody discharge, in contrast to the brisk bleeding of real epistaxis.

In most people the septum is not perfectly straight. Irregularities normally cause no concern unless they are severe enough to interfere with the patency of the airway. Sharp projections, called "ridges" or "spurs," should be recorded. In some cases, the anterior end of the septum may be dislocated and project prominently into one nostril. Crusting often occurs at the site of nasal septum deviation, and evidence of some slight bleeding may also be found there. Perforation of the septum may be of traumatic, surgical, or infectious origin. Perforations commonly found in the anterior septum may be caused by chronic infection along with repeated trauma from picking off crusts.

Normally, the nasal turbinates have a deep pink color, similar to the rest of the nasal mucosa. However, with inflammation, the turbinates may become reddened and swell periodically. (This swelling may cause alternating nasal obstruction, which is especially noticeable at night. The individual turns from one side to the other to obtain decongestion of the previously dependent turbinate.) In allergic states the turbinates become pale and bluish and are often swollen or "boggy." When the septum is displaced to one side, the turbinates on the opposite side tend to swell and fill the cavity. *Nasal polyps* are overgrowths of mucosa that frequently may be seen as smooth, round pale masses protruding from between the turbinates.

Tenderness elicited by palpating over a paranasal sinus indicates disease in that area. Moist secretions seen in the interior of the nose or a stream of mucus on the posterior oropharynx may also indicate infection of the paranasal sinuses. Sinus disease often is accompanied by pain in the orbital area, diplopia, or swelling of the eyelids.

OROPHARYNX

Technique of Examination

This segment of the respiratory system examination is usually done concurrently with the oral examinations, with both the examiner and patient seated, facing each other. After inspecting the various parts of the oral cavity, ask the patient to say "ah," and use the tongue blade to depress the dorsum of his tongue. As he is doing this, observe for uvular elevation and coordinated pharyngeal construction. The tongue blade is best placed on the middle third of the tongue. If placed too far anteriorly, the blade causes the posterior part of the tongue to mound up so as to obscure rather than expose the pharynx. Most patients gag if the blade touches the posterior part of their tongue. While using the tongue blade, the nurse should be careful not to press the patient's lower lip against his teeth (see Fig. 9-2).

Examine the palatine tonsils and estimate their size. Inspect these tonsils and the anterior and posterior tonsillar pillars for signs of inflammation. Examine the lingual tonsils by using a piece of gauze to pull the tongue forward, and looking at them with the hand mirror. Inspect the posterior wall of the oropharynx for color and for the presence of edema, ulceration, and mucopurulent material.

Findings

Uvula.   The uvula is normally the same color or slightly pinker than the soft palate and varies greatly in length and thickness. With inflammation of the pharynx or the tonsils the uvula becomes enlarged and erythematous. This pendulous uvula may fall forward and touch the base of the tongue when the person is lying down, producing an irritating, shallow cough.

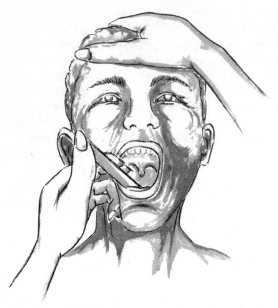

FIGURE 9-2. Examination of the oropharynx. The tongue blade is held so that the thumb pushes the tip upward while the fingers move the middle downward. The resultant motion should depress the tongue and scoop it forward. The left hand is steadied against the cheek while the right hand is used to position the head.

Tonsils. The tonsils should be essentially the same color as the oral mucosa. Normally, the palatine, or faucial, tonsils do not project much beyond the tonsilar pillars. The glossopalatine fold, which connects the tongue to the palate, is known as the anterior tonsillar pillar. Behind it lies the posterior tonsillar pillar. It is sometimes helpful to retract the anterior pillar for a better view of the tonsils.

Following tonsillectomy, lymphoid nodules may remain in the tonsillar fossa and leave a tonsillar tag. The anterior and posterior pillars often also reveal evidence of changes occurring with healing following a tonsillectomy.

The surface of the normal tonsil is relatively smooth but contains indentations, or crypts, in which are found desquamated epithelial cells. If these crypts are deep, plugs of epithelial debris may be seen as white spots on the tonsils. A red zone surrounding the plug, however, suggests infection of the crypt.

Large tonsils are not necessarily diseased and may represent an alteration only if they interfere with respiration or swallowing. With acute tonsillitis, the entire tonsil is reddened, edematous, and displays white or yellow dots or streaks of exudate. Infection may also result in abscesses, forming a large grayish patch on the surface of the tonsils. Both malignant and benign tumors may arise from the tonsils. A physician should be asked to evaluate any alteration of the tonsils.

Posterior Pharyngeal Wall.   The posterior pharyngeal wall is that part of the oropharynx visible through the open mouth, without using mirrors for examination. Small vessels can normally be seen here, on the soft palate and the tonsillar pillars; they usually do not represent inflammatory changes. Irregular spots of lymphoid tissue, pale pink and elevated, are also normal and frequently seen. Observe the posterior pharyngeal wall for soreness or acute pharyngitis, producing edema, redness, and possibly exudation of the mucosa or bleeding. Rhinitis or infection of the paranasal sinuses may cause a stream of mucopurulent material on the posterior pharyngeal wall.

TRACHEA

Technique of Examination

With the patient's head slightly flexed, the trachea may be palpated with the thumb and the index finger just above the suprasternal notch. If the trachea is deviated, the examiner will easily be able to insert his finger between the trachea and the sternocleidomastoid muscle on one side but not on the other.

Findings

The trachea normally lies in midline, equidistant from the insertion of each sternocleidomastoid muscle. Deviation of the trachea indicates that the upper part of the mediastinum is displaced to one side. This may be due to various pathologies but should always be reported to the physician immediately. Aortic aneurysm, enlargement of the thyroid, a mediastinal mass, or gross thoracic asymmetry due to scoliosis may all cause displacement. Pressure produced by pleural effusion or pneumothorax causes deviation of the trachea away from the diseased side, while atelectasis will pull the trachea toward the diseased side.

EXAMINATION OF THE THORAX

Landmarks of the Chest

Nurses must become familiar with landmarks of the chest. This information is needed to communicate effectively the exact position of abnormalities detected and to assist in locating and visualizing underlying anatomic structures of the thorax. Landmarks of the chest consist first of a series of imaginary lines and second, of anatomic topographic landmarks, such as bony prominences, ribs, and intercostal spaces.

Anterior Wall of the Chest.   The locations of two commonly used vertical lines found on the anterior chest, the midsternal and midclavicular lines, are

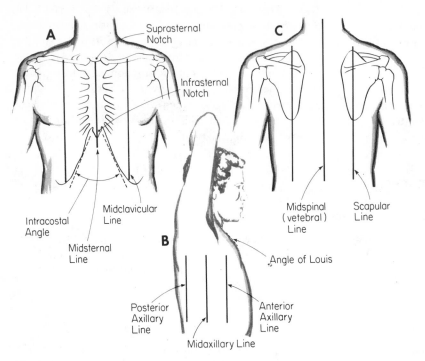

FIGURE 9-3.   Landmarks of the chest. A. Anterior thorax. B. Lateral thorax. C. Posterior thorax.

self-explanatory (Fig. 9-3A). Another important landmark, the sternal angle, or angle of Louis, is also found here (Fig. 9-3B). This is a visible projection of the sternum formed by the articulation of the first and second parts, the manubrium and the body, and is significant for several reasons. It is the location of the second chondrosternal junction and therefore facilitates identification of the second rib and serves as a convenient starting point for counting ribs. The angle of Louis also indicates the point of tracheal bifurcation forming the bronchi. Underneath it is the upper border of the atria of the heart. Finally, the fifth thoracic vertebra is located posteriorly at the same level.

After locating the second rib using the angle of Louis, the examiner should identify the other ribs and the intercostal spaces on the anterior chest. An intercostal space takes it name from the rib directly above it. To count ribs and intercostal spaces, first place the little finger of the left hand on the patient's second right intercostal space, next to the sternum. Next, take the ring finger, place it on the third rib, and allow it to fall down into the third intercostal space. Proceed in the same manner with the remaining fingers. The index finger will be in the fifth intercostal space.

Lateral Wall of the Chest.   Three commonly used lines are found on the lateral wall of the chest, namely, the anterior, posterior, and midaxillary lines (Fig.

9-3B). The anterior axillary line is a continuation of the anterior axillary fold, running downward along the anterolateral wall of the thorax. It begins at the insertion of the pectoralis major muscle. The posterior axillary line is drawn downward from the origin of the posterior axillary fold, which corresponds to the insertion of the latissimus dorsi muscle. The midaxillary line is midway between the other two and runs directly downward from the apex of the axilla. When the patient is in the dorsal recumbent position, the midaxillary line is on the same horizontal plane as the level of the right atrium and thus is often used as a landmark in measuring central venous pressure.

Care must be taken to see that the patient is in the correct position when initially locating these lines. The arm must be abducted directly from the lateral chest, but not more than 90°. It should not extend anteriorly or posteriorly. If the arm is not in the correct position, the relationship of the axilla to the chest wall becomes distorted, and these lines are then improperly located.

Posterior Wall of the Chest.   On the posterior wall of the chest are found the midspinal or vertebral line, running down the spinous process of the vertebrae, and the scapular line, which runs parallel to the spine through the inferior angle of the scapula (Fig. 9-3C). The scapular line is considered a somewhat inconsistent reference because of the mobility of the scapula. For this reason it should be located only when the patient is erect, with his arms at his sides.

Another landmark of the posterior chest is the vertebra prominens, or the prominent seventh cervical vertebra, found at the base of the neck. It can be used to assist in identifying the thoracic vertebrae and also indicates the highest point of lung tissue posteriorly.

Function of Lines and Landmarks

Lines and landmarks are most useful in communicating the exact position of detected abnormalities. Any alteration can be described as being so many centimeters medial or lateral to a line, or in a specific interspace or interspaces. Findings should be recorded in this manner. Nurses should become able to use these terms with facility, both verbally and in writing, and thus contribute to accurate diagnosis and monitoring of alterations.

Landmarks also assist in the location of anatomic structures that lie within the thorax. Anteriorly, the apices of the lungs extend for approximately 1 ½ in. (about 4 cm) above the clavicle on each side and inferiorly to the sixth anterior rib or the sixth chondrosternal junction. Posteriorly, the lung superiorly reaches the seventh cervical vertebrae and inferiorly extends to the tenth or twelfth thoracic vertebra.

On the right side, the dome of the diaphragm is situated approximately at the level of the fifth rib at the midclavicular line. Beneath the right diaphragm is the liver, which extends down to the costal margin. The dome of the left part of the diaphragm is normally about an inch lower. It usually extends to the fifth interspace or the sixth rib at the midclavicular line. The stomach, splenic flexure of the colon, and the left kidney lie below the left diaphragm.

A further series of imaginary lines drawn on the chest help in anatomic interpretation of respiratory system findings. These lines, or fissures, delineate surface areas that correspond to the upper, middle, and lower lobes of the lung. The *long fissure* delimits the lower lobe from the others and extends posteriorly from the fourth thoracic vertebra, obliquely downward, crossing the fifth rib at the midaxilla to the sixth rib anteriorly. The posterior origin of the long fissure is also at the same level as the anterior sternal prominence, the angle of Louis. On the right side, the *horizontal fissure* separates the upper and middle lobes. It extends from the long fissure in the midaxilla to the third intercostal space anteriorly. Locate these fissures in Figure 9-4, and trace them on a friend or patient.

The importance of visualizing the lobes of the lung soon becomes apparent. It is vital that the examiner be aware that the upper lobes are principally located in the anterior chest and that the middle lobe is found only in the anterior chest on

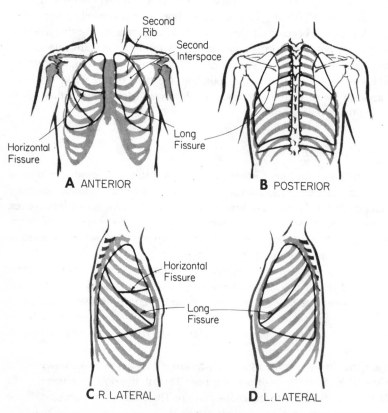

FIGURE 9-4.   Topographic anatomy: location of lobes of the lung. A. Anterior thorax. B. Posterior thorax. C. Right lateral thorax. D. Left lateral thorax.

the right. It is also important to note that the lower lobes correspond to a large portion of the surface area of the posterior chest and that their superior segments extend fairly far upward.

The nurse should employ the anatomic interpretation of her physical appraisal data in selecting the most effective nursing care. For example, with all this information in mind, she would plan positioning of the patient, select a regimen for postural drainage, plan for other types of breathing exercises, and then later use physical appraisal to evaluate the effectiveness of her nursing intervention.

INSPECTION OF THE THORAX

Nurses have been using the tool of inspection extensively for many years and through its use have made valuable contributions to diagnosis and treatment in patients with respiratory alterations. However, nurses are often uncomfortable in just looking at the patient without performing some concurrent motor activity. Still, initial inspection is most profitable in yielding valuable information when done by itself, with full concentration on the observation being made.

General Findings

Normal subjects present a wide range in size and shape of the chest. Posture and dominant use of one side of the body can create slight asymmetry, but general symmetry of the chest and its constituent parts is to be expected. Chest deformities or scars often provide the first clue to the nature of a respiratory difficulty.

The shoulders are usually at the same level, although one may be slightly higher than another. They generally have a convex shape from the neck to their lateral borders. Men usually have prominent clavicles, with depressed supra-clavicular spaces, while in women the clavicles are frequently hidden by adipose tissue, and the supraclavicular spaces are full. Beneath the clavicles the chest wall should be slightly convex and covered by subcutaneous tissue of moderate thickness. The intercostal spaces can be seen as slight depressions beneath the ribs, unless there is considerable adipose tissue. Because of the oblique downward angle of the ribs in traveling from the anterior chest to the posterior chest, the ribs and the intercostal spaces are highest posteriorly, lower laterally, and lowest anteriorly. Since the ribs have also progressively greater oblique angulation from top to bottom, the anterior intercostal spaces are wider than the posterior ones.

Anteriorly, each hemithorax projects further forward than the sternum, which actually represents some depression between the two sides of the thoracic wall. The lower part of the sternum is normally slightly further depressed from the chest wall. The subcostal angle, or the angle formed by the anterior margin of the ribs with the xyphoid at its apex, is normally about 90°, although it can be slightly greater in females and less in males. During inspiration, this angle widens, due to lateral expansion of the thorax.

In a normal adult the entire thorax should have a slightly elliptical shape, and the anteroposterior diameter should be definitely less than the transverse, or side-to-side, diameter. When looking at the posterior thoracic wall, the scapula should be symmetrically located and closely attached to the thoracic wall. Some depression exists between the medial scapular borders and the spine. The range of motion of the scapula should be evaluated. The spine should be straight, without lateral deviation. When viewed from the side, there is a slight anterior concavity of the thoracic spine and a similar but opposite curvature of the thoracic spine.

During inspiration, areas of the thorax should expand and relax synchronously and with equality of movement. Thoracic movement should be observed first as a whole, and then movement of one part in relation to another should be studied. Respirations in the male are usually diaphragmatic; female respirations tend to be more costal. Males also show less movement of the entire chest wall compared with females. Use of accessory muscles or retraction of intercostal spaces should not be detected in any normal patient.

When observing a patient with known emphysema, compare movement of the upper chest with the lower chest, and examine movement of the diaphragm to determine whether or not the patient is concentrating on expanding the lower chest and is using his diaphragm to achieve maximum inspiration.

Specific Findings

Increased Anteroposterior Diameter.   Patients with chronic obstructive pulmonary disease usually have a barrel chest, with an increased anteroposterior diameter, equal to or larger than the transverse diameter. This increase is most commonly due to overexpansion of the lungs with obstructive lung disease but may also be caused by bone structure abnormalities in a patient who has kyphosis (hunchback). Increased prominence of the angle of Louis often accompanies the barrel chest configuration.

Increased Horizontal Slope of Ribs.   Posteriorly, the ribs are normally situated at a 45° angle in relation to the spine. However, in the patient with chronic obstructive pulmonary disease, the ribs are more nearly horizontal, helping to establish the barrel chest configuration.

Use of Accessory Muscles.   A patient who is experiencing labored breathing, in order to aid respiration ordinarily uses accessory muscles such as the sternocleidomastoids, internal and external intercostals, and abdominal muscles, anterior serratus, and scalene muscles. Over a period of time, enlargement and prominence of these muscles, especially of the muscles of the neck and shoulder girdle, develop in patients with chronic respiratory difficulty.

Increased Subcostal Angle.   A widened subcostal angle and a fixed, expanded lower rib margin develop in patients with chronic pulmonary disease. For them, this angle widens little with each respiratory effort.

Unequal Expansion of the Thorax.   Asymmetric expansion of the thorax has many causes. These include massive pleural effusion or atelectasis, especially caused by a mucus plug in a major bronchi, pneumothorax, or any cause of chest pain such as a pulmonary embolus or fractured rib.

In the intensive care setting a patient is occasionally seen who has unilateral diminished chest expansion due to an endotracheal or nasotracheal tube that has been inserted too far and extends beyond the trachea into one of the mainstem bronchi, usually the right. This causes diminished chest expansion in the unaerated side of the chest, and hypoxemia and atelectasis of that lung often result. The nurse who anticipates the possibility of this serious complication can examine the patient with this in mind and, if it occurs, promptly secure medical attention for the patient.

Some abnormalities of chest expansion may not be seen with quiet respirations but will become pronounced with forced inspiration. For this reason, inspection of the chest should be carried out during both quiet and deep breathing.

Retraction or Bulging of Interspaces.   Inspiratory intercostal retractions are seen as sucking in of skin and muscle between the ribs and are often accompanied by retraction of the supraclavicular and substernal areas. These are usually symptoms of obstruction to free inflow of air, resulting in a greater than normal inspiratory effort. This increased inspiratory effort may also occur because the lungs are less compliant (stiffer) than normal, or as a result of excessive negativity of the pleural end-expiratory pressure, as seen in atelectasis.

Intercostal bulging may occur with massive pleural effusion or tension pneumothorax or occasionally be detected on the thoracic wall when a tumor or aortic aneurysm is present. However, bulging is most frequently seen with the forced and prolonged expirations of a patient with asthma or emphysema.

Deformities of Bony Structure of Chest or Spine.   The examiner should note any abnormalities of the thoracic bone structure, since these alterations often interfere with proper posture and adequate chest expansion and can be the cause of respiratory difficulty. Common bone deformities of the thorax and spine are illustrated in Figure 9-5.

Observation of Respirations

Respirations should be observed for three dimensions, namely, rate, rhythm, and amplitude of the respiratory excursion, and counted for a minimum of 15 seconds. The nurse should be aware of the hazards of estimating respirations rather than counting them.

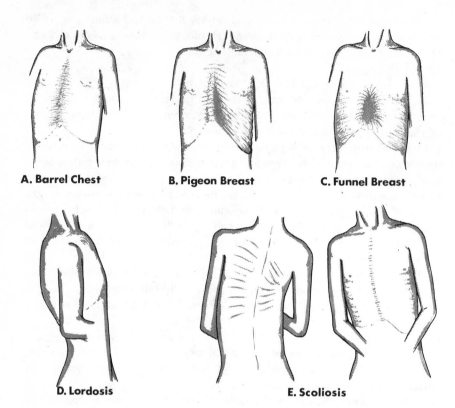

A. Barrel Chest   **B. Pigeon Breast**   **C. Funnel Breast**

D. Lordosis   **E. Scoliosis**

FIGURE 9-5. Deformities of the bony structure of the chest or spine. A. Barrel chest. Hyperinflation or augmented lung volume occurring with respiratory diseases such as emphysema or asthma cause the thorax to assume a permanent inspiratory position, with an increased anteroposterior diameter and increased horizontal slope of the ribs. The transverse diameter may remain the same or also may increase. B. Pigeon breast. Often seen with active rickets. Softening of the ribs causes the sternum to be pushed forward while the ribs slope away at either side. This causes an increase in the anteroposterior diameter at the expense of the width of the thorax. C. Funnel breast. Seen in rickets and in some congenital disorders. In this case the softened ribs allow a depression of the lower portion of the sternum. D. Lordosis. Curvature of the spinal column with anterior convexity, causing thoracic spine to be displaced posteriorly and the lower thorax to be held in the expiratory position. E. Scoliosis. Lateral deviation of the spine. Deviation of the thoracic spine causes a compensating deviation of the lumbar region to the opposite side, resulting in an S-shaped curve. On the side of thoracic deviation the thorax is larger and convex, the ribs separated, and the lung emphysematous. On the concave side the ribs are close together and the chest small.

The normal range for rate is 12 to 18 respirations per minute. Usually, the ratio of respiratory rate to pulse rate is 1:4. In fever, the respiratory rate increases with the pulse rate on an average of four additional respiratory cycles per minute for each 1 degree of elevation in temperature above normal.

The activity of respiratory cycles should occur rhythmically in the normal adult, and the interval between cycles should be equal. Normal respirations are usually two parts inspiration to three parts expiration, but in an adult with emphysema the expiratory time is often prolonged. The amplitude of respiration often reveals as much information as an assessment of the rate. Decreased amplitude may be caused by pain that is intensified with inspiratory effort, such as that occurring with fractured ribs, sprained muscles, or painful skin alteration. A decrease in amplitude may also result from dysfunction of either side of or all of the diaphragm.

The common terms used to describe alterations in rate, rhythm, and depth of respiration are discussed next.

Dyspnea.   Dyspnea can simply be described as "difficult respirations." It is primarily a subjective description, used to characterize the condition of a patient who is experiencing obvious increased respiratory effort, often using accessory muscles. The patient also describes experiencing an uncomfortable sensation of not being able to get enough air, which sometimes persists even with the increased respiratory effort.

Dyspnea naturally varies in degree. Some persons are dyspneic only with moderate amounts of exertion such as climbing one or several flights of stairs; others become dyspneic with such simple activities as walking across the room, taking off a shirt, or carrying on a conversation. Those with severe respiratory dysfunction may experience dyspnea at rest. A notation of dyspnea is often useless information unless the amount of exertion needed to cause it is recorded, as well as the amount of rest to relieve it.

Dyspnea may be either inspiratory or expiratory. *Inspiratory dyspnea* occurs with obstruction to inflow of air, such as with severe laryngitis, a foreign body, or a tumor causing exterior compression on the trachea or larger bronchi. It is often accompanied by intercostal retractions and by the crowing sound of inspiratory stridor. *Expiratory dyspnea* occurs with obstruction of the bronchioles or small bronchi and may be present in patients with asthma, bronchitis, and obstructive emphysema. Expiratory time is prolonged, and bulging of the intercostal spaces may occur.

Tachypnea.   Tachypnea indicates increased respiratory rate, with or without a corresponding increase in depth. It is seen with increased metabolic activity (in fever, pneumonia), in states of alkalosis, and with pleurisy or respiratory insufficiency, either obstructive or restrictive.

Bradypnea, Apnea, and Hyperpnea.   *Bradypnea,* an abnormal slowing of respirations, is the opposite of tachypnea. Agents that depress the respiratory center, such as opiates or brain tumors, produce respirations that are decreased in rate but still uniform and regular in character. Alveolar hypoventilation (see below) can be expected in such a situation. *Apnea* is a temporary cessation of breathing. *Hyperpnea* indicates an increased depth of breathing.

Hyperventilation.   *Hyperventilation* is an abnormal increase in both rate and depth of respiration which, if it results from acidosis, is often called *Kussmal's respiration.* It occurs following intense exertion. Hyperventilation may also occur in highly emotional states.

Apneustic respirations are marked by maintained inspiratory activity unrelieved by expiration. Each inspiration is long and gasping, followed by a short expiratory period. This type of respiration usually follows damage to the pneumotaxic center of the pons.

Pleuritic, or Restrained, Breathing.   As the term indicates, pleuritic breathing occurs during pleurisy, when pain abruptly halts the inspiratory phase of respiration. As a consequence, respirations are shallow but often rapid.

Cyclic respirations.   Cyclic, or periodic, respirations display a patterned cycle of irregularities and are usually the result of central respiratory depression. Two common types of cyclic respirations, Cheyne-Stokes and Biot's, are differentiated by the rhythm of their cycles.

Cheyne-Stokes respirations are characterized by a repeating cycle of gradually increasing then decreasing rate and tidal volume. Each cycle is concluded by a period of quiet breathing or apnea. The patient often lies quietly during the period of apnea but becomes restless when respirations again resume. Cheyne-Stokes respirations are seen in a variety of disease states, including severe congestive heart failure, increased intracranial pressure, cerebral disease, and drug sensitivity. It is important to know that this type of respiratory pattern may also be seen occasionally in children and in adults as they sleep.

Biot's breathing is characterized by alternating periods of regular breathing and apnea but without any consistent pattern of change. Biot's respirations are due to marked depression of the respiratory center and though infrequently seen, may be observed occasionally with meningitis or other forms of central nervous system disease. This is a serious prognostic sign, indicating extensive damage to the respiratory control centers of the brain.

Stertorous Respirations. Stertorous respirations are noisy respirations (snoring sounds) produced by passage of air through secretions that have accumulated in the trachea and large bronchi as a result of the patient's inability to clear them. These respirations are usually seen in a comatose patient whose cough reflex is severely depressed or absent and are often a terminal event. Hence stertorous respirations are at times called the "death rattle."

Sighing Respirations. Sighing respirations are noted when a deep inspiration and then prolonged expiration interrupt the regular respiratory rhythm at frequent intervals. They are usually not a manifestation of organic disease but of emotional tension.

Air Trapping. Air trapping occurs most frequently in patients with emphysema or asthma during times when the flow of air both in and out of the thorax is impaired. Impairment of flow is usually more marked during expiration, making it easier to get air in than out. Patients usually compensate for this by decreasing their velocity of expiration and prolonging expiratory time. However, when they are forced to increase their rate, air becomes trapped in the lungs as more air enters than is allowed to escape during each respiratory cycle. Consequently, the end-expiratory volume steadily rises and a situation described as air trapping occurs.

PALPATION OF THE THORAX

Palpation of the thorax may reveal new findings or confirm or supplement findings from inspection. By simply moving the palm of the hand across the chest, the examiner may detect lumps or masses. Pulsations or areas of tenderness may also be noted. Some special techniques of palpation are also used in the chest examination. Hands are placed on different parts of the chest during the respiratory cycle to determine the amount of thoracic expansion. Normal and abnormal vibrations felt on the surface of the chest are detected by palpation. In addition, crepitation, which is a serious alteration, is sometimes found in the subcutaneous tissue of the thoracic wall by palpation.

Thoracic Excursion

Alterations in thoracic expansion may be first noted on inspection but are often better detected by palpation. The examiner's hands are placed flat against the chest at several locations and, as the chest moves, the hands move also. The amount of excursion is then estimated, using two parameters: the velocity of movement and the distance the thumbs move from each other.

Technique of Examination. First testing excursion of the posterior lower chest, stand behind the patient and place your hands on the lower portion of the rib cage, so that your thumbs are on the spine and your fingers point laterally. Press toward the spine, so that a small fold of skin is found between your thumbs (Fig. 9-6). Normally a 3-in. (7.6-cm) expansion of the thorax is found here as

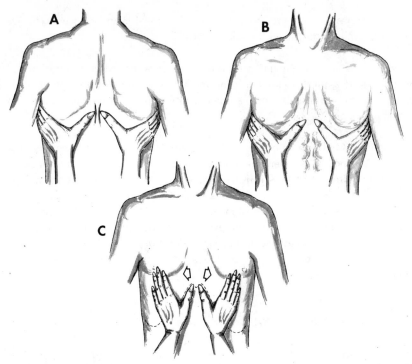

FIGURE 9-6.   Testing inspiratory expansion. A. Testing inspiratory expansion of the posterior thorax. B. Testing inspiratory expansion of the anterior thorax. C. Testing movement of the costal margin.

the patient goes from maximum expiration to maximum inspiration. To test the anterosuperior thoracic wall, remain standing behind the patient and place your hands on the anterior upper thorax, so that your thumbs are along the sternal border pointing toward the xyphoid process and your fingers are spread out over the anterolateral wall. Finally, to test the lower anterior thorax, move so you are facing the patient and place your hands over the lower anterior thorax, thumbs again along the costal margin, but this time pointing upward toward the neck; your fingers should be pointing laterally. In each position, thoracic excursion should be tested with both a normal and maximum inspiration. Abnormalities in expansion are usually more readily detected on the anterior thoracic wall than posteriorly, since the anterolateral wall normally moves more. Although specific areas are tested separately, the entire thorax should be felt to move as a unit and not in several separate movements.

Findings.   It is difficult to describe the correct feeling for normal thoracic excursion. Only by examining a variety of normal healthy people can the examiner acquire an appreciation for the range of normal and be able to detect abnormal findings outside that range. Alterations detected may have various causes; for example, pneumothorax, acute pleurisy, trauma, or thickening of the pleura.

Fremitus

Vocal fremitus, sometimes also called tactile fremitus, is the most common type of palpable vibration and is merely transmission of the vibration of air resulting from phonation. Sounds that are produced in the larynx are transmitted down the tracheobronchial tree to the smaller bronchioles and finally to the alveoli. This vibration is then transmitted to the thoracic wall and the examiner's hand on the chest wall.

Technique of Examination.   To detect vocal fremitus, have the patient speak in a soft voice, repeating phrases such as "99-99," or "1-2-3," or "blue moon," or "how now brown cow." The intensity of vocal fremitus varies with both the loudness and the frequency of the voice. If at first the vibration is slight, ask the patient to speak a little louder. However, once you have begun comparing areas of the chest, the patient should attempt to speak at the same level so as not to introduce an extraneous variable into the evaluation. In persons with a deep voice, the tactile sensation of fremitus is more distinct because of the lower frequency of voice vibrations. There are three commonly used methods of hand placement for detecting fremitus. The open palm may be placed flat against the chest wall. The narrow ulnar aspect of the hand may also be used either with the hand open or with the fingers closed in the palm.

Variations of fremitus normally occur in different areas of the thorax, but corresponding areas should have the same intensity of vibration. It is thus essential to compare corresponding areas consecutively, e.g., to compare the right apex with the left apex, the right middle anterior chest with the corresponding area on the left side (Fig. 9-7). Some prefer to place both hands on the chest at once; others find it best to use one hand and move from area to area. With the first method it is sometimes difficult to detect differences in vibratory levels while using both hands; however, with the second, one may lose the sense of level of vibration in moving from one area to another.

Findings.   The intensity of vibrations felt at any point is dependent on the thickness of the subcutaneous tissue covering the wall of the thorax, and on the distance of the major bronchi from the chest wall at that area. Fremitus is most prominent in regions of the thorax where the major bronchi are closest to the chest wall and becomes less intense as one moves away from these bronchi. Fremitus is least noticeable at the bases of the lungs, an area separated from the bronchi by a large amount of aerated lung tissue. Fremitus of maximal intensity is found at the base of the neck, both anteriorly and posteriorly, at the first and second interspaces lateral to the sternum, at the right apex, and also between the scapulae. Tactile fremitus vibrations are more intense in the thin person than the

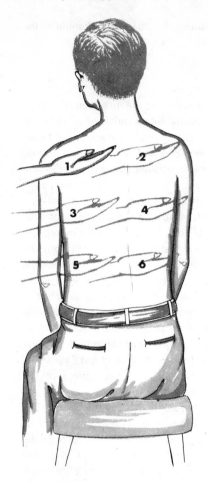

FIGURE 9-7.   Testing vocal fremitus. Method of testing vocal fremitus, using ulnar aspect of hand and comparing contralateral areas sequentially.

very muscular or obese person because of the damping effect of the increased amount of subcutaneous tissue. The examiner should be looking for areas of increased intensity of fremitus, or decreased or absent fremitus. Only gross changes in the pleura and lungs give rise to significant changes in palpable fremitus; small areas of consolidation, tumors, and so on, cannot be expected to cause noticeable changes.

Anything that increases the density of the lung tissue also increases the transmission of vibrations through it. Solid or semisolid material of uniform structure conducts better than a porous structure of solid and air that is constantly undergoing changes in density, such as normal lung tissue. Increased vocal fremitus therefore occurs in conditions that are associated with consolidation of the lungs. However, to produce the increased intensity of fremitus the area of consolidation must be both connected to a patent bronchus and must also extend to the surface of the lung, where vibrations traveling through it can set the thoracic wall in motion.

Decreased or absent fremitus results when something comes between the sound traveling down the tracheobronchial tree and the examining hand on the chest wall. Often, it is an upper airway blockage or an obstruction of a major bronchus. However, air or fluid in the pleural space will diminish the vibrations or make it impossible to feel them.

Vibrations felt on the surface of the chest can result from phenomena other than transmission of vibrations produced in the larynx. *Tussive fremitus* is the vibration of the chest wall produced by coughing. *Pleural friction fremitus,* as its name indicates, results when the inflamed pleural surfaces in acute pleurisy rub together, producing a grating sensation that can be detected by the hand on the chest wall. This sensation is usually felt during both phases of respiration and is most commonly noted on the anterolateral portion of the thoracic wall, where there is the greatest degree of respiratory movement. This palpable friction rub may also be heard on auscultation.

Rhonchal fremitus, in which palpable murmurs or vibrations are created during breathing by air moving through secretions or by an area of stenosis of the bronchi or trachea, is felt by palpating the patient's chest during quiet breathing. Rhonchal fremitus can be differentiated from pleural friction rub fremitus, a more serious omen, by having the patient cough. The rhonchal fremitus should disappear with movement of the exudate, while the palpatory and ausculatory evidence of the pleural friction rub will remain.

Crepitation

Crepitation, the coarse, crackling sensation that is palpated when the subcutaneous tissues contain fine beads of air (also known as subcutaneous emphysema), results from leakage of air through traumatic or surgical wounds in the major airways or the alveoli. This sensation has been described as similar to rolling a lock of hair between the thumb and forefinger or crumpling a wad of plastic food wrap. The crackling sensation, like the "snap, crackle, and pop" of certain cereals, is sometimes actually audible. Immediate action must be taken when crepitation is detected, for it progresses quickly, causing rapid obstruction of the airway. In addition, the puffed subcutaneous tissues make it difficult to insert an endotracheal tube or perform a tracheostomy. This is an emergency situation and medical assistance must be sought at once.

PERCUSSION OF THE THORAX

In examining the thorax, percussion is used both to determine the relative amount of air or solid material in the underlying lung and to define the boundaries of portions of the lung which differ in structural density.

Technique of Examination

Indirect percussion is primarily used in examining the thorax, although direct percussion may be used for examining the area above the clavicles or for defining the cardiac borders. The palmar surface of the distal phalynx of the left middle finger serves as the pleximeter (i.e., receives the blow) and is firmly placed on the chest wall in an interspace, parallel to the ribs. Only the distal phalynx of the pleximeter should rest on the chest wall. If the entire hand is touching the chest, the tone of the percussion note may be muffled. It has been estimated that a strong percussion stroke penetrates for about 6 cm (2.4 in.) beneath the skin through 3 cm (1.2 in.) of thoracic wall and 3 cm of lung tissue. For this reason a more forceful stroke is used to detect changes in density of lung tissue (sonorous percussion) and a lighter stroke to outline the borders of adjacent organs (definitive percussion).

Even when using the more forceful stroke to detect changes in density of lung tissue, many abnormalities may go unrecognized. Any deep-seated mass covered by aerated lung tissue does not cause an audible change in the percussion note. A mass must also be as large as 2 to 3 cm (0.8 to 1.2 in.) in diameter to be detected.

For ease in percussing, the patient's thorax should be at least as high, if not higher, than the nurse's thorax. The room and examiner's hands should be warm. Before starting systematic percussion of the thorax, it is wise to attempt to establish a normal resonant percussion note for the person being examined; this can later be used as a basis for comparison of other notes. Select an area that has little muscular or subcutaneous tissue; the seventh or eighth posterolateral interspace well out toward the axilla gives a good percussion note and is an area usually free from disease.

Begin with the patient in the supine position for percussion of the anterior chest (see Fig. 9-8). His arms should be resting loosely at his sides. Start below the clavicles and use fairly heavy indirect percussion. Percuss downward, interspace by interspace, comparing the sound from each interspace sequentially with that from the contralateral region. Continue downward to the region of hepatic dullness on the right and to the area of tympany, called *Traube's semilunar space,* on the left. The entire thorax should be resonant, with the exception of the area of cardiac dullness. On the right is the transition zone of hepatic dullness from about the fourth to sixth interspaces. This zone is a combination of resonance and dullness, as a portion of the liver lies over a portion of the lung. As you leave the area of the lung, the dullness becomes hepatic flatness. The upper tympanic border is somewhat lower on the left than the upper border of the liver on the right because the left diaphragm lies lower than the right.

Percussion of the other areas of the thorax, such as the anterior apices, the lateral thorax, and the posterior thorax, is most easily done with the patient sitting on a stool. The apices of the lung extend above the clavicle, producing a

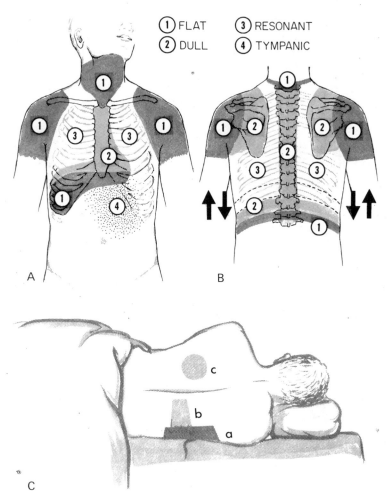

FIGURE 9-8.   Quality of percussion note over the normal chest. A. Anterior chest. B. Posterior chest. C. Effect of lateral recumbent position on percussion note. (a) Zone of relative dullness due to deadening effect of mattress. (b) Zone of dullness due to compression of chest by weight of body. (c) Zone of dullness due to crowding of ribs.

band of resonance which widens at the scapular and clavicular ends. The upper narrow part of this band of resonance is called *Krönig's isthmus.* Percuss the supraclavicular spaces, using indirect percussion. The right apex is best percussed by using your left thumb as the pleximeter while facing the patient. To percuss the left apex, reach around the patient's back with your left arm and use your left middle finger, pointing downward, as the pleximeter.

Percuss the lateral aspects of the thorax by having the patient rest his forearm on top of his head and percuss downward from the axilla.

Next, percuss the posterior thorax with the patient sitting, head and shoulders bent slightly forward in a hunchback position and arms folded in his lap. This position moves the scapulae laterally, since they interfere with percussion of the lung areas they cover. Again percuss downward, interspace by interspace, always immediately comparing the percussion note on the contralateral side. Use lighter percussion for the posterior thorax. During quiet respirations you should find the border of resonance at the ninth rib on the left and the eighth interspace on the right.

Finally, determine the amount of diaphragmatic excursion by comparing the border of resonance at maximum expiration with that at maximum inspiration. Have the patient inhale deeply and hold his breath. Percuss downward, noting the line between resonant lung and dullness of abdominal viscera. Now tell the patient to exhale as far as possible and hold. Again percuss downward to determine the lower border of resonance. The distance between these two points indicates the amount of diaphragmatic excursion, which is normally 5 to 6 cm (2 to 2.4 in.). Diaphragmatic excursion is limited by pleurisy and severe emphysema. In emphysema, the level of the diaphragm will be lower than normal, but with any condition that causes an increase in intraabdominal pressure, such as pregnancy or ascites, the diaphragm will be higher than normal. If there is phrenic nerve damage and diaphragmatic paralysis, the involved side of the diaphragm moves paradoxically upward with each respiration.

Whenever possible, posterior percussion should be carried out with the patient sitting upright. However, where the patient cannot sit up, posterior percussion can be performed in the lateral decubitus position if the examiner is aware of the resulting changes in body structure and percussion notes. The dependent lung is generally somewhat duller. The surface of the bed pressing against the thorax has a damping effect in that immediate area and causes a band of dullness along the chest wall next to the bed. Directly above this there is another area of dullness caused by the body weight compressing the downward lung. In addition, body weight on the mattress causes some degree of sagging, which curves the spine, causing compression of the thoracic wall on the upward side and a similar compression of the underlying upward lung. This results in an area of relative dullness at approximately the tip of the upward scapula. The flexing of the spine also causes the upward intercostal spaces to widen and the downward ones to become more narrow. Curvature of the spine can be relieved to some degree if the pillow is taken away and the head rests directly on the bed.

Findings

The full range of percussion notes that may be heard over the thorax include resonance, tympany, hyperresonance, dullness, and flatness.

Resonance. Resonance is the clear hollow percussion note heard on the thorax over healthy lung tissue. The normal resonant note varies in pitch and amplitude from person to person and across the individual chest; a very bony, muscular thorax has a less resonant note because of the greater amount of solid tissue. Changes in the ratio of air to solid tissue also explain why females often have a lighter, less resonant note (proportionately less aerated long tissue to solid tissue) and children, a more resonant note.

The resonant note is also affected by structures overlying the lung tissue. The apical or superior segments of the lung are covered by fairly thick muscle and bone, resulting in a duller percussion note. However, the base of the thorax has a relatively greater proportion of lung and relatively less muscle and bone — hence a more resonant note. The denser tissues of the scapula, the pectoral and back muscles, and the breasts all tend to dull the resonant percussion note. Therefore, in patients with thick subcutaneous tissues, as in obesity, a more forceful percussion stroke must be used to obtain an adequate diagnostic sound.

In percussing the thorax it is important to note that percussion produces not only a sound but also varying degrees of resistance and vibration which can be sensed by the pleximeter finger. Vibration of the underlying tissues, such as occurs in the thorax, produces less resistance and more elasticity detected by the pleximeter finger. In percussing the thigh, which has little vibration, there is a sense of increased resistance. Percussing the air-filled lung, on the other hand, causes much vibration and decreased resistance. The perimeter finger can also sense changes in relative pitch and duration of the percussion note.

Tympany. Tympany often is found physiologically in the lower left hemi-thorax and the left upper abdomen. Here, it results from air in the stomach, the upper portion of which lies beneath the lower ribs, and possibly from air in the splenic flexure of the colon. Tympany is abnormal when heard anywhere in the thorax other than in Traube's semilunar space, in the left anterior hemithorax and the left upper abdomen. Abnormal areas of tympany may be caused by large emphysematous bullae or collapse of the lung due to pneumothorax.

Hyperresonance. Hyperresonance is usually pathological in the thorax. It is most often caused by the emphysematous lung filled with small air sacs. It may be present also with a small pneumothorax with minimal collapse of the lung, where a combination of resonance and tympany produces it. Physiologically, hyperresonance may occasionally be found in the base of the left lung, due to the same combination of tympany (small amount of air in the stomach) and resonance (lung).

Dullness. Dullness is obtained in percussion over the heart when it is not covered by inflated lung. As indicated in Chapter 2, it is a high-pitched sound, short, soft, and thudlike and does not create a vibrating sensation in the pleximeter finger as with resonance or hyperresonance. These notes are normally elicited over the scapula, areas of the thorax that are covered by thick musculature, the mediastinum, or the upper portion of the liver and spleen — solid organs adjacent to air-containing lung.

Flatness. Flatness or absolute dullness is never normal in the thorax and, when present, indicates massive pleural effusion in which air-containing lung is displaced toward the interior and out of range of the percussion stroke.

AUSCULTATION OF THE LUNGS

Auscultation of the lungs is used to detect and study sounds from the lungs to determine both deviation from normal breath and voice sounds and the presence of abnormal additional or adventitious sounds. Ausculation may elicit new findings or may provide information to supplement or confirm previous observations.

Auscultation is used to detect three different types of sounds. First, breath sounds normally present are auscultated for variations and deviations from their usual characteristics. Second, transmission of the spoken voice and alterations of transmission are observed. Finally, an attempt is made to detect adventitious sounds, or those not heard normally across the chest.

Technique of Examination

Since breath sounds are generally high-pitched, one should use the closed chestpiece of the stethoscope in auscultating the chest. The chestpiece should be held so that the diaphragm is placed firmly against the skin, while the rim of the chestpiece touches the skin lightly. If the chestpiece is held too tightly, the skin is stretched, itself becoming a diaphragm and excluding lower-pitched sounds. For narrower spaces, such as the intercostal spaces or the supraclavicular fossa, the smaller open bell chestpiece may be used, but held tightly against the skin so that the skin can become a diaphragm.

Remember that if the entire rim of the chestpiece does not touch the skin and a leak occurs, extraneous noise in the form of a roaring sound will be heard by the examiner. If the chestpiece is not held firmly, sounds of respiratory excursion, such as movement of intercostal muscles, joints, or skin will be heard and may mimic a friction rub. Movement of the chestpiece over hair on the chest can produce a sound that resembles rales. This can be eliminated by wetting the hair. Breathing on the tubing or sliding one's fingers over the chestpiece may also cause confusing sounds. The examiner should purposely produce all these sounds and become familiar with them so that they can be recognized and eliminated during the chest examination.

Auscultation of the chest must be done in a quiet room. The level of background noise may not seem high, but very little noise will be sufficient to interfere with the low-intensity sounds important to detect on auscultation.

Preferably the patient should be sitting for chest auscultation. If he must remain recumbent, have him turn from side to side to enable auscultation of all areas of the chest. Demonstrate to the patient how to breathe while you are auscultating, having him breathe more deeply than normal and with his mouth open. Keeping his mouth open reduces the noise caused by the turbulence of air passing through the nose and mouth. Respirations slightly deeper than normal make breath sounds more audible, but very deep, strenuous respirations may result in introduction of sounds actually caused by muscle movement. The examiner needs to be aware that there is normally a fourfold increase in the intensity of breath sounds with deep breathing over that in quiet breathing.

Begin auscultation with the anterior chest, first auscultating the apices and then proceeding downward. As with percussion, compare contralateral points sequentially. Auscultate the posterior chest in a similar manner, again comparing contralateral areas as you move downward. When auscultating the back, note where the breath sounds disappear and compare these data with data obtained from percussion and palpation of vocal fremitus to determine where the lung bases lie.

As the nurse listens to breath sounds, she must discipline herself to note systematically the duration of inspiration and expiration, and the quality and pitch of sounds in each area. Particular attention to the expiratory phase is important, since most abnormalities of breath sounds are characterized by changes here. The nurse should identify the breath sounds as vesicular, bronchovesicular, bronchial, asthmatic, cavernous, or absent. Next, she should listen for adventitious sounds such as rales or rhonchi, noting whether rales clear after a few deep breaths or cough. Both the anterior and posterior chest should be auscultated a second time while the patient whispers a phrase the examiner suggests in order to determine the presence or absence of whispered pectoriloquy. The nurse should have the patient speak, to test for bronchophony. Finally, she should listen for friction rubs and other types of abnormal sounds.

Breath Sounds

Breath sounds are essentially the vibrations produced by movement of air through the tracheobronchial tree. What is heard through the stethoscope depends on the place of auscultation on the chest wall and on the resonating and conducting properties of the lung and other tissues between the larger airways.

In listening to breath sounds, four characteristics should be considered:

1. *Pitch.* Normal breath sounds have a rising pitch during inspiration and falling pitch during expiration. In describing pitch of breath sounds, *high* and *low* are used in relation to the pitch of other breath sounds.
2. *Duration.* Ratio of the duration of the two phases of respiration is a distinguishing factor in determining various abnormal breath sounds and should always be noted.
3. *Intensity.* Breath sounds are described as loud or soft in relation to other breath sounds, or inspiration and expiration may be contrasted with one another in loudness. Usually, the longer the phase of respiration, the louder the sound in that phase.
4. *Quality.* This is difficult to describe, but various terms such as *honking* and *wheezing* have been used to indicate quality of breath sounds.

Normal Breath Sounds.   There are only two types of normal breath sounds heard over the thorax, vesicular and bronchovesicular (Fig. 9-9).

Vesicular.   The normal breath sounds heard over most of the lungs are the vesicular breath sounds. They are caused by air moving through the bronchioles and the alveoli and are a result of the turbulence of air as it is distributed to the individual alveoli. Because of the wide distribution of alveoli beneath the chest wall, this respiratory sound is heard over almost all of the chest surface. An expiratory component of the vesicular sound is normally heard over some areas of the chest and originates as the expired air moves out through the bifurcations of the large airways. It is more clearly heard in areas where the tracheobronchial tree lies close to the chest surface, such as in the upper midthorax, anteriorly and posteriorly. Over other areas of the chest the porous lung tissue greatly dampens the expiratory sound. Breath sounds in the normal person are therefore

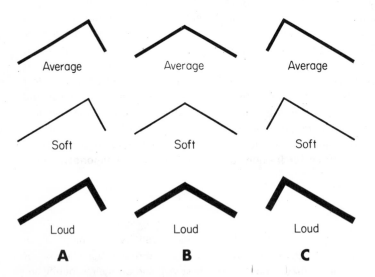

FIGURE 9-9.   Schematic representation of breath sounds. A. Vesicular breath sounds. Inspiration longer, louder, and higher-pitched than expiration. B. Bronchovesicular breath sounds. Inspiration and expiration similar. C. Bronchial breath sounds. Expiration longer, louder, higher-pitched, and with a more tubular or hollow quality than inspiration.

mainly inspiratory and low-pitched. The ratio of inspiratory sound to expiratory sound is 3 to 1.

The vesicular breath sound is a soft, relatively low-pitched sound and has been described as like the gentle rustling of leaves as the air moves through the trees. The inspiratory sound is louder than the expiratory sound, but there is no noticeable pause between inspiration and expiration. Generally, the inspiratory sound lasts three times as long as the audible expiratory sound (Fig. 9-9). As always, great individual variation can be expected both in the intensity and in the relative duration of the two phases.

Bronchovesicular.   The bronchovesicular breath sound is heard where the tracheobronchial tree is close to the chest surface. This sound is caused by a mixture of vesicular sounds and the sound produced as air travels in and out through the tracheobronchial tree.

Bronchovesicular sounds are normally heard on either side of the sternum in the first and second interspaces anteriorly and between the scapulae posteriorly. They may be heard over the apices, often the right more than the left. Their inspiratory phase resembles normal vesicular breathing but is slightly longer and higher-pitched. The expiratory phase is also higher in pitch and increased in duration to the point where it may be longer than inspiration. The expiratory phase may have a slightly tubular quality as compared with the vesicular sound. Actually, the inspiratory and expiratory phases are much alike in duration, pitch, intensity, and quality. Again, there should be little if any pause between phases (Fig. 9-9).

Because of their thinner chest wall, slender adults or children often have louder breath sounds than does the average adult. These sounds have been called "puerile" or "exaggerated" breath sounds and often resemble bronchovesicular sounds in the normal adult.

Abnormal Breath Sounds   Abnormal breath sounds are most frequently characterized by changes in the expiratory phase, although changes in the inspiratory phase may occur.

Bronchial Breath Sounds.   Bronchial breathing is a blowing, hollow, high-pitched breath sound, also sometimes called *tubular breathing*. The inspiratory phase is relatively short, but the expiratory phase is prolonged. The expiratory phase is also louder and higher in pitch than the inspiratory phase, perhaps even rising in pitch. There is a definite short pause between the two phases. A distinguishing characteristic of the sound is that it seems to originate very close to the examiner's ear, almost right at the end of the stethoscope. Bronchial sounds may be louder than normal, but not always.

Bronchial breathing is not normally heard over the lungs. However, a similar sound, called tracheal breathing, can be heard by listening over the trachea just below the larynx. Like bronchial breathing, tracheal breathing has a relatively prominent expiratory phase, but it is louder, harsher, and even more hollow than bronchial breathing. These tracheal sounds have no pathological significance.

Bronchial sounds, on the other hand, always indicate an abnormality. They result from any condition in which the lung tissue is compressed, such as pleural effusion or consolidation, as in pneumonia. Either compression or consolidation causes a denser area which results in greater transmission of sound from the bronchial tree than through the sound dampening air sacs.

Bronchovesicular Breath Sounds.   Bronchovesicular breath sounds have been described as an intermediate between vesicular and bronchial breath sounds. As stated previously, bronchovesicular sounds are normally heard in the upper midthorax. In other areas, if there is both aerated lung and a small degree of pulmonary consolidation or compression, transmission of sounds from the bronchial tree is enhanced to some degree, and abnormal bronchovesicular breath sounds result. If the degree of compression or consolidation is very mild, this sound may be described as vesicobronchiolar; as compression becomes more severe, the breath sounds become truly bronchial.

Asthmatic breath sounds.   Asthmatic breath sounds, like bronchial breathing, have a short inspiratory phase and a prolonged expiratory phase, usually even longer than bronchial breathing. However, there is no hollow or tubular quality to the breath sound. Instead, inspiration is often short and gasping, and expiration has a much higher pitch and is accompanied by wheezing and rhonchi. This type of sound indicates that there is airway narrowing, caused by edema and spasm, as with asthma, presence of foreign bodies or mucus in the airways, or stenosis of the airway. The bronchi still increase in diameter during inspiration, but during expiration the decrease in size is exaggerated and narrowing results.

Decreased or Absent Breath Sounds.   Breath sounds are absent in an area when complete occlusion of the bronchus occurs, although the lung tissue distal to the obstruction may be healthy. Diminished breath sounds not representing a pathological condition in the lung may be due to exaggerated thickness of the chest wall, as in obesity or in those with large thick muscles or large breasts. However, breath sounds may also be diminished in intensity with a variety of alterations. Any cause of generalized shallow breathing, such as the pain of pleurisy or generalized muscle weakness, may result in diminished breath sounds. The dilated air sacs of emphysema cause diminished velocity of air movement and also greater damping of sound transmission, and thus breath sounds are decreased. Any other alteration interfering with the transmission of sound, such as air or fluid in the pleural space, thickened, fibrosed pleura (often following effusion, hemothorax, or empyema, or tumor, will cause decreased intensity of breath sounds on auscultation. Many of these alterations also diminish ventilation in that area of the lung and consequently diminish breath sounds.

Amphoric Breath Sounds.   Amphoric breath sounds (from *amphora,* the Greek word for jar) resemble the sound heard when blowing over the mouth of an empty bottle. The sound has a harsh quality and a fairly high pitch. Expiration is prolonged, as in bronchial breathing, but expiration, unlike that of bronchial breathing, has a lower pitch than inspiration. This sound is heard infrequently but may be heard over an open pneumothorax or a large, thin-walled cavity that has a communication with a bronchus.

Cavernous Breath Sounds. These sounds are much like the amphoric sound, but are relatively low in pitch and hollow. They are like the sound produced by blowing *very softly* over the mouth of an empty bottle.

Cog-wheel Respirations. Cog-wheel respirations are like vesicular breath sounds except that the inspiratory phase is discontinuous and jerky. These interruptions are caused by nonsimultaneous and unequal inflation of the alveoli, such as occurs with pleurisy or muscle weakness.

Voice Sounds

Voice sounds heard on auscultation, called *vocal resonance,* have the same origin as the vibrations perceived as vocal or tactile fremitus. The sound produced in the larynx travels down the bronchial tree and is heard less distinctively as one auscultates toward the periphery of the lung.

When a person speaks in a normal manner, the sound heard on auscultation is soft and muffled as compared with the sound heard directly. The words themselves are not distinct, and one cannot understand what has been said. Often, the patient may be asked to speak in a whisper, since the spoken voice may be too loud for the examiner to detect alterations in the sound transmitted.

Abnormal Voice Sounds. There are several abnormal voice sounds; these furnish clues to pathological conditions in the chest.

Bronchophony. Bronchophony is used to indicate increased clarity and loudness of words, heard as if they were close to the ear. However, the syllables are still somewhat distorted. The word *bronchophony* literally means the sound normally heard when listening directly over a large bronchus. This sound is heard over other parts of the thorax when pulmonary consolidation or compression of lung tissue is present. With those alterations the alveoli lose some of their sound-damping quality, and this causes the increased clarity and loudness of sounds heard on auscultation. Bronchophony is usually associated with increased tactile fremitus, bronchial breath sounds, and dullness on percussion.

Whispered Pectoriloquy. Whispered pectoriloquy describes the transmission of whispered speech to the chest wall in distinct and recognizable syllables. Whispered speech is often more effective than spoken words in detecting abnormalities. Normally, whispered speech is faint and almost inaudible except over the trachea and main bronchi, when it is heard more clearly but still indistinctly. With even small amounts of consolidation, the whispered speech may still be faint, but it is clear, with definite recognition of words. The words may sound as if they were whispered into the end of the stethoscope. This change occurs before brochophony and bronchial breathing develop and consequently aids in early diagnosis of pneumonia.

Egophony. Egophony is another type of auscultated voice sound which may represent consolidation or compression of lung tissue. Normally, when the patient pronounces a long "e" softly, the examiner will hear the long "e" sound. Consolidation or compression of lung tissue alters the character of this auscultated sound, so that the examiner hears a long "a" with the stethoscope. This change from a spoken "e" to an auscultated "a" indicates egophony.

Adventitious Sounds

Adventitious sounds are not normally heard over the chest and, when present, are always abnormal. They are not modifications of breath or voice sounds but are heard in addition to breath sounds, which, in themselves, may be either normal or abnormal. The most common adventitious sounds are the various types of rales or rhonchi and the pleural friction rub.

Rales and Rhonchi. Rales are sounds produced during one or both phases of respiration when there is excess fluid of any sort in the alveoli or in any portion of the tracheobronchial tree. This fluid or exudate may be from inflammation, infection, edema, or retained secretions. Rales of one type or another are the most commonly heard adventitious sounds. Unfortunately, some of the terms used to describe variations of rales have evolved with several meanings and hence are most confusing. An attempt will be made here to identify the most common meaning of the various terms used and to identify other terms that may be used in describing the same sound.

Rales are subdivided into (1) continuous coarse sounds, called rhonchi, and (2) discontinuous crackling sounds, also called rales, the same as the parent term. Rhonchi usually imply the presence of exudate in the larger bronchi, while most medium or fine rales indicate bronchiolar and alveolar disease. Rales are heard mainly or only during inspiration, while rhonchi are heard during inspiration and expiration and may be more prominent during the latter.

Rales are often further divided and described as fine, medium, or coarse (Fig. 9-10). Fine, or crepitant, rales have a high-pitched, interrupted sound, which may be simulated by holding a lock of hair near the ear and rubbing it between the fingers. This sound can also be mimicked by moistening the thumb and forefinger with saliva and separating them slowly near the ear. Medium or crackling rales are both louder and lower-pitched and resemble the "fizz" of a freshly opened carbonated drink or the crackling of rolling a dry cigar between the fingers. Coarse, bubbling, or gurgling rales are lower-pitched and loud. They are at times referred to as the "death rattle," although they may be relieved by vigorous cough or mechanical aspiration.

Fine rales imply alveolar inflammation, exudate, and congestion, conditions found in patients with diseases such as pneumonia, congestive heart failure, and pulmonary edema. Fine rales are produced by the passage of air through secretions and also by the reinflation of alveoli whose walls have adhered together as a result of moisture and secretions. These rales often occur in "showers" at the end of inspiration as the alveoli distend. The fine rales of both

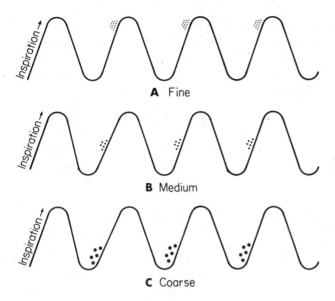

FIGURE 9-10.   Schematic representation of rales. Note that rales consist of a number of
discrete sounds, and that as they progress from fine to coarse, they occur earlier in inspiration. (Adapted from J. A. Prior and J. S. Silberstein. *Physical Diagnosis: The History and
Examination of the Patient* (4th ed.). St. Louis: Mosby, 1973.)

pulmonary congestion and impaired pulmonary ventilation may disappear after a
few deep breaths or coughs, but congestive rales reappear shortly thereafter.

Occasionally, fine rales are heard only after a cough and are then called
latent, or posttussive, rales. To demonstrate these rales, have the patient exhale
completely and then cough without first taking a breath. You should hear a
shower of medium rales on inspiration following the cough. You will probably
have to demonstrate this maneuver to him. These rales, elicited only by
coughing, are often present with a tuberculous lesion.

Atelectatic, or marginal, rales are crepitant-type rales that may be heard with
initial deep breaths in the periphery of the lungs or the dependent portions. The
lungs are never fully expanded during normal respiration, and secretions and
moisture tend to accumulate in the unaerated portions, especially in dependent
ones. These rales are heard only in the periphery with the first few deep breaths
and then disappear after a few breaths as that portion of the lung becomes
aerated. They have no pathological significance.

Medium rales represent a gradation between fine and coarse rales and are
thought to originate with the passage of air through mucus in the bronchioles or
separation of the bronchiolar walls that have adhered, due to exudate. This type
of rales is most commonly heard in bronchitis and pulmonary congestion.

Coarse rales have their origin in the trachea and main and smaller bronchi.
These bubbling, gurgling rales are often heard with the resolution of acute

inflammation, when large amounts of thick exudate are present in the airway. They may diminish or disappear with a vigorous cough that clears the exudate. However, they may also be heard in the acutely ill, moribund patient who has a depression of the cough reflex and accumulation of thick secretion. Coarse rales are also heard with severe pulmonary edema.

A *rhonchus* is a prolonged, continuous rale that has a musical note like that of a reed instrument or the violin. It is present in both phases of respiration, although there may be distinct differences in pitch, intensity, quality, and duration in one phase as compared with the other. If high-pitched, these sounds are called *sibilant rhonchi* and are often wheezing or squeaking. If low-pitched, snoring, or moaning, they are called *sonorous rhonchi.* A dry, coarse rale is interchangeably called a rhonchus by many.

The sound of a rhonchus is caused by an obstruction or narrowing of the tracheobronchial tree (Fig. 9-11). The change may be due to fluid or solid tissue within the lumen (for example, thick wet mucus), in which case the bronchial lumen becomes smaller during expiration and the rhonchi higher-pitched. If this is the case, the rhonchi can sometimes be cleared by several coughs. Narrowing of the bronchial lumen may also result from extrinsic compression on the bronchus, as with enlarged lymph nodes or a mediastinal tumor, or intrinsic narrowing from an endobronchial tumor. Edema of the mucosa and bronchial spasm also cause intrinsic narrowing and may themselves cause rhonchi or exaggerate rhonchal sounds caused by exudate within the lumen. In patients with asthma or emphysema, conditions in which rhonchi are expected, they can sometimes be heard only by having the person exhale as completely as possible as one listens below the clavicle.

Friction Sounds. The pleural friction rub results when inflammation of the pleura causes loss of lubricating fluid so that the opposing roughened surfaces produce a creaking or grating sound when they rub together, rather than sliding silently over each other. This is caused most commonly by pleurisy, often from an inflammation of the lung tissue which has spread to the pleura. It may also be

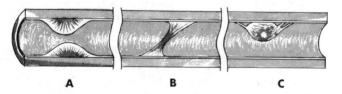

A   **B**   **C**

FIGURE 9-11. Causes of rhonchi. A. Narrowing of entire circumference of lumen, which may be caused by inflammation with edema, stenosis, or tumor. B. Strands of thick secretions, which vibrate with the passage of air. C. Unilateral narrowing of lumen, caused by presence of a tumor or resulting from extrinsic compression by enlarged lymph nodes or tumor. (Adapted from J. A. Prior and J. S. Silberstein. *Physical Diagnosis: The History and Examination of the Patient* (4th ed.). St. Louis: Mosby, 1973.)

caused by a pulmonary embolus, peripheral pneumonia, or trauma to the chest wall that causes changes in the parietal layer. A friction rub may be imitated by placing the palm of one hand over the ear and then stroking the back of that hand with the fingers of the other hand.

The friction rub characteristically sounds close to the ear. It is usually audible in both phases of respiration, although it may be heard only at the end of inspiration. Friction rubs are more commonly heard and are louder in the lower anterolateral chest, where there is greatest mobility of lung tissue. An existing friction rub generally becomes louder with a deep breath or when the stethoscope is held more firmly on the chest wall. A friction rub is almost always accompanied by discomfort.

It may sometimes be crucial to differentiate a rhonchus or coarse rales from a friction rub. A rhonchus will frequently clear with coughing, unlike a friction rub, and is predominantly inspiratory, whereas a rub involves both phases of the respiratory cycle. Also, rubs are usually more localized, are felt or heard unilaterally, and have the characteristic of seeming very close to the surface. In addition, rhonchi do not become louder with pressing harder on the stethoscope. The physician should be notified of the possible presence of a friction rub.

If the nurse finds alterations during the respiratory system appraisal, she should be able to use the data gained to counsel patients in the appropriate help-seeking behavior. It is not necessarily expected, however, that the nurse would use the complete examination at all times or in all situations. It is anticipated that she will be using parts of the examination intermittently to assist her in planning, validating, and evaluating nursing intervention. However, only by habitual and conscientious use of these physical appraisal skills will they contribute to and enhance the nurse's practice.

SUGGESTED READINGS

Broughton, J. O. Physical diagnosis for nurses and respiratory therapists. *Heart and Lung* 1:200, 1973.

DeGowen, E. L., and DeGowen, R. L. *Bedside Diagnostic Examination* (2nd ed.). London: Macmillan, 1969.

Judge, R. D., and Zuidema, G. D. (Eds.). *Methods of Clinical Examination: A Physiologic Approach* (3rd ed.). Boston: Little, Brown, 1974.

Major, R. H., and Delp, M. H. *Physical Diagnoses* (6th ed.). Philadelphia: Saunders, 1962.

Prior, J. A., and Silberstein, J. S. *Physical Diagnosis: The History and Examination of the Patient* (4th ed.). St. Louis: Mosby, 1973.

Sedlock, S. A. Detection of chronic pulmonary disease. *Am. J. Nurs.* 72:1407, 1972.

Carol Gilbert

GLOSSARY

aneurysm Localized abnormal dilatation of the wall of a vessel, usually of an artery.

angina pectoris A paroxysmal, constricting substernal pain often radiating to the left shoulder and down to the hand.

apex of the heart Pointed portion of the heart, usually located near the left fifth intercostal space medial to the midclavicular line.

arrhythmia Any variation of rhythm from the normal (regular) rhythm of the heartbeat.

atrial fibrillation An arrhythmia which has rapid uncoordinated atrial activity associated with an irregular ventricular rhythm.

atrial flutter An arrhythmia in which atrial depolarization is extremely rapid (approximately 300/minute), regular, and uniform in its saw tooth appearance, and the ventricular rate and rhythm varies with the degree of atrioventricular block.

atrial tachycardia An arrhythmia originating in the atria, characterized by rapid, regular beating of the entire heart.

atrioventricular block (AV block) Slowing or interruption of impulse transmission from the atria to the ventricles. *Bundle branch block* occurs when there is impulse transmission alteration in the Bundle of His and may be described as right or left bundle branch block, depending on the origin of the transmission alteration.

base (cardiac) Region of the aortic and pulmonic outflow tracts; usually the second or third intercostal spaces to the right and left of the sternum.

bradycardia Slow heart beat (less than 60 beats per minute in adults).

bruit Extracardiac blowing sound auscultated over a vessel, usually an artery.

diastole Dilatation; period of "relaxation" during which the atria or ventricles fill; corresponding with the interval between the second and first heart sound.

embolism Sudden occlusion of a vessel by a clot or other obstruction carried to its place by the blood current.

gallop rhythm Characteristic cadence created by three heart sounds, in conjunction with a tachycardia.

hypertension Transient or persistent abnormal elevation of blood pressure.

infarct Localized ischemic necrosis of tissue due to obstruction of the circulation.

midclavicular line (MCL) Vertical line midway between the sternal line and the acromioclavicular joint.

murmur Any adventitous auscultatory sound produced by turbulent blood flow within or near the heart.

palpitation Unusually rapid, strong, or irregular heartbeat felt by the patient.

point of maximum impulse (PMI) Commonly synonymous with *apex impulse,* the point of maximal thrusting of the heart against the anterior chest wall during systole.

presystolic Period immediately preceding the first heart sound.

protodiastolic Period immediately following the second heart sound; pertaining to the initial one-third of diastole.

shock   1-Acute peripheral circulatory collapse marked by pallor, coolness and clamminess
of skin, hypotension, weak, rapid pulse, and decreased respiratory depth.
2- Palpable, short, high-frequency vibration over a vessel or precordium.
syncope   Temporary unconsciousness; fainting.
systole   Contraction; period of contraction during which the atria or ventricles eject blood.
Ventricular systole includes the interval inclusive of the first and second heart sound
(used alone, systole generally refers only to ventricular activity).
tachycardia   Rapid regular heart beat (more than 100 beats per minute in adults).
thrill   Sustained high-frequency vibration felt on palpation.
ventricular tachycardia   Arrhythmia originating in the ventricles, characterized by rapid
regular beating of the heart.

In examining the circulatory system it is important to remember that a
complete investigation demands not only an evaluation of the heart but also a
careful appraisal of the peripheral circulation. Problems arising from alterations
in the peripheral circulation, which can be detected easily on physical
examination, may be overlooked by the nurse examiner because of overconcen-
tration on the myocardium. In this chapter the complete evaluation of the
circulatory system will be discussed in terms of techniques of examination and
normal and abnormal findings that often present themselves in adult subjects.

In collecting data for assessment, we usually assume that the person is normal
until the investigation demonstrates otherwise. Because cardiovascular
phenomena are sometimes transient, this mode of thinking may not always be
satisfactory and makes it too easy to miss something. To facilitate the
examination, reverse this process and demand negation of alteration, rather than
presuming normality. Questions should always be on your mind as you examine.
Is the pulse irregular? Is the blood pressure elevated? Is there an extra heart
sound?

Another key factor to be considered is organization. Although necessary for
all areas of physical examination, it becomes especially important here because
of a unique factor involved in circulation, namely, *timing*. For example, while
pulsation is continuous, each individual heartbeat consists of heart sounds that
are finite, necessitating simultaneous use of multiple observational skills to
collect valid data. Again, questions should be kept in mind. What is it I see, feel,
or hear? What is its duration? How can it be described? Planning must be done
to insure a complete and efficient examination. Use of techniques and the order
of the overall examination should be by design, not accident. Start with the
interview. In-depth data collection in this area should provide direction for the
physical examination to follow. Inspection, palpation, and percussion will then
indicate what you should be listening for, and why, when you finally proceed to
auscultation. The order for the overall examination should be as follows:
extremities, neck, and precordium. In this way you move logically from the
periphery toward the center, the heart.

In appraisal of circulation the four techniques of physical examination —
inspection, palpation, percussion, and auscultation — are used extensively.
Because the quality of the data collected for appraisal of the circulatory system

depends on the nurse's ability to use these techniques with ease, they will be discussed first.

TECHNIQUES

Inspection and Palpation

As in any examination, the first concern should be to establish a general picture. Observation of body build, general color, character of respiration, and presence of emotional tension will give this overview (see Chaps. 5 and 6).

Extremities. Examination should include both the arms and legs. As you proceed, compare findings on opposing extremities. Symmetry, or lack of it, may be significant. With the patient in a sitting or supine position, start distally by inspecting the toenails (fingernails) for shape, color, and thickness. Then palpate for capillary refill by pressing the tip of the patient's toenail (fingernail) to produce blanching; release and note the time taken for color to return. Capillary pulsation, while not routinely tested, can be evaluated by using the same maneuver and observing for pulsation before releasing the pressure on the nail. Estimate the skin temperature along the extremities. Palpate with the dorsal surface of the middle phalanges, or with the plantar surface of the fingertips, using a light rapid movement along the extremity (compare temperature gradations along opposing extremities simultaneously if possible). Skin color, hair distribution, and the presence or absence of any atrophy should then be observed.

Observe the pattern of venous circulation. Evaluate the degree of venous engorgement with the extremity in a dependent position and then gradually elevate the limb to heart level, noting the time and angle of dissipation of venous distention. Proceed by observing for the presence or absence of any swelling and then palpate for edema. The maneuver involves using the fingertip of one or two fingers to depress the skin surface over a bony area, removing the finger(s), and noting the appearance of the area immediately and the time taken for the depressed area to dissipate. Measure the limb circumference in centimeters wherever edema is suspected, and compare with the same area on the opposing limb. Note the location of the area measured in terms of centimeters proximal or distal to a bony landmark such as the malleolus or the tibial tuberosity. This notation will help to insure that follow-up measurements are taken in the same place.

Before palpating the arterial pulses, observe for any obvious pulsations. Moving centrally, palpate the arterial pulses — dorsalis pedis, posterior tibialis, popliteal, femoral, radial, and brachial (see Fig. 10-1). In palpating, use the three middle fingers, occlude the vessel completely, then release gradually. Determine the pulse rate, rhythm, force (amplitude), elasticity of the vessel wall, and quality. Elasticity of the vessel wall is established by occluding the vessel with

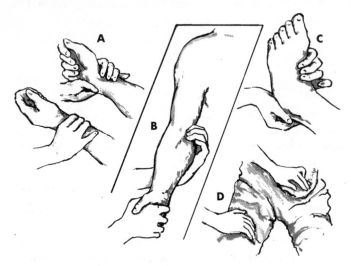

FIGURE 10-1. Method of palpating the arterial pulses of the extremities A. Radial. B. Brachial. C. Dorsalis pedis. D. Femoral. (Adapted from Judge and Zuidema [3].)

one hand while palpating the vessel distal to the occlusion with the other. Using the three-finger technique enhances your ability to obtain the data, especially with respect to elasticity and quality of the pulse. Quality of the peripheral pulses should be noted on a 3+ scale.

Palpation of the abdominal aorta should be done to insure complete examination of the circulatory system. In addition to the data just mentioned, note any deviation of the abdominal aorta from the midline of the abdomen (see Chap. 11).

Neck. While the patient is in a sitting position, observe for obvious pulsations and neck-vein distention. The carotid pulse can then be palpated in this position or after the patient is placed in the supine position. Using the three-finger method, palpate the carotid pulses by placing your fingers medial to the sternocleidomastoid muscle just below the jaw (see Fig. 10-2A). It should be noted that evaluation of pulsations of the neck should be done one side at a time to avoid possible occlusion of blood flow to the cerebrum. Collect data as delineated for the other arterial pulses.

Now, with the patient in the supine position, observe for venous pulsations (see Fig. 10-2B). To be sure that you are observing the venous pulse, palpate a radial or carotid artery with one hand while gently palpating with the other what you consider to be the internal or external jugular vein. Note that in the supine position, the patient's neck veins will be distended and that the venous pulse, undulating and diffuse in nature, differs from the arterial pulse, which is swift and localized. If difficulty is experienced, you can have the patient inhale, hold

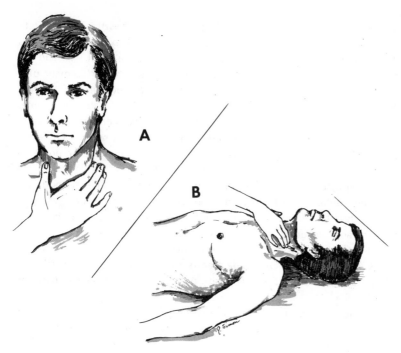

FIGURE 10-2. Method of palpating the pulses of the neck. A. Carotid. B. Jugular.

his breath, and "bear down" briefly. This will cause the neck veins to distend further, as the change in pressure in the chest will diminish blood flow into the heart. Once the neck veins are located, perform the following maneuvers: (1) establish the character of the pulse; (2) observe the effect of respiration on pulsation; (3) observe the effect on pulsation of light pressure applied on the base of the neck; (4) observe the effect of a gradual elevation of the head of the bed to an upright position; and (5) time the pulsations. At present, use of the data on timing of venous pulsations is predominantly diagnostic in nature and falls primarily within the province of the physician. Details on the subject can be found in DeGowin and DeGowin [2], Judge and Zuidema [3], and Kampmeier [4].

Precordium. Position yourself on the right side toward the foot of the patient and observe the anterior chest for any apparent pulsations in both the sitting and supine positions. Notation should be made of the character and location of the pulsations. Record the location of pulsations in respect to the intercostal space (ICS) and midclavicular line (MCL), or sternal border. To identify and number correctly the intercostal space, locate the angle of Louis, which is palpated as a prominence on the upper third of the sternum. Once the angle of Louis is located, move your fingers laterally, to identify the second intercostal space (see

Fig. 9-3B and discussion on the landmarks of the chest). To facilitate demonstration of pulsations on the chest, have the patient exhale and hold his breath. This maneuver reduces the lung volume between the chest wall and the great vessels, making the movement of the heart more obvious. Placement of a tongue blade over the precordium and observing for the movement of the free edge will also help amplify the pulsations (see Fig. 10-3). At the same time, note any bulging or prominence of one side of the chest as compared with the other. Next, palpate the precordium for pulsations, again noting their character and location. The main objective is to identify the apex impulse or point of maximal impulse (PMI).

In performing palpation, both the fingertip and palmar surface methods are acceptable. The application of the palmar surface of the first four phalanges, excluding the thumb, to the chest wall will not only provide for the most comprehensive and accurate data but also is easier to perform (see Fig. 10-4A). Shift your hand from place to place over the precordial area as you palpate. With female patients with large breasts, displace the breast upward with the palpating hand and hold it in this position with the other hand as necessary (see Fig. 10-4B).

The four major areas of interest on the anterior chest are the apex or mitral area, the left sternal border or tricuspid area, the pulmonic area, and the aortic

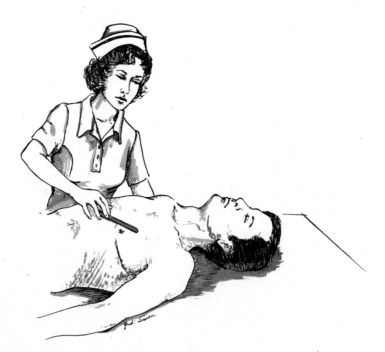

FIGURE 10-3. Method of amplifying the apical impulse using a tongue blade.

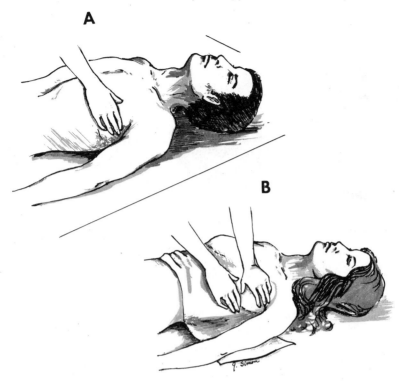

FIGURE 10-4. A. Palpations of the precordium. B. Demonstration of correct positioning of the breast during palpation.

area (see Fig. 10-5). Having the patient exhale and hold his breath will facilitate palpation, as the lungs will be retracted somewhat out of the heart's way, allowing for closer apposition of the heart to the chest wall and eliminating the distraction created by chest movement due to respiration. This technique is very useful when examining a patient with less prominent pulsations.

After palpating in the sitting and supine positions, have the patient turn to his left side. This position makes it easier to locate the apex impulse if it has been difficult to do so with the patient supine. It also assists in the identification of abnormal pulsations, as the heart is now angled more against the chest wall. The sitting position is useful when palpating the pulmonic and aortic areas of the heart. The technique of palpation is of great importance as it allows the identification of pulsations (including those of low frequency and intensity) which may be inaudible on auscultation.

Percussion

Of the four techniques used in the examination of the circulatory system, percussion offers the least information. Chest roentgenography better demon-

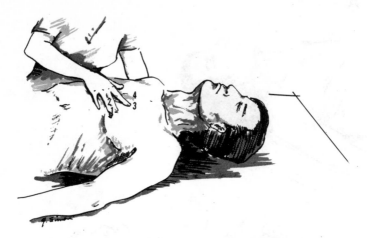

FIGURE 10-5. Demonstration of valve areas on the chest. 1. Mitral or apex area. 2. Tricuspid area. 3. Pulmonic area. 4. Aortic area.

strates the size and contour of the heart. When there is no access to roentgenography, percussion is a useful way to confirm impressions of cardiac size and contour gained by inspection and palpation. Percussion is not used in examination of the extremities or the neck.

Precordium. In examination of the heart, direct percussion (see Chap. 2 for discussion of direct and indirect percussion) can be most useful if guided by the following considerations:

1. Use a light tap rather than a slap (sound changes can be more easily identified with the lighter touch).
2. Place the fingers flat and tangentially along the anterior chest, as it is a convex surface.
3. The movement of your hand should follow the curve of the chest. In addition, when the patient has large breasts you will have a hand free to hold the breast out of the way.

When using indirect percussion, the same guides apply, but examining the patient with large breasts is likely to be more difficult. In indirect percussion, the pleximeter (underlying) finger can be placed either parallel or at right angles to the heart. Either way is acceptable (see Fig. 10-6). Stand to the right side of the supine patient and percuss from the left axillary area to the midline in the sixth, fifth, fourth, and third intercostal spaces. Record the point of change in the percussion note in each space. This information will give you the left border of cardiac dullness (LBCD). Once the left cardiac border is estimated, attempt to locate the right cardiac border by percussing toward the sternum along the second, third, and fourth intercostal spaces on the right anterior chest. Usually, the right cardiac border is not palpable, as it lies below the sternum. Data are

Direct

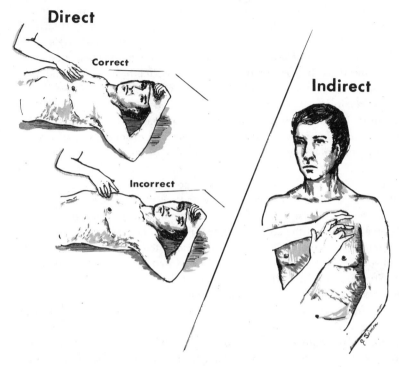

Correct

Incorrect

Indirect

FIGURE 10-6. Direct and indirect percussion of the cardiac border. A. Correct and incorrect method of direct percussion. B. Correct method of indirect percussion.

recorded again in respect to the intercostal space (ICS) and the midclavicular line (MCL), or sternal border.

Auscultation

Auscultation, like percussion, is used predominantly in the examination of the heart, with the notable exception of its use in measuring arterial blood pressure. Before discussing auscultation of the precordium, some comment about arterial blood pressure is appropriate.

Extremities. In measuring arterial blood pressure, several points should be remembered. To insure a true baseline measurement, the patient should be in a stable position, sitting or supine, for at least 5 minutes before the arterial blood pressure is taken. The palpatory technique should be employed prior to auscultation to prevent excessive inflation of the cuff when auscultating. When palpating, inflate the cuff only until the palpable pulse disappears. While an estimation of diastolic pressure is possible by noting the change from *bounding* pulsation to *normal,* the chief concern when palpating is to establish the systolic pressure by noting the first reappearance of the pulse. With the diaphragm endpiece of the stethoscope placed lightly over the brachial artery, cuff inflation should be only 20 to 30 mm Hg above the palpated systolic pressure. Release the cuff pressure 2 to 3 mm Hg at a time. The first sound to reappear, designated phase I Korotkoff, is the systolic pressure. Phase II, the bruit sound, and phase III, the loud sharp sound, will follow as the cuff pressure falls. Phase IV, the muffling or damping of the sound, is considered by the American Heart Association to be the most accurate measure of diastolic pressure. However, many sources still recommend the final disappearance of sound, phase V, as the best index of diastolic pressure. Since the purpose of taking an arterial blood pressure is to determine a baseline for later comparative readings, it is more important for the health team to establish a consistent procedure than it is to debate the appropriateness of using phase IV or V, as either is acceptable.

The final point to consider is cuff size. The rule of thumb is that the width of the inflatable bladder of the cuff should be 20 percent greater than the diameter of the extremity on which it is used [1]. The use of the wrong cuff size can lead to the collection of inaccurate data (usually, elevated results, as the cuff is too narrow). The question of cuff size becomes especially important when dealing with the obese patient or when measuring the arterial blood pressure in the leg. When it is necessary to use the leg, the palpatory technique is usually satisfactory, as it generally is not essential to establish a diastolic pressure. When possible, the cuff should be applied to the calf and the posterior tibial artery palpated. The thigh usually demands a large cuff width that may not be readily available. To insure complete data collection, the arterial blood pressure should be taken in both arms.

Several other extraneous factors can lead to error in measurement, for example:

1. Wrapping the cuff too loosely can give a false result, usually too high.
2. Emotional responses to the situation, the environment or the examiner can also lead to elevated results. To overcome this, take the measurement at least twice during the examination with a minimum intervening time period of 10 minutes.
3. Presence of an "auscultatory gap" can lead to falsely low systolic values. This phenomenon occurs when sounds heard initially, as the cuff pressure is decreased from suprasystolic levels, disappear, only to reappear 10—15 mm Hg lower. Using correct palpatory technique before auscultation is the best defense against this possible error.
4. Presence of feeble Korotkoff's sounds can make auscultation difficult and thus unreliable. Having the patient raise his arm prior to cuff inflation and then inflating the cuff in this position diminishes venous pressure. This may make sounds louder. Once the cuff is inflated, have the patient lower the cuffed arm and proceed as usual. If the sounds are still making measurement unreliable, you may have to accept the results of the palpatory measurement.

Precordium. Auscultation of the heart, while the most difficult of the techniques to master, is the most important of the four. Use of the stethoscope is the only means available to identify many valvular alterations, even with the development and use of cardiac catheterization. Trying to distinguish a sound, its quality, and duration is not easy. While discussion and recordings are helpful, expertise is attained only by extensive practice. The ability to hear sound depends not only on the characteristics of the sound, but also on the examiner's ability to perceive it. If the equipment is inappropriate, the difficulties involved increase dramatically (see Chap. 2).

Sound. Sound has three components: frequency, intensity, and quality. Frequency, commonly referred to as pitch, is the number of vibrations a sound creates per second (noted in cycles per second, or cps). Intensity is the magnitude of the vibration and determines loudness. When overtones are added to the basic frequency of a sound we have the third component, quality. This component allows the listener to recognize the source of a sound, e.g., whether the sound is produced by a violin or a trumpet. Both sounds may be of the same frequency and intensity but because of the overtones, the quality is different, and the careful listener can make the distinction. The hearing ability of the examining nurse is another major consideration and influences the perception of any generated sound. Generally, the human ear can perceive frequencies ranging from about 20 to about 16,000 cps. Sounds below or above these frequencies are difficult or impossible to hear [3]. If a sound's magnitude of vibration (intensity) is too low, the sound may not be heard, even though the frequency is within the audible range. Therefore, the hearing of a sound is a function of both frequency and intensity.

The relationship of intensity and frequency to heart sounds is shown in Figure 10-7. Note that the majority of heart sounds are inaudible and those that are within audible range fall predominantly in the lower frequencies. Furthermore, an examiner's conception of sound can affect what she hears. If inexperienced, the nurse examiner may find the frequency of a sound coloring her perception of its intensity. For example, in loudness comparisons, a high-pitched sound is often described as louder than a low-pitched sound, even when its intensity is actually less than that of the low-pitched sound. This occurs because the listener believes high-pitched sounds are loud and low-pitched sounds are soft. Thus it is important to note carefully what is heard, not only the overall impression of the sound, but also both of its individual components, pitch and loudness.

These factors, along with the masking phenomenon, are what make auscultation so difficult and palpation so important, for even though a sound may be inaudible, it may still be palpable. The *masking phenomenon* is the result of a defense mechanism of the ear, whereby it protects itself from loud (high-intensity) sounds by reducing its receptive ability. Masking comes into play when sounds following a loud one are faint. Because of reduced receptivity, these sounds may not be perceived by the listener.

Heart sounds may create this phenomenon, and so can extraneous room noise. The former must be accepted, but the nurse examiner must work constantly to overcome masking by consciously listening for the low-intensity

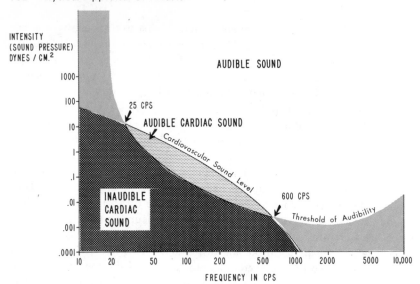

FIGURE 10-7. Comparison of auditory threshold with average intensity of cardiac sound at various frequencies. Note that only sounds of 25 to 600 cps are in the audible range. (Adapted from Judge and Zuidema [3].)

sound which is so easily missed. Room noise can be minimized if not eliminated by preplanning; e.g., closing doors, curtains, turning off air conditioners.

Technique. A major difficulty for the inexperienced nurse is the identification of the first two heart sounds. Two maneuvers are helpful in making this discrimination. First, correlate the auscultated sounds with observation or palpation of the apex impulse or carotid pulse. Both of these are systolic in timing, so it is expected that the first heart sound (S_1) would just precede them since it is produced by the closing of the mitral and tricuspid valves. The second maneuver involves discrimination of the second heart sound (S_2). This is accomplished by listening at the aortic valve area of the chest (see Fig. 10-8). The second heart sound, produced by the aortic and pulmonic valves closing, is invariably loudest in this location. Once you have identified the sound, move the stethoscope slowly toward the apex, keeping this louder sound (S_2) as your focus. You will notice that as you move the stethoscope across the chest this sound decreases in intensity. The former maneuver is also very helpful when timing murmurs or extra sounds, especially when the heart rate is rapid or the quality of sounds is abnormal. Take time to develop skills in the use of these maneuvers. Effective auscultation of the heart requires confidence in your ability to distinguish S_1 from S_2.

While the examination will cover the whole precordium and supracardiac surface of the anterior chest, four areas, the valve areas, have special significance, since sound produced by the valves are heard best in these locations. With the mitral and aortic valves, the area is somewhat distant from the actual valve

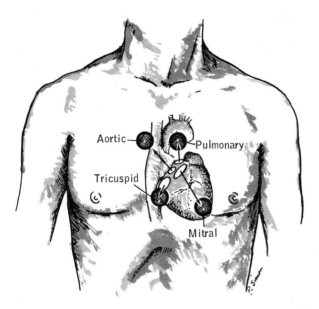

FIGURE 10-8.   Reference points for localizing heart sounds. Diagram demonstrates actual valve locations and the points to which their sounds are usually referred. (Adapted from Judge and Zuidema [3].)

location, as the valves are deep in the chest. Because the tricuspid and pulmonic valves are close to the chest wall, their areas are relatively close to the actual valve location (see Fig. 10-8).

Before beginning to listen, establish a routine. Determine what kinds of data you need to collect and how to proceed; doing this will avoid omissions and facilitate efficiency. The routine should include:

1. *Notation of rate and rhythm.*   Is the rate excessively fast or slow? Is the rhythm irregular in any way? How does the apical pulse correlate with the peripheral pulse?
2. *Identification of the first and second heart sound.* Consider each sound individually and in each of the four areas. Is the sound unusually loud, soft, or accentuated? What is the pitch of each sound? What is the relationship of the first sound to the second in respect to frequency, loudness, and duration?
3. *Identification of extra sounds and murmurs.* Concentrate on systole and diastole separately in each of the four areas. Are there any extra sounds? Where are they heard with maximum intensity? What is the transmission of the murmur?

Listen for one thing at a time. Start at the apex with the patient in the supine position and stand at his left side. Lightly place the bell of the stethoscope endpiece over the precordium. To facilitate good control of the endpiece, place the last three fingers of your right hand (left if you are left-handed) on the chest to allow for pressure variation against the chest wall while the other two fingers hold the endpiece in place

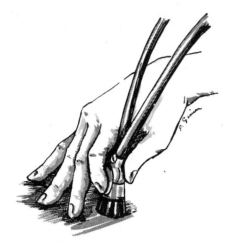

FIGURE 10-9.   Correct method of holding the stethoscope endpiece, permitting use of variable pressure against the chest wall. (Adapted from Judge and Zuidema [3].)

(see Fig. 10-9). Low-frequency sounds are destroyed if too much pressure is exerted. To insure that you are providing yourself with the optimum pressure on the endpiece, start by pressing the bell firmly against the chest wall and then slowly lighten the pressure while listening. The sounds should become louder and then eventually softer as you lift the endpiece off the chest. Using this maneuver will help to develop the desired *light* pressure. The bell endpiece of the stethoscope is used to auscultate the precordium as most heart sounds are of relatively low pitch and this endpiece provides for the best amplification of these sounds. Use of the diaphragm endpiece can be a helpful adjunct in examination as it masks out low-frequency sounds, thus enabling the nurse examiner to concentrate more easily on the high-pitch sounds. This is especially helpful when auscultating the base of the heart where the relatively high pitch sounds tend to originate. However, when using the diaphragm endpiece the nurse examiner must keep its masking effect in mind. When using the diaphragm endpiece a *firm* touch provides the best results (for further discussion see Chap. 2).

Avoid "jumping" from valve area to valve area, or important data will be missed. Instead, move the endpiece in small increments across the chest from the apex toward the tricuspid area, up along the sternal border to the pulmonic area, across the sternum to the aortic area, and then diagonally back across the chest to the apex.

Changes in patient position bring the heart closer to the chest wall, increasing the loudness of certain auscultatory sounds. The left lateral position usually provides for louder sounds at the apex, while the sitting position makes audible some murmurs otherwise inaudible at the left sternal border and base. Exercise can also assist in identifying extra sounds or murmurs; however, it is not usually considered part of the routine examination.

Alterations in respiration can affect the location and identification of sounds and murmurs, which is another reason why listening over the four valve areas alone is not satisfactory. If breath sounds interfere with auscultation, having the patient hold his breath at the end of expiration helps intensify distant or weak heart sounds.

NORMAL AND ABNORMAL FINDINGS

To make proper interpretations of collected data, a thorough understanding of the physiologic interrelationships involved in the circulatory system is essential. While it is not the purpose to detail these interrelationships in this chapter, certain observations about them merit comment here.

The circulatory system is constantly adapting to changes in a person's internal and external environment. These adaptations, which maintain homeostasis, are expected to occur, and from them, the normal range of findings is established; for example, with exercise, an increase in pulse rate is expected. In addition to these variables, individual characteristics influence data interpretation also. Thus an acceptable blood pressure for a 72-year-old man may not be appropriate for a 21-year-old athlete or a 26-year-old pregnant woman. On examination, however, the findings in all three cases may still fall within the normal range, once their individual characteristics and the circumstances under which the data were collected are considered.

Proceeding from the extremities to the precordium, and from inspection to auscultation, the following will serve as guidelines to the detection of normal and abnormal findings.

Extremities

Inspection and Palpation: Normal Findings.   Normally, the fingernails and toenails are convex in shape, pink in color, and smooth in appearance. Capillary refill is immediate, and capillary pulsation is extremely difficult to demonstrate, if possible at all. Generally, skin temperature is warm over the entire extremity. Color and hair distribution are consistent with the rest of the body and symmetrical with the opposing limb. In the dependent position, superficial venous distention is apparent, and venous valves may be identified as nodular bulges. Collapse of the veins will occur when the extremity is elevated to heart level. The vessels themselves are easily movable, flexible, and without tortuosity. Swelling and atrophy are absent.

Normal adaptation as a result of autonomic stimulation can create either vasodilatation or vasoconstriction. In either case, the responses observed in the extremities will be symmetrical. Vasodilatation is demonstrated by warmth, rubor, capillary pulsation more apparent than usual, and throbbing of the digits.

With vasoconstriction, the results are coldness of the extremities, pallor, and collapse of the superficial veins. Warm environment may cause vasodilatation. Vasoconstriction can be induced by smoking, anxiety, or a cold environment.

The normal resting pulse rate in the adult ranges from 60 to 100 beats per minute, with women tending to have higher rates than men. Rates greater than 100 beats per minute may be the result of anxiety and should be rechecked after the patient has been at rest to insure validity. Well-conditioned athletes can, and often do, have rates in the 50s without circulatory compromise. Generally, the rhythm is regular.

Two frequently demonstrated irregularities that are within normal limits are sinus arrhythmia and occasional premature beats. In *sinus arrhythmia,* the pulse rate increases with respiratory inspiration and decreases with expiration. It can be exaggerated with deep inspiration or created by a person with irregular respirations. It can be evaluated by correlation of the pulse rhythm with respiration. It is usually seen in children and young adults and occasionally in older people. *Premature contractions* are usually the result of an early systole, with the pacemaker arising outside of the usual location, the sinoatrial (SA) node. They are common and generally present no problems except for a subjective effect they occasionally have on the people experiencing them, who often make the remark: "My heart skips beats once in a while"; or "Occasionally my heart stops for a second." Keep in mind it is the occasional premature contraction that is considered normal. Any degree of frequency of premature contractions noted in examination or from interviewing should be investigated more closely as pathology may be present.

Force, or amplitude, is the reflection of the magnitude of the pulse pressure, the difference between systolic and diastolic pressure. As pulse pressure is related to stroke volume, any gross changes here will affect the force. Increases in stroke volume cause widened pulse pressure, thus creating an increased force. Exercise, ingesting alcohol, heat, and excitement all create an increased stroke volume.

Elasticity refers to the rebound and expansile action of the vessel wall. Normally, an artery is flexible, nontortuous and nonpalpable after the blood has been forced out of it. Quality (character of the pulse wave) is a function of the rate of change and magnitude of the pulse pressure. It is best evaluated at the carotid artery (discussed in the section on the neck). Symmetry or lack of it is a key concern in evaluating the quality of the peripheral pulses. On a 3+ scale, normal pulses are demonstrated as 2+, absent pulses as 0, thready weak pulses as 1+, and bounding pulses as 3+.

Inspection and Palpation: Abnormal Findings. Abnormal findings reflecting cardiovascular disease and demonstrated by inspection and palpation of extremities are generally: clubbing, cyanosis, edema, varicosities, thrombosis, arterial occlusion, and aneurysm.

Clubbing. Clubbing of the fingers or toes in the early stages is demonstrated

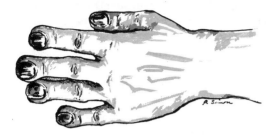

FIGURE 10-10.   Diagram of clubbing. Note the watch-crystal appearance of the nails.

by a flattening of the angle of the base of the nail. Progressively the longitudinal curvature of the nail is increased, giving the finger a drumstick-like appearance (see Fig. 10-10). While the major cardiovascular causes of clubbing are congenital cyanotic heart disease, cor pulmonale, and subacute bacterial endocarditis there are a variety of other causes of clubbing [3].

Cyanosis.   Central or generalized cyanosis is usually caused by congenital heart disease with right to left shunting, pulmonary disease involving arterio-venous fistulas, or incomplete gas exchange. Patients with polycythemia frequently exhibit central cyanosis because of the changes in red blood cell production, even though their oxygen tension is relatively high. The bluish discoloration is observed best in the inner side of the lips, tongue, and conjunctiva. Peripheral cyanosis occurs when there is a drastic decrease in systemic blood flow, usually as a result of a low cardiac output, as in congestive heart failure or peripheral vascular obstruction. In this situation the restricted arterial blood flow leads to an increased extraction of oxygen from the blood in peripheral areas, thus increasing the amount of reduced hemoglobin. The result is localized cyanosis, usually in conjunction with coldness and mottling of the skin. This type of cyanosis is usually seen in the hands, feet, outer side of the lips, and the earlobes. It is demonstrated by a light, one-finger pressure on the bluish skin, producing a blanched imprint which dissipates slowly when the testing finger is removed.

Edema.   Cardiac edema is usually dependent (hands, feet, ankles), pitting, and bilateral in nature. Pitting edema is graded from 1+ to 4+, with 1+ being a slight depression on the skin surface from finger pressure which disappears relatively quickly; 4+ is a deep depression which disappears very slowly. As pitting edema is also graded on a 3+ scale, notation of the scale used, in addition to the grade, will promote better understanding of the findings. While guidelines are available, the grading of edema is still subjective. Comparison of findings with associates and practice are the best ways to develop confidence in one's judgments.

Edema can be demonstrated unilaterally also. In these situations it is frequently the result of some peripheral cause, e.g., occlusion of a deep vein or artery. This edema may be nonpitting or "brawny" in nature. Differences in the circumference of the limb area from one extremity to the other is the key determination to make here. Measurements (in cm) are made, using a bony prominence as a landmark. Record the circumference measurement and the distal, or proximal, distance from the landmark used.

Varicose Veins. Varicosities, which are dilated and tortuous vessels, if present, are usually demonstrated in the superficial leg veins. Because of the vessel distention, blood flow through the affected area is decreased, while the pressure in the vessel is increased. Causation is either primary or secondary in nature. *Primary varicosities* are due to an inherent weakness in the vessel wall and the valves, and are often found to be familial. This alteration is often bilateral. *Secondary varicosities* are usually the result of obstruction.

Varicosities are demonstrated best by inspection of the extremities in the dependent position. In the early stages, vessel distention and tortuosity will be the key signs. The patient may complain of aching pain in the calf which is relieved by elevating the extremity. Night cramping may be experienced also. With further venous insufficiency, the appearance of edema, pruritus, paresthesia, skin ulceration, and dependent cyanosis becomes common. With prolonged venous insufficiency, a brown discoloration of the skin about the ankles (due to iron deposits) may be demonstrated.

Often, the varicosities are found in the greater or lesser saphenous veins, both of which lie superficially. The greater saphenous vein extends from the dorsum of the foot along the medial aspect of the calf and thigh, where it empties into the femoral vein in the groin. The lesser saphenous vein extends from the lateral malleolus along the posterior calf and empties into the deep popliteal vein at the popliteal space. Both veins also connect with the deep system by means of communicating, or perforating, veins. When the valves of these perforating veins are compromised, the saphenous varicosities may fill from the deep veins. Once superficial varicosities are identified, determination is made of the competency of the valves of the perforating veins and involvement of the deep veins.

The *Brodie-Trendelenburg test* [2, 3] is used to evaluate valve competency. With the patient in a supine position, elevate the extremity and drain the venous blood. Stroking the vessels toward the heart will facilitate drainage. Once the vessels are empty, apply a tourniquet to the thigh to occlude the superficial veins. With the patient in the standing position, note the direction and time for venous filling, and then release the tourniquet. The tourniquet should not be left in place for more than 60 seconds. Normally, the veins fill from below in about 35 seconds, and once the tourniquet is released, there is no further vein distention. Valve incompetency is demonstrated by rapid filling of the superficial varicosities from above. Further distention of the veins after the tourniquet is released may also occur.

Deep vein involvement is evaluated by *Perthe's test* [2]. With the patient standing and the superficial veins distended, apply a tourniquet to the midthigh and have him walk for 5 minutes. As the patient walks, the superficial veins will drain if the deep veins are patent. This is due to the pumping effect of the muscles on the deep veins. If the superficial varicosities do not drain, incompetence of the saphenous and perforating veins is present. If the veins increase in prominence and the patient complains of pain, deep vein damage is indicated. The exact level of deep vein incompetence may be determined by the *Ochsner-Mahorner modification* [2] of Perthe's test. After demonstrating deep vein involvement, move the tourniquet distally along the extremity, each time repeating the walking after application until the veins collapse with activity. The level at which the vessels collapse is the point above which deep-vein incompetence begins.

<u>Venous Thrombosis.</u>   Venous thrombosis, an obstructive alteration of the veins, is usually the secondary result of some mechanical, thermal, or chemical injury. Inflammatory venous thrombosis, or thrombophlebitis, may be superficial or deep in nature. Superficial thrombophlebitis produces localized pain, tenderness, redness, induration, and swelling of the affected vein segment. The involved vein is usually thickened and cordlike when palpated. With deep thrombophlebitis there is warmth, tenderness, swelling of the involved extremity (rather than just of the vein segment), and the pain is frequently described as excruciating, piercing, or sharp. In the dependent position, there may be superficial vein distention in the extremity. Arteriospasm with resulting pallor and diminished or absent peripheral pulses may occur. A low-grade fever also may be present.

Asymptomatic venous thrombosis, or phlebothrombosis, frequently involves the deep femoral or pelvic veins. Because of this, it is important to be alert for possible thrombosis, especially in the bed-confined or pregnant patient. Signs suggestive of phlebothrombosis are:

1. Unilateral swelling detected by comparing circumference measurements of the extremities at thigh and calf.
2. Low-grade fever and tachycardia of unknown origin.
3. Minimal ankle edema.
4. Tenderness when the gastrocnemius muscle is compressed anteriorly against the tibia but not when the muscle is pulled away from the tibia.
5. A positive Homan's sign (calf pain on sharp dorsiflexion of the foot).

A positive result on points 4 and 5 must be distinguished from muscle or tendon pain. As you evaluate the venous circulation, it is essential to remember that pulmonary embolism is a major complication of thrombosis.

<u>Arterial Occlusion.</u>   As with the venous system, the arterial circulation can be directly altered either by inflammatory or by degenerative processes in the vessel wall. Whatever the cause, arterial compromise (occlusion) presents signs that involve not only the vessels themselves, such as hardened tortuosity of the vessel in arteriosclerosis, but also of the surrounding tissue. As pointed out in Judge and Zuidema [3], in the investigation of the extremity with possible arterial compromise, the following may be noted:

1. Diminished or absent pulses. Audible systolic bruits extending into early diastole heard over major arteries — femoral or subclavian.
2. Reduced or absent hair peripherally — over the digits and dorsum of the hands or feet.
3. Atrophy of muscles and soft tissue.
4. Thin, shiny, taut skin.
5. Thickened nails with roughened transverse ridges and longitudinal curving.
6. Mild brawny edema.
7. Coolness on palpation.
8. Intense grayish pallor on elevation of the extremity. Dependency after a minute or two of elevation produces a dusky, plum-colored rubor which develops very gradually (in 30 seconds to 1 minute).
9. Flat, collapsed superficial veins.
10. Delayed venous filling time. Empty the superficial veins by elevating the extremity. Prompt filling (less than 10 seconds) occurs normally with dependent lowering.

With prolonged arterial insufficiency, four additional signs indicative of imminent gangrene may be apparent [3] :

1. Bluish-gray mottling of the skin unchanged by position.
2. Early ulceration between or on the tips of the digits.
3. Tenderness to touch.
4. Stocking anesthesia [3] .

In the early stages of insufficiency no apparent signs may be noted, and exercise testing may be valuable in promoting the manifestation of signs of alteration. The changes demonstrated are usually diminished or absent arterial pulses, skin pallor of the distal portion of the extremity, and possible systolic bruits on auscultation over major arteries.

With chronic insufficiency at the bifurcation of the abdominal aorta, sexual impotence and intermittent claudication extending into the buttocks also can occur. Finally, in acute arterial occlusion the onset is usually noted by complaints of intense pain, pallor, cyanosis, absent pulses, and perhaps tenderness and stocking anesthesia are present distal to the occlusion.

Raynaud's disease is a vasoconstrictive alteration of the arteries and arterioles in the hands and feet, usually precipitated by exposure to cold or anxiety. In describing an episode, the patient will usually comment on pain, paresthesia, and color changes that occur. At onset the affected area becomes blue, due to partial occlusion, and progressively becomes white and then red as vasodilatation occurs. Skin ulceration and edema are not common. Because this disease is episodic in nature, it is important to be alert for cues when taking the history and avoid discounting the patient's complaints because they are not readily apparent at the time of examination.

Buerger's disease (thromboangiitis obliterans) combines arterial with venous compromise in addition to nerve involvement. The disease starts with an inflammatory process and develops into arterial occlusion with resultant pain, ulceration, and gangrene. It is more frequently seen in men than women, in smokers than nonsmokers, and most often in persons from 20 to 40 years of age.

Aneurysm.   Aneurysm most often involves the aorta and the popliteal artery. It is usually palpable as a pulsatile swelling along the involved arterial segment, and a systolic thrill may be felt over the area. If the thrill is continuous, an arteriovenous fistula may be present. Rupture of an abdominal aneurysm is commonly accompanied by complaints of persistent and intense back pain. Groin pain, either unilateral or bilateral, may also be present.

Auscultation: Normal Findings.   Like height, weight, or eye color, arterial blood pressure varies greatly among individuals. Two constant influencing factors to be considered are age and sex. Part of the process of aging is progressive arteriosclerotic change. While this process is slower in women than men, the results are the same, namely, increased systolic pressure. While sources differ as to acceptable ranges of values for adults, systolic pressures of 95 to 140 mm Hg and diastolic pressures of 60 to 90 mm Hg are usually considered normal. It is possible to find systolic pressures in excess of 140 mm Hg without associated pathology in the older person. The pulse pressure (difference between systolic and diastolic pressure) should be between 40 and 50 mm Hg.

A difference of from 5 to 15 mm Hg in pressures in the left and the right arm is not uncommon. Comparisons made between pressures in the upper and lower extremities often show a 10 mm Hg difference in the systolic pressure, the higher pressure being found in the lower extremity. Relationships between lying and standing pressures should demonstrate a systolic drop of less than 15 mm Hg on standing, with a corresponding rise of less than 5 mm Hg diastolic pressure.

Bruits, the extracardiac blowing sounds auscultated over vessels, are normal in young adults. They may be heard over the abdominal aorta between the xyphoid process and the umbilicus, in the midline. However, they may indicate vascular disease.

Auscultation: Abnormal Findings.   Abnormalities in arterial blood pressure fall into two general categories: hypertension and hypotension.

Hypertension.   Hypertension is a persistent elevation of arterial blood pressure. Persistence is the key and in many cases is more helpful in making a determination of hypertension than the pressure itself. When the pressure is consistently above 140/90 mm Hg, it is usually considered significant. Episodes of epistaxis, severe headache, and irritability may accompany the elevated pressure. In the presence of an elevated pressure, especially when no other alteration is noted, close questioning of the patient as to family history is important, for essential hypertension has a strong familial tendency. Keep in mind that it is the elevated diastolic pressure more than the systolic pressure that causes increased stress on the cardiovascular and renal systems.

Hypotension. · Hypotension occurs as a result of a decrease in cardiac output, peripheral resistance, or total blood volume. It is often associated with dizziness, blurring of vision, sweating, and occasional syncope. Pressures below 95/60 mm Hg are generally considered significant if the patient's baseline "healthy" pressure was within "normal" limits. For those persons who are hypertensive normally, hypotension may occur with much higher pressures. This example should serve to point out the need to establish norms for patients whenever possible before making decisions as to the significance of data.

Neck

Inspection and Palpation: Normal Findings. On examination, the carotid pulse will present the same information as the other arterial pulses. The additional information the carotid pulse offers is the basic quality of the pulse itself. The character of the pulse wave, or quality, is best evaluated in the carotid, as it is a function of the rate of change and magnitude of the pulse pressure, and these factors can be distorted as one moves to more peripheral pulses. Figure 10-11 shows a sphygmogram of a normal carotid artery in conjunction with a phonocardiogram of normal heart sounds and an electrocardiogram (ECG) of a normal cardiac cycle. Notice that the percussion wave is initiated after the mitral valve (S_1) has closed and systole has begun. This split-second delay represents the time needed to move the pulse wave to the neck. The percussion wave is separated from the dicrotic wave by the dicrotic notch, which is caused by the closing of the aortic valve. The upstroke of the percussion wave normally takes 0.10 second and the rounding of the crest, 0.08 to 0.12 second. While the actual

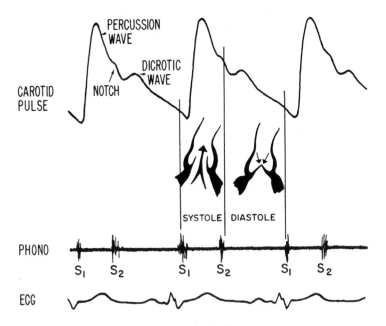

FIGURE 10-11. Characteristic normal arterial pulse wave with simultaneous recordings of a phonocardiogram and electrocardiogram. (Adapted from Judge and Zuidema [3].)

timing of each segment of the wave is important, it is the force (amplitude) of the wave and the relationship of the segments in respect to systole and diastole that is most significant. On examination, then, the pulse wave demonstrated by inspection and palpation should manifest as the relationship of the timing and force of the percussion wave to the dicrotic wave as seen in Figure 10-11. Distinctions between the waves will be hard to make, as differences in the timing and force are small.

The jugular veins of the normal person in the recumbent position are usually obviously distended, and pulsation is easily observed at the base of the neck. In the obese or "bull-necked" person this determination may be difficult to make.

The normal venous pulse is (1) diffuse and undulant in character; (2) decreases in rate with inspiration; (3) is obliterated by light pressure on the root of the neck; and (4) disappears when the patient is elevated to a sitting position, usually by $45°$.

Inspection and Palpation: Abnormal Findings.   Changes in quality of the arterial pulse when determined at the carotid artery provide information about various circulatory abnormalities:

1. *Anacrotic pulse* (see Fig. 10-12) is characterized by a delayed ascending limb of the wave (anacrotic notch) and a broadened summit. While difficult to demonstrate, it can be appreciated on palpation as two beats during each systole, the ascending limb on the wave. This alteration is specific to aortic stenosis.

2. *Bounding pulse* is characterized by a widened pulse pressure in the presence of a normal or slightly lowered diastolic pressure. An increased stroke volume with a diminished peripheral resistence is present also. Common causes of this change in quality are complete heart block, anemia, hepatic failure, and fever.

3. *Water-hammer pulse* (see Fig. 10-12) is an extremly bounding pulse with a low diastolic pressure. It is characterized by a steep ascending and descending limb and a dicrotic notch which is absent or delayed downward. The pulse seems to tap or slap against the palpating hand. This collapsing, shock-like character is reinforced in the radial artery when it is palpated in the elevated extremity. This pulse is a classic sign of aortic insufficiency.

4. *Pulsus alternans* (see Fig. 10-12) is characterized by alternating large and small pulse wave amplitudes in regular rhythm. On palpation it is demonstrated as strong (high amplitude) and weak (small amplitude) pulsation. With a blood pressure cuff, the alternate systolic pressures may fluctuate as much as 25 mm Hg. This phenomenon is common in the presence of left ventricular failure.

5. *Pulsus bigeminus* (see Fig. 10-12) is characterized by two beats coupled, followed by a pause (compensatory pause). The coupling usually is the result of alteration between a normal and premature beat. In addition, the second beat is weak, as the diastolic filling time is reduced. This can be seen with drug overdose (digitalis) or electrolyte imbalance.

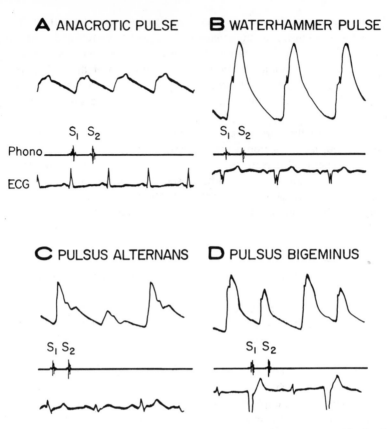

A ANACROTIC PULSE   **B** WATERHAMMER PULSE

S_1 S_2

Phono

ECG

S_1 S_2

C PULSUS ALTERNANS   **D** PULSUS BIGEMINUS

S_1 S_2

S_1 S_2

FIGURE 10-12.   Characteristic arterial pulse wave sphygmograms with simultaneously recorded phonocardiogram and electrocardiogram. A. Anacrotic pulse. B. Water-hammer pulse. C. Pulsus alternans. D. Pulsus bigeminus. (Adapted from Judge and Zuidema [3].)

6. *Pulsus paradoxus* is an exaggeration of the normal pulsation; that is, the pulse is perceptibly weaker on inspiration than expiration, and vice versa. In normal persons, with inspiration there is an increase of the blood volume in the pulmonary system, which results in diminution of stroke volume and therefore of the volume in the peripheral system. With exhalation, the opposite occurs. These differences are slight and not usually demonstrated. Accentuation of the differences occurs when there is an interference in the diastolic filling of the ventricle. This is an important sign of possible cardiac tamponade, constrictive pericarditis, and sometimes of severe pulmonary emphysema.

Auscultation of the arterial blood pressure provides more objective data on pulsus paradoxus. As pressure in the cuff is lowered, the first sounds are heard only during expiration. With further reduction, the sounds are heard on both expiration and inspiration. Differences of more than 10 mm Hg are usually considered significant.

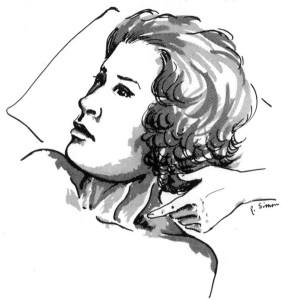

FIGURE 10-13. Demonstration of jugular vein distention in the patient with severe right-sided failure. Note that the patient's head and shoulders are elevated more than 45° from the supine position.

As indications of *localized alteration,* thrills and weakened or absent pulsation are the common carotid findings. Carotid thrill, while common in aortic stenosis, is also an indication of partial carotid occlusion. In the latter, a bruit may be auscultated over the artery. Weakened or absent carotid pulses may be the result of the aortic arch syndrome, a diffuse process involving the aortic arch and its major branches. The syndrome can be caused by aortic aneurysm, aortitis, or congenital anomalies.

Alterations that affect the jugular venous system are demonstrated by venous distention or changes in the venous pulsation. *Jugular venous distention* (see Fig. 10-13) is usually classified as mild, moderate, or severe. Venous engorgement (hypertension) is observed in right-sided congestive heart failure. However, any obstruction of blood flow to the heart can lead to venous hypertension. In long-standing jugular venous hypertension, the veins are not only distended but tortuous in appearance. It is important to remember that distention must be present when the patient is above a 45° angle from a supine position to be considered abnormal.

Precordium

Inspection and Palpation: Normal Findings. What is seen and palpated over the anterior chest varies not only with the size and shape of the chest and amount of subcutaneous tissue but also with position and phase of respiration. Normally, the chest is symmetrical and without bulges or depressions. In the young asthenic (thin) person the apex impulse is usually sharp, localized, and quick or prominent in nature. In the older person it can be less prominent and quick because of decreased elasticity of the chest wall. The apex impulse generally is visible and palpable at the fifth or sixth intercostal space medial to the midclavicular line in the recumbent or sitting position. It may be found at the fourth intercostal space and somewhat more laterally in the short, deep-chested (hyperasthenic) or pregnant individual. The apex impulse may not be demonstrated either by inspection or palpation in the obese person.

Inspection and Palpation: Abnormal Findings. Abnormalities in precordial movement often represent hypertrophy of one of the ventricles. *Left ventricular hypertrophy,* commonly caused by aortic stenosis and hypertension, is demonstrated by an apex impulse that is displaced downward and laterally (see Fig. 10-14A). The impulse is systolic and has a sustained, forceful and thrusting nature described as a *heave* or *lift.* A palpable presystolic component or sound may occur, resulting in a double impulse (see Fig. 10-14A). Use of the tongue blade technique shown in Figure 10-14B can facilitate its demonstration. With *left ventricular dilatation* a second impulse may occur, but it is protodiastolic. (see Fig. 10-15). *Right ventricular hypertrophy* presents a similar heaving impulse located over the precordium, just left of the sternum at the fourth or fifth intercostal space.

Impulses other than the apex or PMI can be identified. Pulsations can be demonstrated in the second or third intercostal space in pulmonary artery dilatation. Shock, palpable heart sounds (resulting from increased aortic or pulmonary pressure), and thrills (palpable murmurs produced by turbulence within the circulatory system) may be encountered. The presence of a thrill indicates a murmur, but absence of a thrill does not preclude the existence of a murmur.

Percussion: Normal Findings. Because of differences in body build and cardiac movement with respiration, specific measurements relating the normal left border of cardiac dullness can be misleading. Any individual characteristic or event, (e.g., respiration) that causes elevation of the diaphragm will move the heart to a more horizontal position without necessarily indicating an alteration. In the asthenic patient the left border of cardiac dullness (LBCD) in the fifth, fourth, and third intercostal spaces is usually found to be 7 to 10 cm, 5 to 7 cm, and 2 to 4 cm from the midsternal line respectively (see Fig. 10-16). The right border of cardiac dullness (RBCD) is usually not percussible, as it lies beneath the sternum in the normal person.

Percussion: Abnormal Findings. The most frequent abnormalities in the precordium are related to cardiac enlargement. As Figure 10-17 illustrates,

A   LEFT VENTRICULAR HYPERTROPHY

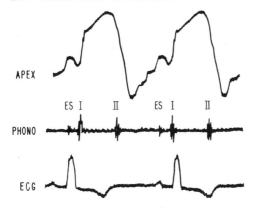

APEX

PHONO

ECG

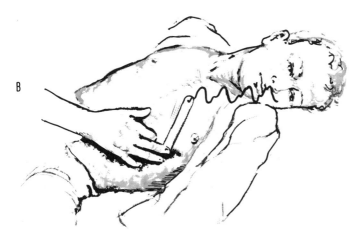

B

FIGURE 10-14.   A. Kinetocardiogram from patient with left ventricular hypertrophy. Note the presystolic extra sound, which correlates with presystolic component (a wave). B. Double apex impulse amplified by tongue-blade method. (From Judge and Zuidema [3].)

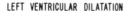

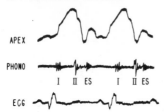

LEFT VENTRICULAR DILATATION

APEX

PHONO

       I   II ES   I   II ES

ECG

FIGURE 10-15. Double apex impulse with left ventricular dilatation. Sustained systolic component is followed by a smaller movement in early diastole. Notice the presence of a protodiastolic extra sound in this case. (From Judge and Zuidema [3].)

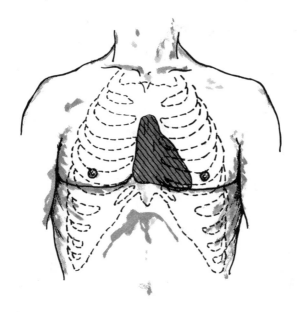

FIGURE 10-16. Characteristic configuration of the areas of cardiac dullness in the normal heart. Notice the relation of the cardiac borders to the intercostal spaces.

enlargement can be distinguished as to left or right ventricle by shape. In left ventricular enlargement, the displacement is downward and lateral, usually about the fourth, fifth and sixth intercostal spaces, creating a boot-shaped heart. With right ventricular enlargement the displacement is more lateral, showing changes in the third and fourth intercostal spaces. Pleural effusion, when considerable, is demonstrable and tends to create a triangle effect, with dullness to the left and the right of the sternum.

Auscultation: Normal Findings. The intensity (loudness), frequency (pitch), duration, and quality of the sounds heard are affected by such factors as

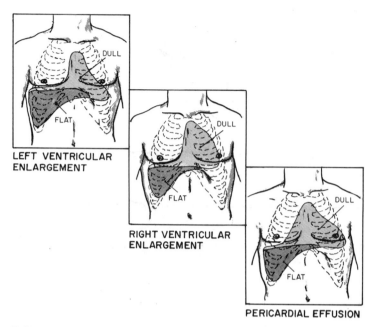

LEFT VENTRICULAR
ENLARGEMENT

RIGHT VENTRICULAR
ENLARGEMENT

PERICARDIAL EFFUSION

FIGURE 10-17. Characteristic configuration of the areas of cardiac dullness in left ventricular enlargement, right ventricular enlargement, and pericardial effusion. (Adapted from Judge and Zuidema [3].)

location of the stethoscope in relation to the valves, patient position, respiration, age, and body build. Sounds which are loud and clear in the young athlete may be almost inaudible or muffled in the older or obese person. Furthermore, listening at different locations on the same person will demonstrate differences in sound. While individual characteristics form the basis for differences in the former situation, relative proximity of the valves to the anterior chest wall and the stethoscope in part determine the explanation in the latter.

Figure 10-18 illustrates the relationship between the cardiac cycle and the normal heart sounds in respect to their origin. The sounds of greatest importance are the first (S_1) and the second (S_2) sounds, since they divide the cardiac cycle into systole and diastole.

The physiologic third sound is a ventricular filling sound occurring in early diastole and is occasionally audible during periods of rapid filling. The physiologic fourth sound occurs late in diastole, just prior to the first sound. It is related to atrial contraction and is normally inaudible.

The illustrations in Figure 10-19 diagram the normal heart sounds at the valve areas, showing intensity (loudness) by height and the duration by width. The terms at the right of the diagrams are phonetic representations describing cadence.

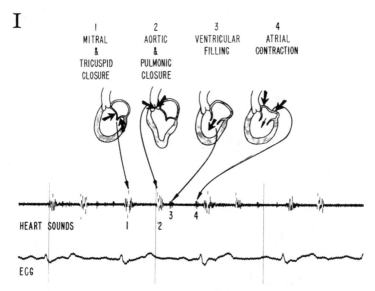

FIGURE 10-18. Origin of heart sounds with correlation to the phonocardiogram and electrocardiogram. (From Judge and Zuidema [3].)

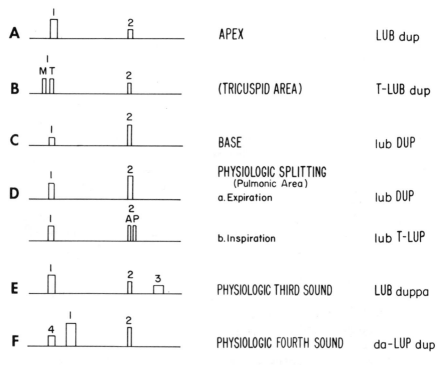

FIGURE 10-19. Normal heart sounds in respect to valve area with phonetic representation included. (Adapted from Judge and Zuidema [3].)

The *first sound* (S_1) is louder, longer in duration, and lower in pitch than the second sound at the apex (see Fig. 10-19A). The mitral valve closes from 0.02 to 0.03 seconds before the tricuspid valve. Splitting of the first sound is therefore normally common, particularly in the tricuspid area (see Fig. 10-19B). Because the closing of the tricuspid valve usually is not heard well at the apex, a single-component first sound due entirely to the mitral valve is generally heard there.

The *second sound* (S_2) results from the combined closure of the aortic and pulmonic valves. This sound is almost always louder than the first sound at the base (see Fig. 10-19C). The aortic component is widely transmitted to the neck and over the precordium. As a rule, it is entirely responsible for S_2 at the apex. The pulmonary component is softer and is heard normally only at and near the second left intercostal space (pulmonic area). Splitting of the second sound is therefore best detected in this region.

Transient splitting of the second sound may be demonstrated in most normal persons at the end of inspiration (see Fig. 10-19D). Closure of the aortic and pulmonic valves during expiration is synchronous, or nearly so, because right and left ventricular systole are approximately equal in duration. With inspiration, venous blood moves into the thoracic cavity from the large systemic venous reservoirs. This increases venous return and prolongs right ventricular systole by temporarily increasing right ventricular stroke volume, thereby delaying closure of the pulmonic valve. At the same time, venous return to the left side of the heart diminishes, due to the increased pulmonary capacity during inspiration. This in turn shortens left ventricular systole and permits earlier closure of the aortic valve. These two factors combine to produce transient "physiologic splitting" of the second sound.

The *physiologic third sound* is a faint, inconstant, low-pitched sound audible at or near the apex (see Fig. 10-19E). It is heard best when the patient is lying on his left side and frequently disappears when he sits up. It varies in intensity with respiration, usually becoming louder with expiration. It is common in children and young adults but is rarely heard in older individuals.

The *physiologic fourth sound* is a low-pitched, short sound heard best at the apex with the patient lying on his left side (see Fig. 10-19F). This sound is rarely heard in the normal person.

Murmurs are gentle blowing sounds produced by turbulent blood flow within or near the heart. The *functional, or innocent, murmur* is commonly heard in children and young adults. This murmur is systolic in timing and is characteristically soft, short in duration, and variable. It is usually heard best at the pulmonic area or at the left sternal border. These murmurs vary with position and respiration and are not associated with any demonstrable heart disease (see Fig. 10-20).

Auscultation: Abnormal Findings. Abnormal findings on auscultation consist of abnormal heart sounds, murmurs, and friction rub.

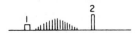

FIGURE 10-20.   Representation of a functional systolic murmur. (From Judge and Zuidema [3].)

Abnormal Heart Sounds.   Abnormal *first heart sounds* are either accentuated in nature, as in hyperkinetic disorders (e.g., fever or mitral stenosis), or they are diminished (e.g., low output failure or heart block). In either case, an irregular rhythm usually is present.

Changes in the *second sound* also involve accentuation or diminution. With accentuation, pulmonary or systemic hypertension may be present. A diminished or inaudible second sound is associated with aortic or pulmonary stenosis.

Delayed closure of the pulmonic valve, usually due to overfilling of the right ventricle causing prolongation of systolic ejection time, results in a persistent splitting of the second sound. This is commonly associated with pulmonic valve stenosis and atrial ventricular septal defects. Right bundle branch block also may cause a persistent splitting.

Reversed or paradoxical splitting of the second sound results from delayed ventricular stimulation, as in left bundle branch block or prolonged left ventricular ejection time. In this situation the splitting occurs with *expiration* and disappears with inspiration as the normal mechanism of delayed pulmonic valve closure on inspiration compensates for the altered left ventricular activity (see Fig. 10-21).

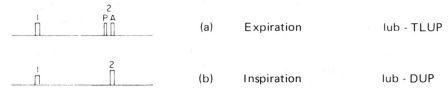

(a)   Expiration   lub - TLUP

(b)   Inspiration   lub - DUP

FIGURE 10-21.   Abnormal heart sound. Representation of revised splitting of S_2. (From Judge and Zuidema [3].)

Ventricular gallop is a pathological appearance of the third heart sound, usually in the presence of an increased heart rate. Because it occurs early in diastole, it is also called a *protodiastolic sound*. It is heard best at the apex with the patient in the left lateral position. The sound occurs as a result of an overdistention of the ventricle in the rapid filling segment of diastole. Consequently, it is usually found in the presence of mitral insufficiency or ventricular failure. To facilitate distinction between normal and abnormal third sounds, remember that the normal third sound disappears when the patient is in the sitting position. With disease, the third sound persists (see Fig. 10-22).

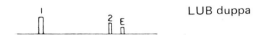

LUB duppa

FIGURE 10-22.   Abnormal heart sound representation of a protodiastolic extra sound. (From Judge and Zuidema [3] .)

Atrial gallop is the pathological manifestation of the fourth sound. This sound, also called a *presystolic extra sound,* is dull and low-pitched and is heard best at the apex with the patient in the left lateral position. The sound occurs in the presence of forceful atrial contraction where there is resistance to ventricular filling late in diastole, such as in left ventricular hypertrophy. It is also seen with pulmonary stenosis (see Fig. 10-23).

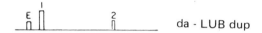

da - LUB dup

FIGURE 10-23.   Abnormal heart sound representation of a presystolic extra sound. (From Judge and Zuidema [3] .)

Murmurs.   Except for the functional or innocent murmur previously mentioned, all murmurs should be considered abnormal. To make proper interpretations of information collected in respect to murmurs, the nurse examiner must understand the (1) production, (2) transmission, and (3) character of the murmur.

1. *Production.*   Turbulence in blood flow can be produced by: (a) increasing the rate or velocity of the blood flow; (b) increasing or decreasing the diameter of a vessel or area through which the blood flows; (c) decreasing the viscosity of the blood; or (d) altering the normally smooth inner surface of the vessel wall. Blood flow velocity is a key determinant of intensity (loudness) and frequency (pitch) of the murmur. Increase the velocity of the flow (e.g., as in exercise), and the murmur becomes louder and higher in pitch.

2. *Transmission.*   Murmurs, like all sounds, are loudest at their point of origin, and the closer the site of origin to the anterior chest wall, the louder the sound on auscultation. Frequency (pitch) is also affected by the amount of interposed tissue the sound must pass through before reaching the chest wall. Another factor affecting the frequency of a murmur is related to the transmission of the sound within the cardiovascular system itself. As a sound moves against the stream, as in regurgitation, high frequencies tend to be preserved while low frequencies are damped out. When moving downstream with the flow, the opposite is true. Consequently, many murmurs sound very different when auscultated from different locations on the chest.

3. *Character.*   Description of a murmur should take into account and include in the record the following six categories: timing, location, intensity, frequency, duration, and quality.

- **Short Duration**

  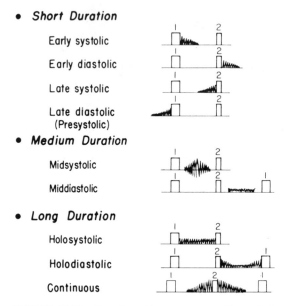

  Early systolic

  Early diastolic

  Late systolic

  Late diastolic
  (Presystolic)

- **Medium Duration**

  Midsystolic

  Middiastolic

- **Long Duration**

  Holosystolic

  Holodiastolic

  Continuous

FIGURE 10-24.   Duration of heart murmurs. (From Judge and Zuidema [3].)

a. *Timing* refers to the placement of the sound in relationship to the cardiac cycle — systolic, diastolic, continuous.
b. *Location* is the point of maximal intensity of the murmur, using the valve areas and the intercostal spaces for accuracy of reference points.
c. *Loudness* is graded on a six-point scale, with grade I/VI being barely audible and increasing in loudness to VI/VI, which is audible without a stethoscope.
d. *Pitch* is noted as low, medium, or high.
e. *Duration* is noted as short, medium, or long in timing (see Fig. 10-24).
f. *Quality* refers to crescendo (increasing in intensity) or decrescendo (decreasing in intensity) and overall presentation, namely, blowing, harsh, rumbling, rasping, musical, ejection, regurgitant.

Murmurs are classified as systolic or diastolic and within these two groups are described as to quality.

1. *Systolic ejection murmurs* are produced by the forward movement of blood through the pulmonic and aortic valves. They begin after the first sound, swell and fade in a crescendo-decrescendo fashion peaking in early or middle systole and terminating before the second heart sound. They tend to be of medium pitch, short in duration and do not override either the first or second sound. Examples of this type of murmur are the murmur of aortic and pulmonic stenosis and the functional or innocent murmur.

2. *Systolic regurgitant murmurs* are produced by the backflow of blood from the ventricles into the atria or through a septal defect. Because the blood moves from an area of high to low pressure, these murmurs tend to be high-pitched and

longer in duration, usually holosystolic (pansystolic), that is, they extend through the entire systolic period. They tend to override the second and the first sounds. Their intensity tends to remain constant, occasionally increasing late in systole. In mitral regurgitation, the murmur is usually blowing in quality and loudest at the apex. With tricuspid regurgitation, the murmur tends to increase in intensity on inspiration. Septal defect murmurs are usually coarse in quality.

3. *Diastolic regurgitant murmurs*, as in systole, are high-pitched, long, usually holodiastolic (pandiastolic), and transmitted in the direction of regurgitant blood flow. Examples are the murmurs of aortic and pulmonic regurgitation.

4. *Diastolic filling murmurs* are low-pitched, localized, and rumbling. They tend to be middiastolic. In mitral stenosis, an opening snap of the mitral valve is often heard, and the murmur has a decrescendo quality. With tricuspid stenosis, the timing and quality are similar; however, the murmur tends to be high in pitch.

<u>Pericardial Friction Rub.</u>   Pericardial friction rub is a grating-like sound resembling the rubbing together of two pieces of sandpaper. It has also been described as a "leathery" sound, suggestive of the squeaking of a shoe. Its appearance is a sign of pericardial inflammation. Friction rub may be heard over any part of the precordium but is usually demonstrated at the left sternal border. Occasionally it is loud and continuous throughout systole and diastole; however, it is more commonly muffled, high-pitched, and transient in nature. The quality of the sound can be created by moving the stethoscope endpiece lightly over a "hairy" skin surface while auscultating.

REFERENCES

1. Burch, G. E., and DePasquale, N. P. *Primer of Clinical Measurement of Blood Pressure.* St. Louis: Mosby, 1962.
2. DeGowin, E. L., and DeGowin, R. L. *Bedside Diagnostic Examination* (2nd ed.). New York: Macmillan, 1969.
3. Judge, R. D., and Zuidema, G. D. (Eds.). *Methods of Clinical Examination: A Physiologic Approach* (3rd ed.). Boston: Little, Brown, 1974.
4. Kampmeier, R. *Physical Examination in Health and Disease* (3rd ed.). Philadelphia: Davis, 1964.

SUGGESTED READINGS

Ask-Upmark, E. *Bedside Medicine Selected Topics* (2nd ed.). Stockholm: Almquist & Wesell, 1969.
Hopkins, H. *Leopold's Principles and Methods of Physical Diagnosis* (3rd ed.). Philadelphia: Saunders, 1965.
Feinstein, A. R. *Clinical Judgement.* Baltimore: Williams & Wilkins, 1967.
Hochstein, E., and Rubin, A. *Physical Diagnosis: A Textbook and Workbook in Methods of Clinical Examination.* New York: McGraw-Hill, 1964.

206 Physical Appraisal of Adults

Kampmeier, R., and Blake, T. M. *Physical Examination in Health and Disease* (4th ed.). Philadelphia: Davis, 1970.

Major, R. H., and Delp, M. H. *Physical Diagnosis* (6th ed.). Philadelphia: Saunders, 1962.

Prior, J. A., and Silberstein, J. S. *Physical Diagnosis: The History and Examination of the Patient* (3rd ed.). St. Louis: Mosby, 1969.

PHYSICAL APPRAISAL OF THE ABDOMEN AND THE MALE GENITOURINARY SYSTEM

11

Candace M. Burns

GLOSSARY

anuria Total suppression of urinary secretion.

ascites Free fluid in the abdominal cavity.

ballottement Palpation technique to detect a floating enlarged organ when accompanied by ascites.

borborygmus Sounds produced during hyperperistalsis.

burning Urethral irritation with sensation similar to voiding hot water.

dyschezia Difficult or painful defecation.

dysphagia Difficulty in swallowing.

enuresis Voiding involuntarily or during sleep.

fluid wave Transmission of an impulse through fluid in the abdomen.

frequency Felt need to void often.

guarding Tension of the abdominal musculature over an area of tenderness.

hematuria Blood in the urine.

linea alba A vertical, tendinous line between the rectus muscles, extends from the zyphoid to the symphysis pubis.

megacolon enlarged or dilated colon.

nocturia Excessive urination during the night.

oliguria Deficient secretion of urine.

paradoxical (overflow) incontinence Loss of urine due to chronic urinary retention or secondary to a flaccid bladder causing constant dribbling.

pneumaturia Gas or air in urine.

polyuria Excess in amount of urine voided.

pyuria Pus in the urine.

rushes Accentuation of normal bowel sounds but longer and higher-pitched.

strangury Difficult, painful passage of urine accompanied by spasm.

stress incontinence Involuntary urinary discharge resulting from an intravesicular pressure increase as in sneezing, coughing, or straining.

succussion splash Sound created by moving air and fluid in a hollow organ.

tinkles Very high-pitched bowel sounds, musical in quality.

urgency Sudden strong desire to urinate.

This chapter presents various aspects of the physical examination currently not generally performed by most nurses. At present only a few female nurses are carrying out complete genitourinary examination of male patients, and these nurses usually are functioning in some specialized clinician role. However, with little controversy male nurses in a wide variety of clinical settings have employed and continue to employ successfully the various techniques of physical examination. As these techniques are learned and utilized by more nurses and as more liberalized views and expectations as to the role of the female nurse emerge, this situation will change rapidly.

EXAMINATION OF THE ABDOMEN

Physical examination of the abdomen differs from examination of other body areas in several features. Auscultation is generally less important in examination of the abdomen than in the thorax. Palpation of the abdomen provides less exact and useful information because the abdominal contents are separated from the examiner's hands by a thick muscular wall.

Order of the Examination

Although the same four basic techniques (i.e., inspection, palpation, percussion, and auscultation) of examination are employed by the nurse examining the abdomen, auscultation should in this instance be performed before palpation and percussion, since the latter two may alter bowel sounds that might normally be heard, creating a false impression. For example, a "normal" abdomen may suddenly present hyperactive bowel sounds after stimuli from palpation, or percussion, or both.

Positioning and Draping the Patient. Correct positioning of the patient is important for proper examination. The optimal position is to have the patient supine, with his hands at his sides. Do not allow the patient to put his hands behind his head; this causes contraction of the abdominal musculature, making it difficult to palpate the abdomen. Relaxation of the abdominal musculature is essential for successful palpation. The following techniques may be employed to assist the patient to relax.

The head should lie flat, preferably on a small pillow, and the knees kept slightly flexed to help prevent tensing of the abdominal musculature. The nurse examiner should stand at the right side of the patient, regardless of whether she is right-or left-handed. When examining for the presence of a hernia, bulges of the abdominal wall or psoas sign, it is most desirable to have the patient standing. Abdominal organs will drop in the upright person due to gravity, thus increasing pressure on the mass and causing its descent and easier detection. The patient should be draped to provide for his modesty and comfort and ease of examination.

Landmarks

Certain specific landmarks are generally used to describe findings. These landmarks are identified in Figure 11-1. The examiner should be familiar with them as they will assist her in describing findings in a clear, concise manner and will support uniform interpretation. In descriptions of physical appraisal findings, the abdomen is frequently divided into sections. Two methods are seen most often. The first method divides the abdomen into quadrants by drawing a line from the tip of the sternum to the pubic bone through the umbilicus. These

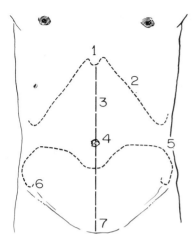

FIGURE 11-1.   Anatomical landmarks.   1.   Tip of sternum-epigastric hollow.   2.   Costal margin.   3.   Midline extending from sternum to pubic bone (os pubis).   4.   Umbilicus. 5. Anterosuperior iliac crest.   6.   Superior margin of os pubis.   7.   Symphysis.

four sections are namely; right upper quadrant, left upper quadrant, right lower quadrant, left lower quadrant. Figure 11-2 shows the quadrants and the abdominal organs usually located in each and should serve as a guide for the physical appraisal. The second method of division, used less often than the quadrant method, sections the abdomen into nine areas.

Inspection

Inspection is an important part of the physical appraisal and is too often rushed or entirely omitted. With the patient properly positioned, the nurse notes the presence or absence of distention, symmetry, and midline protuberances. These are best seen by the nurse first standing and then sitting to one side and looking across the surface of the patient's abdomen. Standing may help the nurse detect unusual abdominal shadows and movement; the sitting position provides a plane horizontal to the eye. Asking the patient to take a deep inspiration will help accentuate an enlarged liver, spleen, or distended gallbladder, making detection easier.

Inspection of the abdominal skin for scars, dehydration, malnutrition, venous patterns, and discolorations can provide an abundance of information about the patient's general state of health. Scars may yield pertinent clues about previous trauma or surgery and may signal the possibility of adhesions or bowel obstruction.

Venous Patterns.   Normally, the venous pattern is very faint with blood flow centrifugal from the umbilicus. The venous pattern becomes more prominent

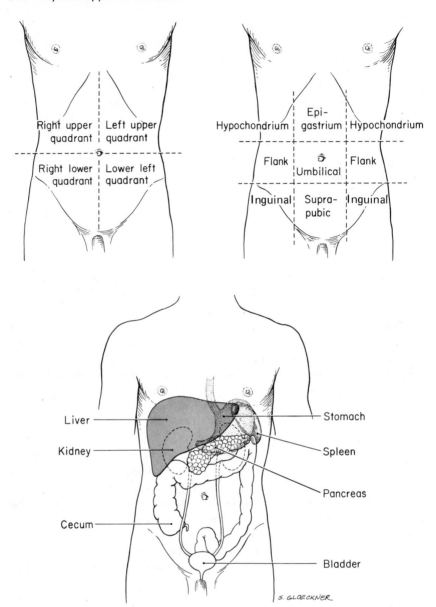

FIGURE 11-2. Topographic anatomy of the abdomen. [Figs. 11-2 to 11-5 modified from R. D. Judge and G. D. Zuidema (Eds.). *Methods of Clinical Examination: A Physiologic Approach* (3rd ed.). Boston: Little, Brown, 1974.]

with thin skin and with decreased elasticity of the skin, as in aging. Irregular patches of faint pigmentation on the abdomen, flank, and back may be indicative of von Recklinghausen's disease.

Because of obstruction in large intrabdominal or intrathoracic venous channels, a collateral circulation may develop in the veins of the abdominal wall. To determine the direction of flow, the nurse should compress and "strip" the veins and observe their refill. In obstruction of the superior vena cava, the blood from above finds its way to the heart via the inferior vena cava; thus the blood flow is downward. In portal obstruction, the flow is commonly upward to anastomose with part of the veins in the attachment of the diaphragm. When describing venous patterning, it is important to record the flow pattern in a diagram.

Umbilicus. The position and shape of the umbilicus is important to note. Normally, it is a flat sphere with a long vertical axis and is positioned midway between the xyphoid process and the pubis. Intraabdominal hemorrhage may cause discoloration of the umbilical area from the blood pigments reaching it via lymphatics in the medial umbilical ligament. This often is referred to as "Cullen's sign." Bluish, periumbilical patches frequently occur with pancreatitis. A yellow-tinged navel may be due to free bile in the peritoneal cavity. Reddish or purple mottling due to circulatory collapse also may develop. The mottling blanches with pressure, and the blanching lasts only a second or so.

Pelvic or lower abdominal masses may displace the umbilicus cephalad; masses of the upper abdomen may displace it caudally, as ascites also does. The umbilicus may protrude, due to an umbilical hernia. It may become dirty, infected, or lose mobility and become fixed as with malignancies, presenting as a hard, button-shaped mass. The umbilicus is a frequent site of fungal infection. When any abnormal findings are detected, prompt referral to a physician is indicated.

Hair Distribution. The nurse should observe and describe the distribution of the abdominal and pelvic hair. Disturbances of hormonal balance may alter the distribution of pubic hair to patterns characteristic of the opposite sex (see Chap. 6). A female-type hair distribution found in a male may be an indication of cirrhosis and failure of the diseased liver to conjugate estrogenic substances. A typically masculine hair distribution in a female may suggest an adrenocortical or genital abnormality. Sparse or absent hair associated with thin, smooth skin may be due to pituitary insufficiency. When such observations are made, the patient should be referred to a physician for follow-up.

Respiratory Movement. The abdomen and the liver, spleen and gallbladder typically follow thoracic respiratory movement due to the pull of the diaphragm. In general, females usually breathe with costal movements only, while males (breathing quietly) breathe abdominally. Decreased respiratory movement occurs with increased rigidity of the abdominal muscles or undue distention. An ulcer perforated into the peritoneal cavity will usually result in little or no respiratory movement of the abdomen. Frequently, appendicitis with local peritonitis will cause immobility of the hypogastric region.

Abdominal Contours. A flat abdominal contour is seen when the anterior wall extends in a horizontal plane from the level of the costal margins to the pubic bone. This is often seen in the young, athletic, well-nourished person or in the spare elderly person. A round abdomen is convex to the horizontal plane as the body is observed from the side. In the supine patient the height of the convexity is in the area of the umbilicus, whereas in the erect patient, gravity will cause a shifting of this point to a lower position between the umbilicus and pubis. The round abdomen, characteristic of young children (see Chap. 15), is seen more commonly in the female than in the male and is due to excess subcutaneous fat or to lack of activity, or of muscle tone, or both. The aged frequently have this abdominal contour, due to these factors mentioned, as well as to kyphosis of the dorsal segments of the spine. The scaphoid abdominal contour, when viewed laterally, presents as a concavity to the horizontal plane and may be seen in patients of all ages.

Abdominal Distention. *Abdominal distention* is an abnormal state that requires further assessment. Distention may be localized or generalized, often resulting from gas in the intestines, fluid in the abdominal cavity, or tumor. Generalized distention is abdominal protuberance. If due to gas, the flanks do not bulge, and the lateral walls slope toward the midline as toward a rigid pole. The percussion note is resonant, bowel sounds are usually increased, and the patient may be nauseated and vomit. When the distention is due to fluid, the weight of the fluid causes the flanks to bulge (unless the abdominal musculature has *excellent* tone), resulting in a more flattened anterior abdominal area than seen in the abdomen distended with gas. If the patient is relaxed, requesting him to roll from side to side will demonstrate a protuberance on the dependent side of the abdomen as the fluid shifts from side to side. There will be no change in the area of maximum distention if the abdomen contains gas. This maneuver is known as *shifting dullness.* The air-filled bowel will float on the fluid so the difference between the dullness of fluid and the tympany of air is readily detected by percussion.

To elicit a *fluid wave,* one hand is placed on the lateral aspect of the abdomen while the other hand taps the opposite side of the abdomen gently but sharply. If fluid is present, a wave will be seen as the fluid transmits the impulse through the abdomen (see Fig. 11-3).

The *puddle sign* indicates the presence of small amounts of intraabdominal fluid. To test for this sign, request the standing patient to assume a hand-knee position for several minutes. This will encourage any fluid present to "puddle" around the umbilicus. Then the examiner should percuss around the umbilicus to detect small (several hundred milliliters) amounts of fluids. Ascites occurs for

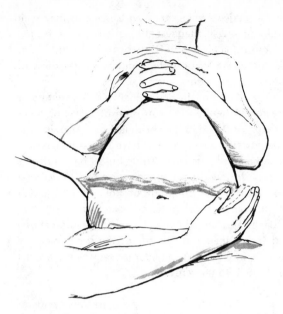

FIGURE 11-3.   Eliciting a fluid wave to demonstrate the presence of intraabdominal fluid.

a variety of reasons, and its causes will not be detailed here. Whenever fluid is detected, the patient needs referral to a physician for further evaluation.

An extremely large amount of feces in the colon may cause abdominal distention, as in megacolon.

Localized distention may be caused by an enlarged organ, a tumor, localized fluid, or distended loops of bowel. A bulging will be evident in one specific area of the abdomen and not in other areas. For example, an enlarged spleen may cause the left side of the abdomen to be distended, whereas hepatomegaly (enlarged liver) may cause right-sided distention. An ovarian cyst may cause asymmetrical fullness in one or the other lower quadrants. Large hyper-nephromas or polycystic kidney may fill one or both sides of the abdomen.

Bowel contours should also be noted. Peristaltic waves may be visible through the abdominal wall (e.g., in mechanical obstruction). The bowel is frequently distended with gas, and this distention is obvious in the peristaltic waves observable.

An enlarged abdomen due to obesity cannot truly be classified as distended. Yet it is important to note that this is a common cause of abdominal enlargement. Folds or aprons of fat are usually deposited in the suprapubic or flank areas. When obesity is caused by hypopituitarism, the body fat is centrally rather than peripherally distributed. Results elicited may be similar for abdominal fat as for fluid. Doubt as to the cause of abdominal distention may require that paracentesis be performed by a physician.

It is important to observe the patient while straining, since this may yield information concerning the abdominal wall. Request the patient to rise from a supine to a sitting position without using his hands. Diastasis recti (separation of the rectus abdominalis in the midline) may be noted, indicating weakness of supporting tissue between the longitudinal rectus muscles.

Hernias. Hernias result from weakness of the abdominal wall or structure or undue stress on the wall or region. A hernia is a protrusion of bowel or other tissue through an abdominal hiatus, enclosed in the peritoneal sac. An epigastric hernia occurs in the midline, penetrating the linea alba above the umbilicus, and frequently contains omentum rather than intestine. An umbilical hernia occurs through a weakness at the site of former (fetal) umbilical vessels. A femoral hernia occurs in the femoral canal at the midpoint of Poupart's (inguinal) ligament and is most common in women. Inguinal hernias occur more often in men. A direct inguinal hernia penetrates the abdominal wall at the internal ring and appears as a variable-sized tumor medial to the site of the deep epigastric artery. An indirect hernia enters the internal ring and later moves down the canal to protrude through the external ring into the scrotum.

Abdominal Pulsations. An abdominal pulsation may be readily evident. Pulsation of the abdominal aorta may be observed in the midline, cephalad to the umbilicus, and is systolic in timing. Pulsations from the normal aorta may be transmitted to the abdominal wall and may be difficult to separate from the expansile pulsation of an abdominal aneurysm (a local enlargement with a pulsation). One method of determining whether the pulsation is expansile or transmitted is to hold two matchsticks lightly over the pulsating mass. If their motion is in a vertical direction only, it is probably a pulsation transmitted from the aorta. Horizontal movement of the matchsticks indicates that the pulsation is possibly exspansile. Although this simple test is by no means precise, it may be informative during an initial assessment. Findings indicative of any abnormality should be immediately reported to a physician.

Pigmentation. The linea alba, usually seen as a narrow furrow above the umbilicus and invisible below it, may become notably pigmented, or hairy, or both during pregnancy. Lineal albicantes, which are striae produced by stretching of the skin and rupture of elastic fibers of skin, may be seen. They may result from any rapid increase in abdominal size such as that caused by weight gain, fluid, and pregnancy.

Pain. The patient's description of pain experienced may be helpful and should be carefully elicited. Facial expression, posture, restlessness, or immobility observed prior to and during the examination may yield useful data. The nurse must determine such facts as where the pain is, where it started, and where it radiates. Often, the manner in which the patient points to painful areas is helpful in identifying the source of the pain. For example, pain with peptic ulcer is usually localized, and the patient will use one finger to point to the specific area. Functional distress is more diffuse, and the patient moves his hand across the abdomen, unable to localize it in any one site.

Palpation

General Guides.   Palpation is used to confirm and amplify findings from inspection. The nurse should position herself at the right side of the patient and palpate with uniform pressure. Her hands should be warm, since cold hands will be uncomfortable for the patient and may cause abdominal tensing. Fingers are to be held together; nails should be trimmed and smooth. To make accurate measurements, centimeters rather than finger breadths are used, since finger size varies greatly among examiners.

Light palpation — just indenting the skin — should be used initially to detect tenderness. Soft organs may be detected in this manner, and distended hollow visceral organs may be missed if only deep palpation is used.

In moderate palpation, used to detect enlarged organs or masses, the side of the hand is used rather than the fingers to prevent digging the fingertips into the patient and producing involuntary guarding. Organs that move with respiration (e.g., liver, spleen) are first palpated with normal respiratory effort and then with deep inspiration. An organ undetected with normal respiration may be felt on deep inspiration.

Deep palpation is used to detect tenderness and organs not found with light or moderate palpation. Retroperitoneal masses such as the kidneys may be felt in this manner.

Various methods of bimanual palpation are used. Using both hands placed on separate parts of the abdomen enables the nurse to delineate the extent of an organ or mass and to measure the dimensions with the fingertips. This technique is useful in detecting a pulsatile mass. Pulsations felt in the fingertips of both hands indicates that the organ itself is pulsating rather than that the pulsation is being transmitted from the aorta. Placing one hand anterior and one posterior to the organ or mass serves to "trap" the organ and is a very useful technique to determine size, consistency, texture, etc. of the organ. For example, in palpating kidneys, the right hand presses down from the anterior and the left hand presses up from the posterior. In attempting to detect minimal descent of an organ (e.g., liver, spleen), the nurse may find it useful to place one hand next to the other for palpating.

Palpation to detect *rebound tenderness* is an important maneuver when examining the abdomen. To elicit this sign, one hand is pressed slowly into the abdomen and then quickly withdrawn. Discomfort is elicited when the hand is suddenly withdrawn rather than with the downward pressure.

General Survey.   A general survey of the entire abdomen should be done with light palpation, using the distal phalanges of the fingers of the examining hand (the right hand of a right-handed person). Systematically explore the abdomen with light pressure to detect an increase in abdominal muscle tone, enlarged solid organs (liver, spleen, kidneys, uterus), or hollow organs (bowel, stomach, bladder, aorta). Deliberate, firm, but gentle pressure is used to avoid tickling or sudden jabbing thrusts. It is best to examine areas of suspected or known discomfort last. Determine the area of greatest tenderness and location of possible resistance. In general, the degree of resistance (rigidity) is proportional to the degree of peritoneal irritation. An exception to this is the rigidity with peritonitis, which is initially very intense and then decreases or even ceases within a short period. Note the size and shape of the resistance, the character of its limits, its relation to the surrounding area, and whether it is in connection with an organ or corresponds to an enlargement of an organ. The relationship of resistance to respiratory movements should also be noted in terms of directions and limits of movement. The nature of the resistance should be described, e.g., soft, elastic, compact, cartilaginous, glandulous, tumorous, or fluctuating. Muscular resistance may also be due to increased tone of the abdominal musculature or reflex action spasm. Resistance should also be palpated from the vagina or rectum.

Guarding. Guarding may be voluntary or involuntary. Voluntary guarding is a conscious response by the patient on palpation over a painful abdomen; involuntary guarding is a reflex contraction of abdominal muscles and is not responsive to conscious effort on the part of the patient. Involuntary guarding often indicates the presence of a more serious pathological condition. Rigidity is an extreme form of guarding and may be seen in conjunction with absent bowel sounds.

Organ Survey. Deep palpation is utilized to determine abnormality of organs where tenderness indicates underlying disease (e.g., tender liver edge, spleen, gallbladder). If an abnormality is felt, note its size, movement with respiration, tenderness, position, consistency, and attachment to underlying tissue, viscera, or both. Examination should also include palpation of the left supraclavicular space since this may reveal an enlarged lymph node, an important sign of possible intraabdominal malignancy. A systematic survey of the following is made by deep palpation.

    Abdominal aorta. Deep palpation of the epigastric area may reveal the aortic pulsation. The examiner's fingers will feel the thrust of the systolic pulse against the rigid spine.

    Colon. In the older person, or one with lax abdominal muscles, the examiner may be able to outline the transverse colon across the abdomen just above the umbilicus. It is soft and movable. The sigmoid colon forms a ropelike structure in the left lower quadrant almost parallel to Poupart's ligament. Occasionally, the cecum and ascending colon can be palpated in the right lower quadrant.

    Urinary bladder. Normally, the bladder, a pelvic organ, cannot be palpated unless distended well above the symphysis pubis.

Liver.   The left hand should be placed under the patient's flank, fingers extended, palm side up, and lying parallel to the ribs. The hand is placed so the patient's eleventh and twelfth ribs lie on the nurse's hand. By creating upward pressure with this hand, the liver can be pushed toward the anterior abdominal wall. The right hand is placed flat on the abdomen, fingers in the long axis of the body and in the right upper quadrant, about midway between the costal border and the level of the umbilicus. The patient is then instructed to take a deep breath. The right hand should move with the abdominal wall as the patient inspires. With the descent of the diaphragm on deep inspiration, the liver moves downward. If it is to be palpated, one can feel it slip under the palpating fingers as they move with the abdominal wall (see Fig. 11-4).

The edge of the normal liver is usually sharp, regular, and relatively straight in contour. To determine the size of the liver, measure in centimeters the distance it reaches below the costal margin and the total span by percussion of the thoracic cage with deep inspiration. The normal liver may be felt to descend to 1 to 2 cm below the costal margin. Normal liver size is about 10 to 12 cm.

Note whether the entire border is palpable (indicating diffuse enlargement). Also note any complaints of tenderness as the edge slips under the right hand, consistency, presence of nodes, and irregular or systolic pulsations or both. Nodules may be felt when the palm of the hand is placed over the liver surface as the patient takes a deep breath. Nodules on the liver wall can be felt as they move; whereas nodules on the abdominal wall cannot.

Ballottement is performed when ascites is present. The anterior wall is depressed with the fingertips over the suspected organ enlargement. Fluid will be

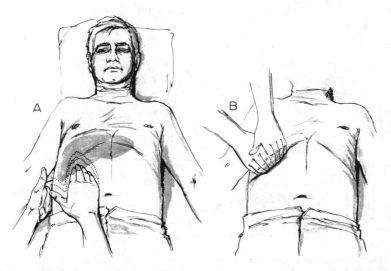

FIGURE 11-4.   Techniques of palpating the liver. A. The anterior hand should parallel the rectus muscle. B. The hooking technique is occasionally preferable.

more readily displaced than a solid organ; therefore, when the fingers strike a floating organ, a distinct solid mass will be felt.

Spleen. To palpate the spleen, the left hand reaches across the abdomen and is slipped under the flank. Fingers of the right hand are directed obliquely upward and laterally under the left costal margin. On deep inspiration, the right hand should move with the abdominal wall. The tip of the spleen may be felt as it is pushed downward by the descending diaphragm. The spleen edge will resemble a firm edge, similar to that of the liver. A normal spleen is rarely palpable, and its consistency is softer than that of the liver. Spleen size is more difficult to determine, but centimeters of descent below the costal margin should be recorded when possible.

Kidneys. Kidneys usually can be felt with bimanual palpation at the height of inspiration only in the young person, multiparous woman, or aged person with relaxed abdominal walls (see Fig. 11-5). The right kidney lies slightly lower than the left and is the most commonly palpated. The left hand should be placed under the flank, parallel to and just below the twelfth rib. The right hand is placed on the abdomen so the fingertips are in the lower quadrant below the level of the umbilicus. The fingers must press deeply and move with the abdominal wall on deep inspiration. The kidney is felt as a solid, firm, but elastic mass.

To palpate the left kidney, the left hand reaches across the abdomen to be placed under the flank and similar technique is employed.

The differences in palpation of an enlarged left kidney and the spleen are:

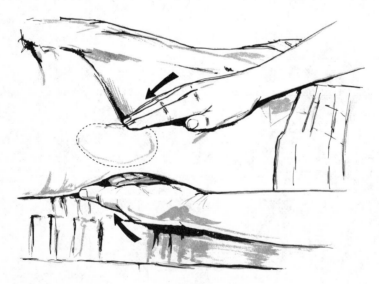

FIGURE 11-5. Palpation of the kidneys.

1. The splenic notch can be felt, whereas, no kidney notch can, since blood vessels fill this space.
2. The spleen has a sharper outline than the kidney.
3. The spleen is usually enlarged anteriorly, whereas the kidney rarely is.

Inguinal rings.   Palpation is especially important in detecting dilatations. Patient may be supine or erect; the latter is usually preferred. The index finger is pressed upward through the scrotal wall along the spermatic cord into the external inguinal ring. Normally, the nurse should feel the sharp edge of the aponeurosis of the external oblique muscle (about the size of the tip of the index finger).

Gallbladder.   Light palpation is best used in attempting to palpate this fluid-filled, hollow organ. It is difficult to palpate.

Aorta.   Normally, the aorta is palpable as a pulsatile, slightly tender epigastric structure less than 4 cm in diameter.

Stomach.   The normal stomach cannot be palpated even after meals. Gastric carcinoma may cause a left upper quadrant mass when the distal half of the stomach is involved.

Pancreas.   The pancreas cannot be detected by palpation due to its small size and retroperitoneal position. Even pancreatic masses are often undetected.

Percussion

General Guides.   The purpose of percussion is to extend information gained by inspection and palpation or to substitute for palpation in certain circumstances. Using percussion, the nurse is able to outline air-containing or solid structures by the changing sounds. The normal percussion note over the abdomen is tympanic, except for dullness over the liver. Percussion is useful to delineate borders and contours of solid organs, i.e., liver, spleen. The technique employed is identical to that used in percussing the chest (see Chap. 9). Percussion should be light, so that small differences in densities may be perceived. A change in relative versus absolute dullness may be overlooked with too vigorous percussion.

General Survey.   Just as with palpation, percussion should be systematic and orderly. First, percuss down the lower left thoracic border wall in the midaxillary line. Normally, this produces a resonant note over the lung. Below the level of the hemidiaphragm, there is normally a tympanic note, due to colon at the splenic flexure. Next, percuss down the right midaxillary line. The upper limit of liver dullness is usually detected at the seventh rib or interspace. Third, percuss to determine the lower limit of liver dullness by percussing down the right side of the chest in the midclavicular line. Normally, the lower limit of liver dullness is the costal margin. Last, percuss for the presence or absence of ascites. Percussion of a distended abdomen can assist the nurse in differentiating between fluid and gas. As described earlier, the percussion note will change to dull when percussing the dependent side or at the umbilicus (see shifting dullness and puddle sign, pp. 212 and 213). To detect distended loops of bowel filled with fluid or gas, the nurse can percuss with quick, repeated, slightly forceful taps at the left iliac fossa. Audible, one-wave "splash" sounds follow each tap rather than multiple waves, as with ascites.

Normally, when the spleen is percussed in the left axillary line and in the lowest intercostal space, the percussion note is resonant due to the gastric air bubble. When the spleen is enlarged, the percussion note will be dull because of stomach displacement. Free air from perforated air-filled viscera (duodenum) will rise to the highest possible point, frequently between the liver and anterior ribs. This will change the percussion note from dullness to tympany when the liver is percussed.

Auscultation

General Guides. The diaphragm of the stethoscope is used rather than the bell, in order not to miss the usually faint peristaltic sounds. The stethoscope is placed lightly on the abdomen, and each quadrant is auscultated for several minutes. Interpretation of bowel sounds requires persistent practice and a fundamental knowledge of what causes the sounds. The nurse must auscultate the abdomen of many normal patients to establish a set of norms to serve as a basis for comparison. Any intestinal sound requires that both air and fluid are in interphase in the lumen of the intestine. Alone, neither will produce a sound. A normal peristaltic wave produces audible sounds of air and fluid moving along a tube.

General Survey. The "auscultation center" is about 1 to 2 cm below and to the right of the umbilicus. At this point the active sounds of the bowels (especially the small intestines) are most audible. After examining this area first, proceed to auscultate the remainder of the abdomen. Under normal conditions, the best time to hear peristalsis is between meals or at night. Normal tones occur at intervals of about 3 to 5 seconds and are of short duration (about 0.5 second). They are low but distinct dry, rumbling sounds with only slight fluctuations of intensity. The sounds should not be bubbling, squelching, or dissonant in either tone or intensity. After a large meal, normal peristaltic sounds are multiplied, condensed, louder and damped, and there is an increased rate of peristaltic movement. If abnormal bowel sounds are detected, the nurse should try to determine the point of greatest intensity.

Significant abnormal findings are usually at *two extremes:* (1) absent sounds when motility is inhibited, as in inflammation, gangrene, reflex ileus; and (2) a marked rush of persistent activity with waves of loud "gurgling" and "tinkling" sounds (borborygmi), as with gastroenteritis or diarrhea.

Esophageal bleeding frequently causes hyperperistalsis; intraabdominal bleeding often results in a "silent" abdomen. Active bowel sounds are rare or absent for one to three days after abdominal surgery, but an abdomen silent for longer than three to four days may indicate a complication, and physician referral is necessary. Active peristaltic sounds may be decreased or entirely subdued by ascites, but a moderate amount of fluid will intensify the sounds of the intestines floating on the fluid. A peritoneal friction rub may be heard over the liver or spleen and usually indicates juxtaposition of two irritated or inflamed surfaces. It usually occurs over an abdominal organ, and the rubbing is associated with respiratory movement.

Rushes, tinkles, and succussion splash may occur with various types of bowel obstruction and should be brought to the attention of a physician. A bruit may be heard over vascular structures. The epigastric area is the most frequent site for auscultating the aorta.

EXAMINATION OF MALE GENITOURINARY SYSTEM

Penis and Scrotum

Examination of the male genitalia is based primarily on inspection and palpation. The prepuce of the uncircumcised male should be retracted around the head of the penis. Normally, this should be accomplished with ease. A small amount of thick white secretion (smegma) is normally present between the prepuce and the glans. The shaft of the penis varies in size and is not considered abnormal unless very small and infantile in appearance. The urethra opens at the tip of the head of the penis. Ideally, the examiner should observe the patient void to examine the urinary stream. In adulthood, a poor urinary stream may indicate urethral stricture or prostatic obstruction.

Phimosis is an adhesion of the prepuce to the head of the penis, making it difficult or impossible to retract. Paraphimosis is an inflammation of the prepuce due to retraction that forms a tight ring around the penis, causing painful swelling of the glans. Edema of the penis is commonly seen with fluid retention due to dependent positioning. The penis should be examined from the tip to the base of the shaft for healed scars or any active lesions. An indurated, painless ulcer is characteristic of syphilis, while superficial ulcers of vesicles may indicate herpesvirus infection.

The urethra should be examined for *hypospadias,* the abnormal positioning of the urinary meatus on the ventral surface of the shaft, or *epispadias,* an opening on the dorsal surface. Usually surgically corrected in childhood, these conditions are rarely seen in adults. The urethra should be observed for the presence of any discharge. A thick, purulent discharge may be due to gonorrhea and should be cultured. A thin, mucoid discharge may indicate urethritis.

The scrotum is examined and the testes palpated. An asymmetrical position of the testes is normal, the left testes being slightly lower in the scrotum than the right. The normal size of the testes varies but the largest should be about 2 centimeters in diameter and of firm consistency. Tenderness is normally present when anything but very light palpation pressure is used. The epididymis surrounds the testes laterally and may be palpated with ease. The spermatic cord extends from the epididymis to the inguinal canal, where it is palpated between the thumb and forefinger as a thin cord. Testicular masses are frequently malignant. Atrophy may occur with other disease, e.g., mumps and liver disorders. Orchitis, or inflammation of the testes, is very painful, and the patient will present with this complaint.

Cystoceles, which are scrotal cysts filled with clear fluid, present as rounded, nontender masses and may be detected by transillumination. This is done in a very dark room, using a flashlight positioned under the scrotum. The entire cyst will "light up" as the light shines through the fluid. A *varicocele* is enlargement of the veins accompanying the epididymis and spermatic cord. A *spermatocele* is a cystic, localized enlargement of the spermatic cord or epididymis. Patients with any such abnormalities should be referred to a physician.

Inguinal Region

Femoral pulses should be palpated first to detect evidence of aortic disease. Lymph nodes in the groin area are palpated and often felt as "shotty," firm, freely movable, half-centimeter masses.

The inguinal canal begins with the internal ring and extends in continuity with the scrotum. The external inguinal ring is the opening between the scrotum and the inguinal canal. The spermatic cord and accompanying vessels enter the inguinal canal at this point. To examine the inguinal ring for hernias, it is preferred that the patient be in a standing position. The index or little finger is directed upward from the distal aspect of the scrotum, turning the scrotal skin inward like the finger of a glove. The internal inguinal canal is a natural opening in the abdominal wall and is felt at the end of the canal as a fibrous circle of tissue with a soft center. Requesting the patient to "strain" as in defecating will increase the intraabdominal pressure and accentuate any weakness of the internal ring or abdominal musculature. Straining is preferred to having the patient cough, since the intraabdominal pressure is increased only momentarily with coughing and makes a thorough examination more difficult.

Other than increased or decreased femoral pulses or enlarged lymph nodes, the most frequently encountered abnormality in the inguinal region is a hernia (see Fig. 11-6). An indirect inguinal hernia is a herniation along the path of the spermatic cord. Both direct and indirect hernias may involve a variety of organs, including the mesentery, small bowel, colon, and urinary bladder. Incipient hernias are felt as a bulge at the internal inguinal ring when the patient strains down in a standing position. This small bulge may not be felt on the outside and may never progress to a true hernia. A small hernia produces a large bulge at the

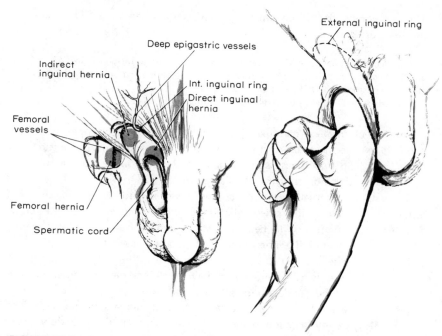

FIGURE 11-6.   Inguinal hernias. [Figs. 11-6 and 11-7 reprinted from R. D. Judge and G. D. Zuidema (Eds.).   *Methods of Clinical Examination: A Physiologic Approach* (3rd ed.). Boston: Little, Brown, 1974.]

internal ring. It is felt by the examining hand placed externally over the area of the internal ring. Large hernias usually descend into the inguinal canal to variable distances and frequently enter the scrotum. A strangulated hernia is a medical emergency requiring prompt referral to a physician. Hernias may also be described as indicated in Table 11-1.

A direct inguinal hernia occurs when the herniation is directly through a defect or weakness in the abdominal wall rather than along the inguinal canal. A small direct hernia differs from a small indirect one by invaginating into the scrotum. With the examining finger at the internal ring, the bulge can be felt pressing against the length of the finger rather than the fingertip. Direct hernias may produce scrotal masses and become incarcerated and strangulated.

Table 11-1. Types of Hernias

Reducible	Can be returned into the abdominal cavity
Incarcerated	Nonreducible, entrapped
Strangulated	Blood flow to the bowel has been impaired

Rectum and Prostate

The positioning of the patient for rectal examination varies. There are four possible positions:

1. Left decubitus position with the patient's knees drawn up to the abdomen.
2. Standing position with the elbows flexed and resting on the bed or table.
3. Supine position with the knees spread apart.
4. Knee-chest position with the patient's head turned to one side.

To inspect the external area, spread the patient's buttocks apart with both hands to expose the anal area for examination. Requesting the patient to "bear down" will help to emphasize the anatomy and cause the normal anal sphincter to contract and demonstrate intact innervation.

To palpate internally, the examining hand should be gloved and well lubricated. Explain to the patient what is going to be done and the sensations he will feel (e.g., pressure), to help him stay more relaxed. Begin with gentle pressure of the ball of the index finger and gradually insert the tip of the finger as the sphincter relaxes. At this point, it may be helpful to tell the patient that he may feel the urge to have a bowel movement. Ask him to tighten his anal sphincter so that you can determine sphincter strength.

A bidigital examination may also be performed in the sphincter area. The thumb of the examining hand is pressed toward the index finger, and the tissue of the perianal area is palpated between the digits for masses or irregularities. Enlarged bulbourethral (Cowper's) glands can be detected in this manner.

The prostate gland is located anterior to the mucosa of the anterior rectal wall. The posterior aspect of the gland protrudes into the rectal ampulla, which allows this portion of the gland to be examined for abnormalities. The size of the normal prostate gland varies but averages 4 cm in diameter (see Fig. 11-7). It is divided into two lobes by a vertical median fissure. It should be of firm consistency and without "bogginess." The patient should not complain of tenderness when the normal gland is palpated; however, he may feel the urge to urinate. The seminal vesicles extend above the prostate gland and are normally not palpable.

The rectum normally can be palpated to a depth of 10 cm. The rectal valves normally are felt as protruding intrarectal masses. The lateral walls may be palpated by feeling the sides of the rectum. The examiner should be able to palpate the ischial spines and the sacrotuberous ligaments. The posterior wall of the rectum normally follows the curve of the sacrum and coccyx and feels very smooth.

External *hemorrhoids* can be identified by inspection of the anal area. Requesting the patient to "bear down" may make a visible hemorrhoid more prominent. Hypertrophied anal papilla resemble hemorrhoids, but there are no dilated veins. Perianal skin may be irritated or inflamed. Thickening of the surrounding skin may occur secondary to chronic scratching and pruritus ani. The pilonidal sinus is a tract into the skin overlying the tip of the coccyx. Normally, it contains hair. When it becomes obstructed and infected, a pilonidal cyst or abscess occurs.

Palpation of the anal sphincter may detect hypertonicity. This usually occurs due to tension or local irritation, as with anal fissure. Hypotonicity or a weak anal sphincter may be due to previous surgery or underlying neurologic disease. A perianal abscess may be found by bidigital palpation of the circumference of the anal sphincter.

Rectal masses are often malignant; approximately one-half of all carcinomas occur in the colon and rectum. A rectal shelf may be palpated as a stony hard mass above the prostate on the anterior rectal wall. This shelf usually occurs with metastatic carcinoma to the pelvic floor. Any abnormalities detected by the nurse requires prompt referral of the patient for further evaluation by a physician.

Hesitancy and straining while voiding are early signs of prostatic obstruction. Loss of force and decrease of the caliber of the stream occurs as urethral resistance increases, despite increased transvesical pressure. Terminal dribbling also increases with obstruction, and acute urinary retention may be seen in the

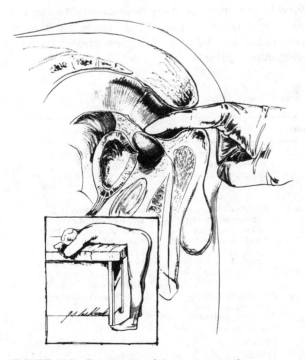

FIGURE 11-7.   Examination of the prostate gland.

patient who is unable to void. He will have increasing suprapubic pain with urgency and be able to dribble only small amounts of urine. Chronic urinary retention involves little or no pain. There is a great deal of hesitancy in starting the stream and a marked decrease in its force and caliber. Constant dribbling (paradoxical incontinence) may also occur.

In benign prostatic hypertrophy the gland may be palpated as diffusely enlarged, without masses. Atrophy of the prostate occurs with loss of secondary sex characteristics. Tenderness on palpation is a common finding. Extreme tenderness may occur with urinary abnormalities. The gland may feel soft and "boggy" with prostatitis also.

Carcinoma of the prostate may be felt as a mass or node on the posterior lobe of the gland. Advanced tumors usually feel stony hard, are irregular, and not tender.

PAIN IN GENITOURINARY DISEASE

Pain is an important complaint of many patients with genitourinary alterations. In general, the patient may complain of two types of pain, localized or referred. Localized pain is felt in the region of the involved organ. Referred pain originates in a diseased organ but is felt at some distance from the organ. It is also important for the nurse to remember that many genitourinary diseases are painless due to the slow progression of the disease (e.g., carcinoma, chronic pyelonephritis, and tuberculosis). Table 11-2 gives a brief description of types of pain that the nurse may encounter in patients.

Table 11-2. Pain Characteristics of Selected Genitourinary Organs

Organ	Type	Duration	Location	Possible Causes
Kidney	Dull	Constant	Costovertebral angle, lateral; lateral to sacrospinalis muscle	Acute pyelonephritis with sudden edema Acute urethral obstruction with sudden renal back pressure
Urethra	Severe	Colicky	Back; may radiate from costovertebral angle to lower anterior quadrant of abdomen (radiates to vulva in females)	Acute obstruction (e.g., stone or blood clot) (Severity and colicky nature of pain is due to hyperperistalsis and spasm of smooth muscles in attempts to overcome the obstruction.)
Vesicle	Severe		Suprapubic; usually referred to distal urethra; related to urination	Overdistended bladder in acute urinary retention
Testicle	Severe Dull ache		Testicle Testicle	Trauma or infection Varicocele

SUGGESTED READINGS

Buckingham, W. B., et al. *A Primer of Clinical Diagnosis.* New York: Harper & Row, 1971.

Campbell, M. (Ed.) *Urology* (2nd ed.). Philadelphia: Saunders, 1963.

Cope, Z. *The Early Diagnosis of Acute Abdomen.* New York: Oxford University Press, 1968.

Endre, K. *Physical Diagnosis of Acute Abdominal Diseases and Injuries.* Budapest: Academy Press, 1964.

Macleod, J. *Clinical Examination.* London: Livingstone, 1964.

Mills, P. *The Significance of Physical Signs in Medicine.* London: Lewis, 1971.

Newsam, J. E., and Petrie, J. J. B. *Urology and Renal Medicine.* Edinburgh and London: Livingstone, 1971.

Smith, D. *General Urology.* Los Altos, Calif. Lange Medical Publications, 1972.

Winter, C. *Practical Urology.* St. Louis: Mosby, 1969.

PHYSICAL APPRAISAL OF THE FEMALE REPRODUCTIVE SYSTEM   12

Jo Waylan Denton

GLOSSARY

adnexa The uterine appendages, the ovaries, uterine tubes, and ligaments of the uterus.

amenorrhea Absence of menses.

anteflexion of uterus The normal forward curvature of the uterus in which the upper part is bent forward.

atrophic vaginitis A nonspecific vaginal infection in which the epithelium may be spotted with small petechiae.

caruncle A small red eminence on the mucous membrane of the urinary meatus.

chronic cystic mastitis Inflammatory condition of the breast characterized by diffuse nodularity and cystic changes.

cul-de-sac A blind pouch posterior to the uterus.

cystocele Hernial protrusion of the urinary bladder through the anterior vaginal wall.

dysmenorrhea Painful menstruation.

dyspareunia Difficult or painful intercourse.

enterocele Hernial protrusion of part of the intestine through the posterior vaginal wall.

fibroma Fibroid tumor derived from connective tissue.

fornices The recesses formed between the vaginal walls and the vaginal part of the cervix. The areas are termed *anterior* or *posterior,* depending on their relation to the cervix.

greater vestibular (Bartholin's) glands. Two small mucous glands on the inner aspect of the labia minora in front of the hymen.

gynecomastia Hypertrophy of breast tissue in the male, which causes resemblance to a female breast.

hypermenorrhea Abnormally increased volume of menstrual flow.

introitus The entrance into the vagina.

kraurosis vulvae Dryness, shriveling and increasing fibrosis of the vulva and the vaginal vestibule, vulvovaginal stenosis. This condition frequently occurs in conjunction with leukoplakia.

leiomyoma Fibroid tumor of the uterus.

lesser vestibular glands Numerous minute mucous glands opening on the surface of the vestibule between the orifices of the vagina and the urethra.

leukoplakia The appearance of white, thickened patches on the vulvar surface. This condition frequently occurs in conjunction with kraurosis vulvae.

mastitis Inflammation of the breast, usually due to pyogenic infection.

menarche Beginning of the menstrual function.

menopause Termination of menses.

multipara Woman who has given birth to more than one child.

nabothian follicles Dilation of the mucus-secreting glands of the cervix caused by obstruction of their orifices and retention of the mucous secretions.

parametrium The loose connective tissue and smooth muscle lying beside the cervix and lower segment of the body of the uterus.

paraurethral (Skene's) glands Numerous mucous glands in the wall of the female urethra.

polymenorrhea Abnormally frequent menstrual flow.

polyp   Protruding growth from any mucous membrane such as that of the cervix.
primigravida   Woman pregnant for the first time.
primipara   Woman who has given birth to one viable infant.
rectocele   Hernial protrusion of part of the rectum through the posterior vaginal wall.
retraction   Dimpling of the nipple or skin overlying the breast tissue.
retroversion of uterus   Abnormal position of the uterus in which the entire uterus is tilted backward.
uterine prolapse   Protrusion of the uterus through the vaginal orifice. *First-degree prolapse* The cervix lies between the level of the ischial spines and the vaginal introitus. *Second-degree prolapse*   The cervix protrudes through the introitus. *Third-degree prolapse*   Both the cervix and the body of the uterus have passed through the introitus, and the entire vaginal canal is inverted.
vestibule   The area between the inner surfaces of the labia minora and below the clitoris which forms the entrance to the vagina.

Investigation and examination of the female reproductive system reveals considerable information on the status of the lower urinary tract and the lower abdomen, as well as the reproductive organs. The number of physiologic functions related to the genital area — micturition, defecation, menstruation, ovulation, copulation, impregnation, and parturition — makes a regular, thorough examination of this area exceedingly important. Examination of the female genitalia should, without question, be a part of every woman's annual physical examination.

The current sexual revolution and increasing frankness in relation to sexuality might lead one to anticipate only minimal reluctance from women in seeking or experiencing examinations of the reproductive system. However, it is important to remember that attitudes and behaviors developed over many years do not change quickly. Thus one must anticipate and respect a spectrum of reactions to and concerns about the history and the physical examination. Nurses have a vital role in educating women as to the importance of regular examinations and the necessity of early reporting of any alterations they themselves notice. Hopefully, the practice of having annual pelvic examinations will be conveyed from mothers to daughters, so that pelvic examinations will be a routine part of the health maintenance practices of each new generation of women.

HISTORY AND GENERAL ASSESSMENT

A thorough evaluation of the female reproductive system involves exploration of the woman's relevant history and observation of some general characteristics. The following should be included:

1. *General body stature.* Is the woman generally of a female body build?
2. *Secondary sex characteristics.*
   a. Distribution of facial and axillary hair.
   b. Pitch of voice.
   c. Breast development (see below for a thorough discussion).

3. *Family history.* Is there any history of cancer or other reproductive disorders, especially in the mother?
4. *Obstetric and surgical history.*   Determine gravidity and parity. Has she had any abortions? If so, what type? What was the precipitating factor? Has she had previous gynecologic surgery, and if so, were there any complications?
5. *Menstrual pattern.*
   a. *Menarche.* At what age did she experience menarche? Were there any associated problems?
   b. *Menstrual periods* Determine the interval between periods, the duration, and the amount of flow. What is the color of the menstrual discharge? Do clots occur? What is the date of her last menstrual period?
   c. Does dysmenorrhea or intermenstrual bleeding occur?
   d. *Menopause.* If she has experienced menopause, at what age did it occur? Was it natural, or was it artificially induced as by surgery or irradiation? Were there any associated problems? If she has not yet experienced menopause, what are her expectations regarding it? Does she have any questions as to what she may anticipate?
6. *Vaginal discharge.*   Have her describe any vaginal discharge she has been having. Determine the amount (number of pads), character, color, odor, presence of tissue, and any precipitating factors.
7. *Sexual history.* How is her relationship with spouse or partner? How frequently does she engage in intercourse? Is it satisfying for her? Does she experience dyspareunia? This is a particularly important area to explore with the postmenopausal woman for whom menopausal dyspareunia is frequently a problem.
8. *Knowledge of own health care.*
   a. Has she had routine pelvic examinations and Papanicolaou smears? How often? When was her last one?
   b. Does she do monthly breast self-examinations?
   c. What method of contraception does she or partner use? Is it satisfactory to both? Does she need further contraceptive information?

BREAST EXAMINATION

A thorough, systematic examination of both breasts and surrounding lymphatic drainage sites is necessary because of the high incidence of disease in this organ. The breast is the most common site of cancer in the female [2, p. 209].

The woman should disrobe to the waist so that both breasts can be exposed simultaneously for comparison. Good lighting is important to assure observation of areas of retraction. The woman is examined in both the sitting and the supine positions. Inspection is followed by palpation.

Inspection

Inspection of the breasts includes attention to symmetry, position and size, superficial appearance, nipples, and any skin retraction present.

With the woman in the sitting position, it is not uncommon to notice some asymmetry in the size and position of the two breasts. Generally, this is due to developmental differences, but it might indicate an abnormality such as a cyst, tumor, or inflammation.

In the thin, flat-chested woman, the nipple with its areola will be approximately over the fourth intercostal space in the midclavicular line. With the accumulation of fat, there may be some dropping of the nipple below the fourth intercostal space. In most women, the breasts extend in area from the third to the sixth ribs. However, with obesity, the loss of breast hypertrophy after lactation, or increasing age, the breasts sag and the nipples drop lower. The atrophy of breast tissue and muscular supports beginning at menopause results in the sagging, limp breasts of the aged female.

The skin overlying the breasts should be carefully observed. The examiner should look for local areas of erythema and signs of edema. The latter is manifested by hair follicles and follicular openings that are more pronounced or noticeable than usual.

The nipples should be carefully examined for bleeding, discharge, retraction, or ulceration. It is particularly important to note the color of any discharge, which may range from clear yellow to blue or green. Some asymmetry in the size and shape of the nipples is not necessarily abnormal. Inversion of the nipples may be present but is significant only if it is of recent origin.

Careful inspection for skin retraction, or dimpling, is one of the most important aspects of the breast examination, and good lighting is essential for this purpose. Dimpling, which appears in different degrees, can be found on any part of the skin of the breast or nipple. It can occur with inflammation, but most often it denotes a malignancy.

To demonstrate best an early stage of retraction, the woman can perform a variety of movements to place pull on the suspensory ligaments (Fig. 12-1A). After she has been examined while sitting erect, ask her to raise her arms directly overhead. Also she can cause contraction of the pectoral muscles by placing both hands together in front of her and pushing them against each other (Fig. 12-1B). A second way this can be accomplished is by her placing her hands on her hips and pushing forcibly against them (Fig. 12-1C). The latter two methods exaggerate any retraction that is present. The woman should continue one of these actions until all areas of both breasts have been inspected for retraction.

Observation of the axillary and supraclavicular regions is also important, to check for bulging, retraction, discoloration, or edema. These are the most important lymphatic drainage areas for the breasts.

Palpation

After the thorough inspection, the breasts, axillae, and supraclavicular regions should be systematically palpated. There is a wide variation in the consistency of normal breast tissue. Such factors as age, obesity, stage of the menstrual cycle, and pregnancy contribute to this variation. As the examiner becomes more experienced in the physical examination, she will gain an appreciation for the range of normal breast size and consistency. In young women, the breasts tend to be firm, somewhat elastic in consistency, and cone-shaped, with the border

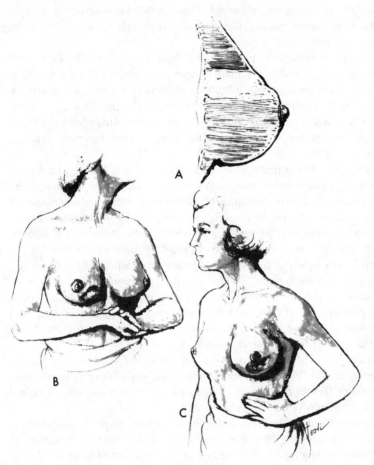

FIGURE 12-1.   Demonstration of skin retraction. A. Diagram showing how shortening of Cooper's ligaments may produce skin retraction. B. Method of bringing out skin retraction by pressing hands together. C. Method of bringing out skin retraction by pressing against the hip. (Reprinted from Judge and Zuidema [1].)

clearly delineated. The young breast may be particularly sensitive to palpation, especially at the time of its growth at puberty or just prior to the menstrual period. The breast tissue of the older woman is commonly stringy and nodular. The older breast develops an irregular consistency, with disappearance of the sharply delineated borders. Large breasts may become pendulous.

As palpation begins, the nurse should remember the monthly cyclic physiologic changes that occur in the breast. The breasts become engorged, lobular, and sensitive prior to the menses and decongest promptly thereafter. As a result of years of such cyclical changes, nodules may develop, giving the breast a granular consistency. During pregnancy, the breasts become firmer and larger, and the lobulations become more distinct. These well-defined lobules may easily be confused with tumor masses. Detailed recording and follow-up to assure appropriate medical attention is mandatory.

For thorough examination, palpation of the breasts should be performed with the woman seated and then supine. In both positions, the breasts should be examined with the woman's arms at her side and then with her arms overhead. (Fig. 12-2). When examining the woman in the supine position, use a small pillow under the shoulder on each side as it is examined. This allows the breast to rest more symmetrically over the chest wall, permitting more accurate examination.

Palpation begins in the upper, lateral quadrant of each breast where most tumors occur. The examination must be systematic to assure that the breasts are completely examined. The palpation can be done in a clockwise direction until the entire breast is examined, or palpation can proceed in and out, laterally to medially, forming a pattern like spokes of a wheel. If the woman complains of tenderness or a lump in one breast, that area should be palpated last.

Palpation begins lightly and gently, using the palmar aspect of the fingertips, with a rotary to-and-fro motion. Following light palpation, each area is more deeply explored. It is important not to compress a portion of the breast tissue between the fingers of one or both hands, as this may give the erroneous impression that a lump is present. To avoid this, the breast tissue should be compressed gently but firmly against the chest wall (Fig. 12-2).

After examination of the breast tissue, attention is focused on the nipple. Any subareolar masses, induration, loss of elasticity, dry scaling, or excoriation should be noted. Gentle pressure or a stripping action should be used to see whether or not a discharge can be elicited.

The examiner should note the consistency and elasticity of the breast tissue and nipples, the texture of the skin, and any masses detected. If a mass is located, it should be characterized according to the following features:

1. *Location.* The exact location of the mass must be designated. One method is to consider each breast as if it were the face of a clock with the nipple as the central point and the numbers of the clock placed clockwise in a 1 to 12 position. Thus a lesion can be stated to be along a specific axis, e.g., the 9 o'clock axis. Also, the mass should be located as to its distance from the nipple. It is often helpful to draw a circle and make a sketch of the mass, illustrating it on the proper axis.
2. *Size.* The size of the mass should be estimated as accurately as possible in three dimensions. It is particularly important to describe it in centimeters of length, width, and thickness for comparison with future progression or regression of the mass.
3. *Contour.* A description of the surface of the mass should be made. Is it regular and smooth or irregular and infiltrating?
4. *Consistency.* Determine the firmness or softness of the mass. It may be described as soft, cystic, moderately firm, firm, or stony hard.
5. *Tenderness.* Determine if the lesion is tender and, if so, to what degree.
6. *Mobility.* Determine if the lesion is freely movable, movable only in certain directions, or fixed. Is mobility of the mass limited by fixation to deep structures, to the skin, or to surrounding breast tissue?

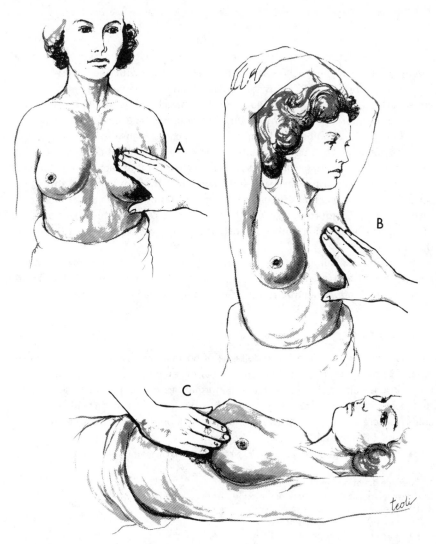

FIGURE 12-2.   Positions used for palpation of the breast. A. Erect with arms at sides.
B. Erect with arms raised overhead. C. Supine. (Modified from Judge and Zuidema [1].)

7. *Discreteness.* Determine if the boundaries of the mass are easily detected, or if it is difficult to differentiate the margins of the mass.

After completion of the examination of the breast, the axilla should be carefully palpated. Thorough examination can be made with one hand while the examiner's opposite hand holds the ipsilateral arm of the woman, who may be either sitting or supine. The axilla should be thought of as having an apex and three walls: anterior or pectoral group, central group, and posterior group (Fig. 6-6). Cup the examining hand slightly and reach as high into the apex of the axilla as possible. Then pull the hand downward, exerting gentle pressure against the thorax with the fingertips. Repeat several times so that each area is palpated with the woman's arm at her side and again while the arm is moved through a full range of motion. This is done to uncover any lesions hidden under muscle or fatty tissue. It is important not to abduct the arm too far, for this tenses the skin of the axilla, interfering with deep palpation and possibly causing the woman discomfort.

Following examination of the breasts and axillae, both supraclavicular regions should be palpated. By deeper palpation check the deep jugular chain of nodes, as these are frequently routes of metastatic spread of breast cancer.

Significant Findings

As discussed earlier, there is a wide range of normal characteristics of the female breast. Experience in inspection and palpation of the breast will best help the nurse in developing skill in detecting abnormalities. Differentiating the nodules that occur with aging from tumor masses is one of the most difficult skills. Of course, where there is any question, the woman should be referred to a physician for biopsy of the lesion.

A thorough physical examination provides the following information:

1. Presence, location, and number of masses.
2. Consistency, size, tenderness, and mobility of mass(es).
3. Retraction or dimpling of skin over mass.
4. Displacement or retraction of nipple.
5. Palpable regional lymph nodes, if any.

These characteristics will be discussed here only in relation to the most common alterations.

Benign lesions, such as lipomas or adenofibromas, are most often soft and cystic, smooth-surfaced, with well-defined borders, and easily movable. In contrast, malignant lesions are generally firm with uneven surfaces, infiltrating, have irregular margins, and are often fixed to other structures as they become invasive. Tenderness is rarely found with a malignant lesion. An inflammatory process often demonstrates symptoms similar to those of a malignant lesion, having an irregular contour, a firm consistency, and being firmly or moderately firmly fixed to surrounding structures. One differing feature, however, is that inflammatory lesions are usually moderately to markedly tender.

Chronic cystic mastitis is an exceedingly common breast lesion characterized by multiple nodules diffusely located in both breasts. The breast tissue is usually thickened and may be tender to palpation. Occasionally, the process may be fairly localized. In either event, the woman should be referred for diagnostic biopsy.

Mastitis is a generalized inflammation of breast tissue, usually occurring during lactation. The involved breast tends to be red, edematous, and tender; chills and fever often accompany the inflammation. The usual cause is a pyogenic infection.

Any discharge from the nipple should always be considered significant and reported to a physician. Bloody or dark discharge can indicate intraductal papilloma or Paget's disease, a malignant disease of the nipple and areola.

Male Breast

Examination of the breast in the male is just as important as it is in the female. Carcinoma of the breast does occur in males, though much less frequently than in females.

In examination of the male breast the same procedure is followed as in examination of the female breast. In the young, moderately thin man, the nipple and areola are found approximately in the fourth intercostal space, midclavicular line. With the accumulation of fat or with increasing age, this anatomic relationship is usually lost, with the nipple dropping below the level of the fourth intercostal space.

Carcinoma of the male breast usually occurs as an irregular, hard nodule underlying the areola, causing retraction of the nipple and fixation to the skin and deep tissues. The paucity of breast tissue accounts for the early metastasis to axillary lymph nodes.

Gynecomastia is usually unilateral and noninflammatory. In the young male, the breast has a glandular consistency and is conical in shape. With age, the nodularity increases, making differentiation from a neoplasm more difficult, and biopsy is necessary. Systemic disease, such as cirrhosis of the liver, may cause bilateral gynecomastia. In such cases the liver is no longer able to detoxify estrogens.

Self-examination of the Breast

Nurses play an exceedingly important role in instructing women in the technique of self-examination of the breast. The importance of regular examinations cannot be underestimated, and every woman should know and practice the technique. Additionally, mothers should begin teaching their daughters to do self-examination as soon as they begin to have significant breast development.

Ideally, the examination should be performed immediately following each menstrual period. Temporary changes preceding the menstrual cycle give the breasts a nodular consistency and increase their sensitiveness to palpation. Following menopause, breast self-examinations should continue on a regular basis. The woman should be taught to look for the following: any dimpling or puckering of the skin; retraction of either nipple; any thickening or change in consistency; or any alteration in symmetry, size, contour, or position. Also to be reported are pain, swelling, inflammation, or discharge. If she has some nodules that have been checked by a physician, they should be followed closely for any changes in characteristics.

After being given information as to what findings are important, women should be taught how to observe and how to palpate the breast.

Observation. The woman should place herself before a mirror with her arms at her sides. She should carefully examine her breasts in the mirror for symmetry, size, and shape, searching for any evidence of puckering, dimpling of the skin, or retraction of the nipple. She should then raise her arms above her head and again study her breasts in the mirror, looking for the same physical signs. She should also be alert for any evidence of fixation of the breast tissue to the chest wall. This may be displayed as she moves her arms and shoulders.

Palpation. Palpation should be performed in the reclining position. This position permits the breasts to spread over a greater area and thins the breast tissue, making accurate palpation easier. A small pillow or folded towel should be placed beneath the shoulder on the side of the breast to be examined. This raises that side of the body and distributes the weight of the breast tissue more evenly over the chest wall. The arm on the side to be first examined is placed at her side, and the breast is gently examined with the flat surface of the fingers of her opposite hand. The technique calls for gentle palpation of the breast tissue against the chest wall, usually beginning on the outer half of the breast and systematically covering the entire half of the breast, paying particular attention to the upper outer quadrant where the axillary tail of breast tissue is thickest and where many tumors occur. She should then raise the arm above her head and thoroughly examine the inner half of the breast, beginning at the sternum.

When the entire breast has been carefully palpated, the axilla should be examined carefully. With the arm on the side being examined again resting at her side, she should cup her examining hand and reach as high into the apex of the axilla as possible. Exerting gentle pressure against the thorax she should pull her hand slowly downward. Repeating several times she should check in order: the anterior group, the central group, and the posterior group. Each of these areas should be palpated again while the resting arm is taken through a full range of motion, to uncover any lesions that might have been hidden by fatty or muscle tissue. She should be reminded not to abduct the arm too far, for this interferes with deep palpation and may cause her some discomfort.

Following palpation of the one breast and axilla, the pillow is placed beneath the opposite shoulder, and the woman investigates the second breast and axilla in exactly the same manner.

Palpation of the breast and axilla should be thorough and unhurried. Every portion of the breast must be deliberately and carefully examined if small lesions are to be detected.

The woman should be instructed to place the greatest emphasis on the regions where most breast cancers develop, namely in the axillary tail of the breast and beneath the nipple. If the technique is to have any meaning she must establish a definite habit pattern and conduct a thorough examination at monthly intervals. The method will be effective only if used regularly [1, p. 311].

PELVIC EXAMINATION

As discussed earlier, the pelvic examination should be a part of every woman's physical examination. Preparation for the examination includes both emotional and physical aspects. The degree of fear and embarrassment, of course, varies from person to person; but the nurse can anticipate that nearly all women will experience some degree of apprehension. Cultural background and untoward experiences during previous examinations are often contributing factors. Thorough explanations of your actions and of what the woman can expect to feel will help her to relax sufficiently for satisfactory palpation with only minimal discomfort.

Certain basic items of equipment are needed for the routine pelvic examination. These are:

1. Examination table with stirrups
2. Instrument table and stool
3. Sink
4. Portable, easily adjustable light source
5. Assortment of bivalve vaginal specula of various sizes
6. Sponge forceps and cotton sponges
7. Lubricant
8. Rubber gloves
9. Cotton applicators
10. Glass microscope slides
11. Specimen bottles and fixative solution or fixative spray

The woman should not have douched for at least 24 hours prior to the pelvic examination. Douching will interfere with proper evaluation of vaginal discharge, cytologic studies, and cultures or stained smears for microorganism identification if necessary. She should void immediately prior to the examination, since an empty bladder makes palpation easier, eliminates possible distortion of the position of the pelvic organs caused by a full bladder, and obviates the danger and embarrassment of incontinence during examination. Since collection of a urine specimen is often indicated at this time, it should be routine. It is desirable that the rectum be empty, but it is not always mandatory. It may sometimes be necessary to have the woman return for examination after emptying the lower bowel by enema or laxative.

Positioning and Sequence

Proper positioning of the woman and good lighting are essential for an accurate examination. Avoiding unnecessary exposure and assuring privacy add to her comfort. The most satisfactory draping is a square sheet. For the common lithotomy position, she holds one corner over her xyphoid process, and the corners adjacent to this are placed over each knee. The fourth corner hangs between her legs and over her perineum. This fourth corner is turned back on her abdomen during actual examination of the perineum.

Pelvic examination may be performed with the patient in one of the following positions:

1. *The lithotomy position* is the most practical. With the woman lying on her back, the thighs are flexed and abducted, the legs are flexed, and the feet are supported in stirrups. Both legs are manipulated at the same time to prevent strain to the lower back.

2. *The left lateral prone (Sims) position* has the woman lying on her left side with her chest inclining toward the table. Her left arm is behind her, her right thigh is flexed about 90°, and the left thigh is slightly flexed. This position is reserved primarily for women who have ankylosis of the hips or knees and those who are too weak for the lithotomy position. Also, it provides closer observation of the urethra and the anterior vaginal wall, especially if these areas are obstructed from view by uterine displacement when the lithotomy position is used. A single-blade retractor is placed in the vagina, retracting the posterior vaginal wall.

3. *The knee-chest position* with the patient on her arms and knees and buttocks uppermost may also be used for closer observation of the urethra and anterior vaginal wall. However, many women find this an uncomfortable position.

4. *The standing position* is used to evaluate hernias, uterine prolapse, relaxation of the vaginal walls or pelvic supports, and stress incontinence of urine.

For complete pelvic examination, the following sequence is suggested:

1. Examination of the abdomen
2. Inspection and palpation of vulva and perineum
3. Collection of specimens for cytologic examination
4. Inspection of the vaginal walls and cervix
5. Bimanual examination
6. Rectovaginal abdominal examination

Examination of the Abdomen

The pelvic examination begins with the examination of the abdomen, utilizing the usual four methods: inspection, palpation, percussion, and auscultation as is discussed in Chapter 11. Inspection may reveal enlargement or obvious tumors. Characteristics of such masses or areas of tenderness should be determined by palpation. Palpation of the inguinal lymph nodes should always be included.

Percussion aids in differentiating free fluid and encysted fluid within the abdomen. Usually, the tympanitic bowel floats on free fluid and is found in the midline or the most distensible part of the abdomen. In contrast, encysted fluid, whether it be that within a pregnant uterus, a distended bladder, or a large ovarian cyst, presents dullness in the midline and tympany in the lateral portion of the abdomen. Shifting dullness is characteristic of free fluid. A tense cyst may be differentiated from a solid tumor by demonstration of a fluid wave within it.

Auscultation of the abdomen provides detection and evaluation of bowel sounds, bruits, and fetal heart sounds.

Inspection and Palpation of Vulva and Perineum

The perineum is as tender and sensitive as any area examined during physical assessment. Anyone placed in the lithotomy position and then touched abruptly on the perineum will experience the anal sphincter reflex. The external anal sphincter and portions of the levator ani will involuntarily contract, creating a barrier to comfortable examination. Thus the examiner's initial contact with the perineum should be at some distance from the labia and should be firm but gentle.

The pattern of pubic hair distribution should be that of a female, namely, an inverted triangle with its base anterior. The labia majora are usually plump and well formed in the normally developed adult female. They are free from erythema, edema, lesions, varicosities, hydroceles, tumor masses, or lacerations that may distort the normal configuration.

The labia minora are parted, with the examiner noting the clitoris, the vestibule, the urethral meatus, and the introitus. The size and development of the clitoris normally is variable, but true enlargement of the organ is obvious. The area of the vestibule between the inner surfaces of the labia minora and below the clitoris is the most common site of granulomatous and ulcerative venereal lesions in younger women and of malignant changes in the elderly. It should be checked carefully for erythema and ulcerations. The orifices of the lesser vestibular glands and the paraurethral (Skene's) glands are barely distinguishable unless infected. The external urethral meatus should be free from inflammation, tumor, and prolapse of the urethral mucous membrane. No discharge should be expressed from the urethra or the paraurethral glands when the examiner gently presses on the undersurface of the urethra and slowly withdraws her finger.

In examining the introitus, the examiner notes its general appearance. In the nonparous individual, the labia minora lie together in the midline. If there is relaxation or laceration of the perineal muscles, the labia gape and fall to either side. The hymen or hymeneal remnants appear just inside the introitus. In the virgin, this structure is variable in thickness and in its restriction of the opening of the vagina. It normally will admit one finger, sometimes two fingers, or may be impenetrable. The remnants of the ruptured hymen also normally vary in thickness and size in the nonvirgin.

The ducts of the greater vestibular (Bartholin's) glands open into the margin of the vaginal orifice just outside the hymen on either lateral side, slightly posterior to the horizontal midplane. They should be checked carefully for inflammation and swelling but are normally not palpable. Palpation of enlargements on the surfaces of the labia and within the labia is accomplished by inserting the index finger into the vagina while exerting counterpressure with the thumb on the suspicious area.

Collection of Specimens for Cytologic Examination

Insertion of the bivalve Graves' speculum enables the examiner to obtain epithelium for cytologic examination, as well as inspect the vaginal walls and the cervix. The examiner must be adept at using the speculum to avoid unnecessary discomfort for the woman. The specula come in three different sizes, and the size of choice depends on the woman's size and parity. The posterior blade is fixed and the anterior blade movable. The two blades are held together by a thumbscrew on the handle of the anterior blade. Loosening the thumbscrew allows the tips of the blades to come together. Depressing the anterior handle separates the blades, and tightening the screw holds the blades in position. Informing the woman of your actions and telling her what feelings to anticipate are particularly important during this phase of the examination. Instructing her to breathe deeply and slowly through her mouth will help her relax.

To avoid interference with cytologic studies, the speculum should be lubricated only with warm water. For the right-handed examiner, the speculum is held in the right hand, and the labia are separated with the thumb and index finger of the left hand. With the first joint of the thumb against the underside of the thumb rest to hold the blades tightly together, the speculum handle is turned 45 to 60° to the examiner's right (counterclockwise), so that the blades are held obliquely. The tip of the speculum is inserted into the posterior part of the vaginal introitus that has been exposed, avoiding pressure on the external urethral meatus. If the flat surfaces of the blades are horizontal, the introitus may be stretched; if the blades are vertical, the suburethral area can be damaged.

As soon as the broad portions of the blades have passed the introitus, the speculum is rotated so that the blades are horizontal, and the handle is elevated so that the speculum is advancing at a 45° angle toward the examining table. Again, exert slight posterior pressure during this maneuver to avoid the sensitive area of the urethra. When the speculum is fully inserted, the blades are opened by pressing down on the thumbpiece to elevate the top blade, while the hand lifts on the handle to lower the fixed posterior blade. In this way the blades move away from each other, and the cervix and vaginal walls are exposed (Fig. 12-3).

Another method of speculum insertion is to introduce one or two fingers of the left hand through the introitus and depress the perineal body backward. The posterior blade of the speculum is introduced into the vagina over the top of the fingers. This method also avoids pressure on the urethra.

Because of its extreme value in the early detection of uterine cancer, a simple screening test, the Papanicolaou smear, must be considered a routine part of the pelvic examination. There are several methods for obtaining cells for the study, but only one method will be discussed here. Regardless of the method used, obtaining an adequate and representative sample of the endocervical epithelium is essential. Since this test is for the identification of epithelial lesions, the specimen should be obtained before the vagina and cervical face are wiped off or disturbed by bimanual examination.

The two slides and fixative, whether a solution of ether alcohol or a spray, should be readied before the specimen is obtained. With the speculum in position, exposing the cervix, use the handle of an Ayres spatula or a cotton-tipped applicator to collect a smear from the posterior fornix of the vagina. For the cervical smear, reverse the spatula and place the longer arm of the tip in the cervical os and rotate the blade a full circle. To avoid causing the woman unnecessary discomfort, the applicator should be inserted gently and not too far. The two slides should each be spread evenly and prepared with the fixative.

Abnormal cervical epithelium can also be detected by Schiller's test in which Lugol's iodine solution is applied to the cervix. Normal cervical epithelium contains considerable glycogen and is immediately stained dark brown. Abnormal epithelial cells are devoid of glycogen and therefore do not stain. Areas that remain unstained may be areas of glandular erosion, but the tissue certainly must be studied microscopically for the possibility of cancer.

Inspection of the Vaginal Walls and Cervix

After the specimens have been obtained, the cervix can be visually inspected with the speculum in position. The vaginal walls can be inspected as the speculum is withdrawn.

The normal cervix is 2.5 to 3 cm in diameter and extends into the upper vagina about the same distance. It is normally much smaller in the aged female, coinciding with uterine hypoplasia. The cervix is cylindrical in shape and points posteriorly; but if the uterus is displaced, as it is in about 20 percent of women, the cervix will point anteriorly [2, p. 327]. The cervix should be the normal pink epithelial color and should be free from lacerations, ulcers, erosions, and new growths. It should be sponged vigorously and examined for any signs of

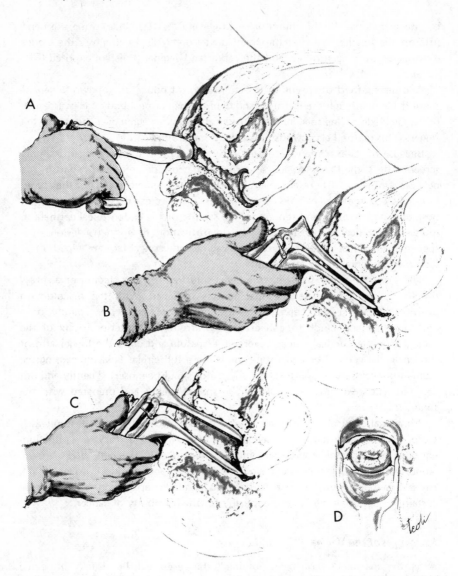

FIGURE 12-3. Insertion of vaginal speculum. A. Blades held obliquely on entering vagina. B. Blades rotated to the horizontal position as they pass the introitus. C. Blades separated by depressing thumbpiece and elevating handle. D. Normal parous cervix. (Reprinted from Judge and Zuidema [1].)

bleeding. Ulcers or erosions usually present a beefy red color and have regular margins. Early carcinoma is difficult to differentiate visually from an erosion, though the margins are more likely to be irregular and the area may bleed easily. A cyanotic, bluish appearance of the cervix (Chadwick's sign) is an early indication of pregnancy.

Inspection of the cervical os includes the size, shape, and color of the os as well as observation of any discharge or polyps present. The normal os of the nulliparous adult female is small, closed, and usually in the horizontal plane. In the parous female, the os is more likely to be larger, with possibly some curvature and small, healed lacerations on it. There should be no discharge or polyps exuding from the cervical os. If there is a discharge, attention to its quantity, consistency, color, and odor are important. Chronic infection of the endocervical canal is accompanied by a thick mucous or mucopurulent discharge. In such a condition the cervix is enlarged and edematous in appearance, and nabothian follicles may be visible on the vaginal portion of the cervix. A cervical polyp generally appears as a dark, cherry-red mass, 1 to 3 cm in diameter, extending through the cervical os. It is smooth and uniform in contour and bleeds easily.

The lateral vaginal walls visible through the open speculum and the fornices should be inspected as to texture, color, support, and discharge. A more detailed inspection of the vagina may be made as the speculum is withdrawn. The normal vaginal epithelium of the adult appears thick and heavy and is obviously distensible because of its elasticity and its many folds. The color is normally pink and uniform. Any abnormal redness or blueness should be noted. If a discharge is present, again determine its characteristics and source — vaginal mucosa, cervical os, or both. Infection by *Candida* organisms, which are fungi, produces a thick, white, patchy, curdlike discharge that clings to the vaginal wall. Bacterial invasion of the vagina produces a thin, yellow purulent material. In *Trichomonas* vaginitis the discharge is thin, yellow, often frothy, with a characteristic musty odor. Further, the vaginal wall may have a "strawberry" appearance, with small red spots seeming to show through the vaginal epithelium. A gonorrheal infection presents a situation similar to that seen with a *Trichomonas* infection, except that gonorrhea develops rapidly and typically produces a severe inflammation of the urethra and the greater vestibular (Bartholin's) glands, as well as of the vagina and cervix. The urethra and Bartholin's glands usually are not infected by *Trichomonas* organisms.

The anterior and posterior vaginal walls are inspected by rotating the speculum in the long axis of the vagina. The remainder of the vagina can be viewed as the blades are withdrawn. After the blades of the speculum clear the cervix, release the thumbscrew of the speculum and hold the speculum partially open by the thumb to allow the rest of the vagina to be viewed.

The integrity of uterine supports and the vaginal walls can be evaluated by asking the woman to bear down when the speculum has been withdrawn to the midpoint of the vagina. There should be no protrusion of the cervix nor bulging of the anterior or posterior vaginal walls. If the uterine supports are relaxed, varying degrees of uterine prolapse will occur. The cervix will protrude into the open speculum and may follow it to the introitus. Where there is relaxation of the anterior or posterior vaginal walls, a cystocele or rectocele bulges into the vaginal cavity. Vaginal palpation, as discussed below, gives additional information on the presence of a cystocele, rectocele, or prolapse of the uterus.

Bimanual Pelvic Examination

The uterus and adnexa are palpated by the bimanual procedure, which involves placing two examining fingers in the vagina and a hand on the abdomen. The hand should move at least three-quarters of the way to the umbilicus to assure that all the organs to be palpated are brought within reach of the intravaginal fingers. If the hand is too close to the symphysis pubis, the abdominal wall is pressed down in front of the uterus, and one is unable to feel the intrapelvic structures (Fig. 12-4A). Opinion is divided as to whether the intrapelvic portion of the examination should be done with the right or the left hand. This author believes the examiner should use the hand with which she feels she can best palpate the internal organs. Indeed, the examiner may find that to achieve a thorough examination, it may often be necessary to change the intrapelvic hand, since the adnexal regions can often be felt best with the hand of the same side, for example, right hand for right adnexal region. Also, there are differences of opinion as to whether one or two fingers should be used intravaginally. It is advisable for the examiner to be skilled in the use of the one-finger examination in order not to be handicapped in the examination of the virginal or elderly woman. However, whenever possible, the examiner is encouraged to use the two-finger technique because it permits a longer reach into the fornices and more thorough palpation of the internal genitalia. As with other skills, the examiner develops expertise in the bimanual examination only with considerable experience in doing it.

Helping the woman remain relaxed during the bimanual examination will definitely increase the likelihood of a thorough examination. Encourage her to breathe slowly through her mouth, relax her abdominal muscles and the abductor muscles of the thighs, and to keep her knees as far apart as possible. The examiner begins with gentle pressure on the abdomen to prevent tightening; deeper palpation follows as the woman becomes accustomed to the palpation. She should continue to be informed of the examiner's actions and of what she will be experiencing. She will experience some pressure, but, unless abnormalities exist, she should not experience pain if she is relaxed.

Before the lubricated fingers are introduced into the vagina, spread the labia apart with the other hand to avoid the discomfort of pulling pubic hair into the vagina. The examining hand is held with the palmar side superior, the thumb is hyperextended, the third and fourth fingers are completely flexed, and the first and second fingers are extended straight. With the fingers intravaginal, any

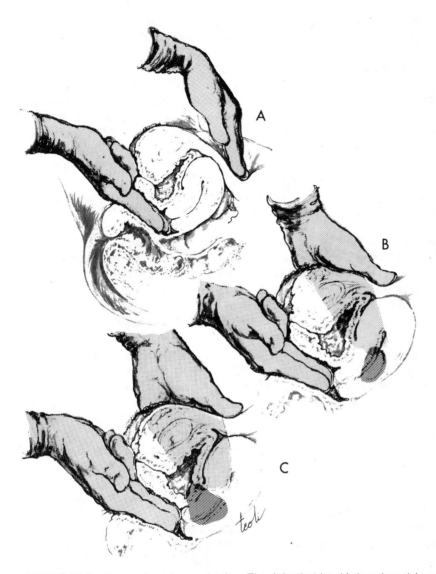

FIGURE 12-4. Bimanual pelvic examination. The abdominal hand brings the pelvic contents to the intravaginal fingers. A. Palpation of the uterus. B. Palpation of the right ovary. C. Palpation of the right parametrial tissues. (Reprinted from Judge and Zuidema [1].)

firmness, tenderness, induration from scars, or adhesions present can be felt. The amount of relaxation of the vaginal walls can be noted. Congenital abnormalities are quickly evident.

By maintaining slight pressure against the posterior portion of the vagina, the examiner avoids pressure on the bladder, which is normally sensitive. Inflammation of the bladder or bladder neck causes marked sensitivity on palpation. If the bladder is tender, there is frequently an associated reference of pain to the region of the umbilicus. The normally smooth bladder should be checked for tumor induration or stones. Though the anterior rectal wall and the rectovaginal septum may be examined at this time, a better evaluation can be made later by the rectovaginal examination.

The cervix will be easily palpable. Note its size, shape, position, mobility, regularity, and consistency. In the normal adult, the length of the cervix is one-half the size of the uterine body. The external os of the cervix is normally small (3 to 5 mm) in diameter. Normally, the cervix feels like a firm, smooth rounded button with a central depression. Invasion by a carcinoma makes the cervix hard and gives it a granular feeling. Nabothian follicles are felt as small, firm nodules. Cervical polyps feel like soft, spongy masses. Lacerations, especially from childbirth, may be responsible for areas of deformity.

The position and direction in which the cervix may point are variable. As a general rule, the cervix points the opposite way from the fundus, so that in the normal position the cervix points posteriorly from the top of the anterior vaginal wall, and the fundus points anteriorly. If the cervix points anteriorly, the fundus will most often be retroverted and found in the cul-de-sac, a condition occurring in 20 percent of adult women. [2, p. 322]. The normal cervix lies in the midplane of the pelvis with no displacement from the normal axis of the vagina, which is downward and backward. Changes in the axis and position of the cervix are usually caused by a tumor or an intrapelvic organ displacing the body of the uterus as well as the cervix. Normally, the cervix is freely movable for 2 to 3 cm in any direction. Motion of the cervix should not produce pain. Malignant infiltration or pelvic inflammatory disease may cause fixation of the cervix.

The position, size, shape, consistency, and mobility of the uterus should be determined. With the vaginal fingers placed in the posterior fornix, it should be possible to push the uterus forward and upward while the abdominal hand palpates for the fundus in the midline above the symphysis. A circular motion of the abdominal hand helps in penetrating the normal resistance of the abdominal wall. The normal, nonpregnant uterus is approximately 5 to 6 cm in length, with a smooth, firm surface. Softening of the lower uterine segment is an early indication of pregnancy (Hegar's sign). Irregular enlargement of the uterine body is suggestive of fibroid tumors. In either anteflexion or retroversion, the uterine body should be freely movable. The woman may experience some discomfort when attempts are made to move the retroverted uterus, but this should not occur with the anteflexed uterus (Fig. 12-4A).

Palpation of the adnexa is the most difficult part of the pelvic examination, especially for the beginner and occasionally for the expert. The normal tube is usually not palpable, and in many instances, neither is the normal ovary. This is particularly true in obese women. The ovary is about 3 by 4 cm in size, soft in texture, and normally sensitive to pressure. It lies deep in the pelvis above the lateral fornix of the vagina and is best palpated by the vaginal fingers. To palpate the woman's right ovary, the abdominal hand is brought forward and inward just inside the anterior superior iliac spine while applying deep pressure in a direction slightly toward the midline. At the same time, the vaginal fingers in the lateral fornix should be directed slightly laterally and anteriorly to feel the ovary being pressed toward the palmar surface of the vaginal fingers by the abdominal hand. The same movements are employed in examining the left ovary on the other side. However, if the examiner is not satisfied with her examination of the left ovary, she may wish to change hands, using the left fingers intravaginally and the right hand on the abdomen. Any significant enlargement of the ovary, abnormal tenderness, masses, or indurations should be noted (Fig. 12-4B). When the normal tube is palpated medially to the ovary, it is approximately 4 mm in diameter, and has the consistency of a piece of rubber tubing. Marked tenderness of the adnexa is a characteristic finding in acute inflammatory changes caused by tuboovarian infections. In such instances, the tube and ovary usually cannot be differentiated by palpation but appear to be a single, tender, indurated area.

The parametrium (tissue beside the cervix and lower segment of the corpus of the uterus) is usually pliable, soft, and nontender. This tissue is palpable in the lateral and posterior fornices of the vagina. It contains the vascular supply and the lymphatics which drain the cervix; therefore it is indurated and tender if the cervix is inflamed (Fig. 12-4C).

Before removing the intravaginal fingers, the hand should be rotated and fingers pressed into the cul-de-sac to check for the presence of masses or any irregularities.

Rectovaginal Abdominal Examination

The pelvic examination is completed by rectovaginal abdominal palpation (Fig. 12-5). The middle finger is gently inserted in the rectum and the index finger into the vagina. The rectovaginal septum can be palpated, and nodules, scarring, or induration noted. The vaginal posterior fornix and cul-de-sac can be better evaluated between rectal and vaginal fingers. With pressure from above, using the abdominal hand, the posterior wall of the uterus may be palpated with the rectal finger. By moving both fingers laterally, the adnexa and parametrial tissues may be palpated again.

For the young woman experiencing her first pelvic examination, the sensation she experiences on removal of the examiner's rectal finger may closely resemble the feeling of defecation. Telling her to anticipate this sensation will allay any fear that she, in fact, may have expelled some stool.

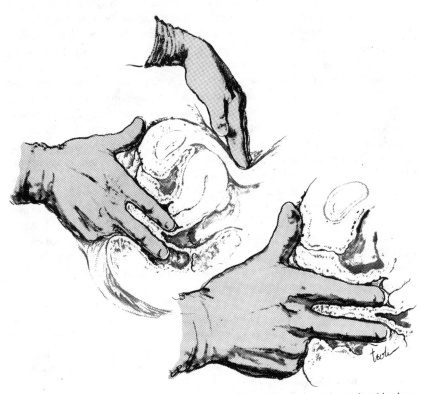

FIGURE 12-5. Rectovaginal abdominal examination. Indicates how the perineal body may be depressed to allow deeper entry into the pelvis. Note that one finger is inserted into the vagina and one into the rectum. (Reprinted from Judge and Zuidema [1].)

THE POSTMENOPAUSAL WOMAN

The health professions are becoming increasingly aware of the special problems experienced by the postmenopausal woman. This seems to be due both to the increasing number of women in this category and to a willingness to deal with conditions that previously were accepted as a normal part of aging for which treatment was believed to be of no benefit. In the gynecologic appraisal of the postmenopausal woman, the nurse should evaluate changes, both in the perineum and throughout the entire body, that may be resulting from the lowered estrogen level of menopause. These changes are the normal physiologic results of aging. In some cases, simple actions like using a lubricant during intercourse to decrease menopausal dyspareunia can offer some relief. In other situations, the knowledge that the changes one is experiencing are normal is sufficient to allay a woman's fears.

Systemic effects which the examiner should evaluate are related primarily to bone structure and the vascular system. A decreased serum estrogen level has been shown to increase the rate of osteoporosis, which may be responsible for the frequent complaint of back pain from the postmenopausal woman. Similarly, the changes in estrogen and follicle-stimulating hormone levels upset the balanced hormonal control of the vascular system, thus giving "hot flashes" a definite physiologic basis. Hypertension may also occur, as estrogen seems to have an inhibiting effect on the development of atherosclerosis.

Observing changes of appearance and structure, one sees atrophy and loss of fullness in breast tissue as well as in the genital area. The atrophy of breast tissue and muscular supports allows the breasts to sag and the nipples to drop far below the fourth intercostal space. The vulva loses its contour and becomes thin, due to reabsorption of fatty tissue. The vaginal mucosa becomes thinner and smoother, while the vagina decreases in length and width. With increased fibrotic tissue, much of its elasticity and ability to expand are lost. This loss of expansion may necessitate the use of only one finger intravaginally during a bimanual examination. In appearance the vaginal folds have disappeared, and the epithelium has a thin, velvety appearance. Examination of the uterus and adnexa will reveal a smaller and firmer uterus and cervix, resulting from tissue hypoplasia. The ovaries and tubes atrophy also and will be nonpalpable.

There are several alterations frequently seen in this age group. *Atrophic vaginitis* is a nonspecific vaginal infection in which the epithelium is frequently spotted with small petechiae. If this condition is exaggerated enough to result in shrinking and fibrosis, it is known as kraurosis vulvae. The white, slightly raised plaques of leukoplakia are also seen commonly in the postmenopausal group. Kraurosis vulvae and leukoplakia frequently occur together.

The postmenopausal woman may also develop a prolapsing or outpouching of the mucous membrane of the urethra. When the membrane is prolapsed to any extent, it frequently becomes infected, inflamed, and tender.

Weakening of the vaginal walls, as well as of the broad and round ligaments supporting the uterus, occurs to differing degrees in this age group, but many have some degree of uterine prolapse or development of a cystocele, rectocele, or enterocele.

The nurse may often find it worthwhile to explore with a women her expectations or reactions to menopause. Numerous, inaccurate "old wives' tales" still exist about "the change." This time in one's life often involves many changes, but it need not be a depressing experience. Understanding why physiologic alterations are occurring should help one accept them.

NURSING IMPLICATIONS

It seems obvious that the gynecologic appraisal involves more than just the actual pelvic examination. It provides an excellent opportunity for health teaching, as well as for giving the woman a means of discussing concerns that may be related to the female-male relationship and interpersonal relationships within a family or with close associates. She should have the opportunity, if desired, to discuss her feelings or concerns about her sexuality, her role in society, her role as a wife, her role as a mother in helping adolescent daughters deal with their own evolving sexuality, and her reactions as she anticipates and experiences menopause and postmenopause.

Even though the general public is becoming increasingly knowledgeable about health matters, the nurse should not miss opportunities to emphasize important areas of health teaching. The opportunity given by the gynecologic examination enables her to stress the necessity for regular examinations of the breasts — which mothers should teach to daughters as soon as breast development begins — perineal cleanliness, and regular pelvic examinations and Papanicolaou smears — all practices that should be started by their daughters by the mid-teens or certainly by the late adolescent years. The importance of the nurse's role in these areas of health teaching cannot be overemphasized.

REFERENCES

1. Judge, R. D., and Zuidema, G. D. (Eds.).   *Methods of Clinical Examination: A Physiologic Approach* (3rd ed.). Boston: Little, Brown, 1974.
2. Prior, J. A., and Silberstein, J.   *Physical Diagnosis: The History and Examination of the Patient* (4th ed.). St. Louis: Mosby, 1973.

SUGGESTED READINGS

Behrman, S. J., and Gosling, J. R. G.   *Fundamentals of Gynecology* (2nd ed.). New York: Oxford University Press, 1966. Pp. 413-431.

DeGowin, E., and DeGowin, R.   *Bedside Diagnostic Examination* (2nd ed.). New York: Macmillan, 1969. Pp. 239-250, 583-604.

Kampmeier, R., and Blake, T.   *Physical Examination in Health and Disease* (4th ed.). Philadelphia: Davis, 1970. Pp. 269-284.

DETECTION OF ALTERATIONS IN NEUROMUSCULAR FUNCTIONING

13

Margie J. Van Meter
Elisa A. Diehl

GLOSSARY

active range of motion Limits of motion through which a joint may be moved by those muscles which cross the joint.

ankylosis Complete loss of motion of a joint.

aphasia Loss of the power of expression by speech, writing, or signs, or of comprehending spoken or written language, due to injury or disease of the higher cerebral centers concerned with expression and comprehension.

arthritis Inflammation of a joint.

ataxia Failure of muscular coordination; irregularity of muscular action.

atrophy Wasting away of or diminution in the size of muscle.

bursa Potential space often filled with fluid found between tissue layers which move upon each other.

cavus foot Foot deformity in which a very high arch is present.

chorea Constant rapid and jerky, but well-coordinated involuntary movements.

clonus Muscle spasm in which contraction and relaxation alternate in rapid succession.

consensual Similar reaction of both pupils to a stimulus applied to only one.

contractures Fibrosis of tissues supporting a joint, or disorders of the muscle fibers, limiting normal motion of the joint.

contralateral Pertaining to the opposite side.

crepitation Grating or crackling noise produced by rubbing together the ends of a fractured bone.

decerebrate posturing Hypertonic extension of the legs, internal rotation of the shoulders, arms extended at the elbows, and hyperpronated fingers hyperextended. Legs are extended at hip and knee, with plantar flexion of ankles and toes.

decorticate posturing Spontaneous spasms of rigidity consisting of flexion of the arm, wrist, and fingers, with adduction of the upper extremity and extension, internal rotation, and plantar flexion in the lower extremity.

dermatome The area of skin supplied with sensory nerve fibers by a single posterior spinal root.

dorsiflexion Backward flexion or bending.

dysarthria Imperfect articulation in speech.

dysphagia Difficulty in swallowing.

dysphasia Incomplete degree of aphasia.

eversion Position achieved by turning a part away from the midline of the body.

extinction Failure to perceive one of two identical bilateral simultaneous stimuli; if sensory perception is otherwise intact, extinction or suppression may indicate parietal cortex dysfunction.

fasciculation Visible spontaneous contraction of a number of muscle fibers supplied by a single motor nerve filament.

graphesthesia Sense by which figures or numbers written on the skin are recognized.

hemiparesis Muscle weakness affecting one side of body.

inversion Position achieved by turning a part toward the midline of the body.

ipsilateral Pertaining to the same side.

joint effusion Excessive fluid within a joint.

kyphosis Curvature of the spine, the convexity of which is posterior.

language Systematic means of communicating ideas or feelings by the use of conventionalized signs, gestures, marks, or especially articulated vocal sounds.

lower motor neuron Peripheral neurons whose cell bodies lie in the ventral gray columns of the spinal cord and whose terminations are in the skeletal muscles.

meniscus Fibrocartilaginous structure found between the articular surfaces of certain joints.

nystagmus Involuntary repetitive rapid movement of the eyeball.

paresis Weakness or partial paralysis.

paresthesia Abnormal sensation such as burning or prickling.

passive range of motion Limits of motion through which a joint may be moved without use of the muscles which cross the joint.

plegia Complete paralysis. *hemiplegia* Paralysis of one side of the body and the limbs on that side. *paraplegia* Paralysis of the legs and lower part of the body, caused by disease or injury of the spinal cord. *quadriplegia* Paralysis of all four limbs.

pronation Position of the forearm achieved by turning the palm down; position of the foot achieved by turning the sole down.

proprioception Perception of movements and position of the body and joints.

sensory level Level below which there is a decrease or loss of sensation corresponding to the level of dysfunction of the spinal cord.

stereognosis Faculty of perceiving and understanding the form and nature of objects by the sense of touch.

supination Position of the forearm achieved by turning the palm up; position of the foot achieved by turning the sole up.

supine Position of lying on the back, face upward.

tic Spasmodic movement or twitching, as of the face.

tremor Involuntary trembling or quivering.

upper motor neuron Neuron in the cerebral cortex which conducts impulses from the motor cortex to the motor nuclei of the cranial nerves or to the ventral gray columns of the spinal cord.

The intent of this chapter is to help the nurse practitioner determine abnormal from normal responses in the neuromuscular physical appraisal of the patient; to monitor for progression or regression of symptoms of neuromuscular alterations; and to be able to describe the normal and the abnormal clearly. It is not intended that the content presented here will enable the nurse examiner to localize lesions. Additional knowledge is needed to correlate sensory changes, motor weaknesses, pathological reflexes, and the patient's subjective symptoms, which is essential in localizing the site of the lesion in the nervous system.

To achieve the intent of the chapter the basic parameter will be identified and a detailed description of each manuever used for these tests will be given. This approach has been used for the following reasons: There are few nurses skilled in the neuromuscular examination to serve as preceptors, so the nurse developing her skills needs textual references to help her analyze her particular problems in technique and to develop her skills with a minimum of direct supervision. The preceptor can then be used to validate the interpretation given to the patient's responses. The nurse can become confident in evaluating the responses elicited in testing because she has learned how to examine the patient carefully.

The patient who is a vague historian and with vague complaints will then not remain such an enigma to the nurse who is skilled in obtaining and evaluating objective data. When a patient coming for evaluation of his hypertension regimen who has had a benign brain tumor removed complains of a headache and nonspecific left shoulder and left ankle symptoms, the nurse can systematically assess objective functioning and symptoms and be comfortable in referring or not referring him to the physician.

MENTAL STATUS

The higher cerebral functions of orientation, mentation, and language are a beginning consideration in the neurologic examination. It is necessary to determine whether or not alterations in these functions have occurred, so that their effect on responses will be recognized and misinterpretation of the responses avoided.

Orientation and Memory

Orientation and memory can be ascertained by the behavior and answers given during the history-taking interview. If the patient's behavior is suggestive of confusion or forgetfulness, further investigations should be made in these areas. Tact is required when the mental incapacities of an alert person are being considered or exposed. The patient might be asked if he has noticed any difficulty with his memory before he is asked if he remembers your name, or what your role is, or what day, month, or year it is. It is helpful to begin with an explanatory statement to the alert patient indicating that you are aware of the simplicity of the questions you are going to ask but for the sake of thoroughness, you want him to respond to them.

Recall ability is tested by asking the patient why and on what day he came to the hospital, who visited him last night, or what he had for breakfast. The patient who cannot answer these questions may still be able to recall where he was born and other events of the distant past because remote memory may be intact.

Specific exercises can be utilized for testing recall and concentration. Give the patient an address, a color, and an object to remember. Have him repeat them immediately and instruct him to remember them. Later in the interview ask him to recall them.

A series of randomly selected digits may be given at the rate of one per second. A normal person can repeat a series of six to seven digits in order and a series of four digits in reverse order.

Direct testing can also include the serial 7 test. In this test the patient is asked to subtract 7 from 100, then 7 from the remainder (93), then 7 from 93, and so on. Prior mathematical skills irrespective of education must be taken into account when evaluating the patient's performance.

Estimation of intellectual abilities can be made from the patient's vocabulary, the way he presents material having to do with his illness, his occupation and activities and from direct questioning. Included in the factors that influence testing results in this area are the ability to conceptualize, the level of education, life experiences, and social and cultural background. It is expected that a person can name several past presidents of the United States in order and name five large cities and five countries.

Interpretation of sayings such as "Cheaper by the dozen," or "A stitch in time saves nine" indicates the level of ability to understand and to make abstractions. Persons with impaired mentation will make literal interpretations or will be unable to do much more than rephrase the words. Cultural and social factors may influence the patient's interpretation of the saying. Educational level also can be an important factor in developing a person's ability to conceptualize.

Grammatical structure and vocabulary can be observed during the interview. There may be only simple words used. Sentence structure may consist only of essential words, e.g., subject and verb, or may be more complex, with many descriptive words and phrases included. Talking may consist only of a minimal response to questions asked or may be spontaneous, with additional information voluntarily supplied.

Language Function

Assessing the ability of a person to communicate with others is necessary but complex. In order to determine the presence of language impairment, the patient's ability to communicate must first be determined.

The two main components of speech are the ability to receive incoming verbal or written symbols and the ability to communicate, or to send messages. Between these receptive and expressive components is the interpretation of the message. Language symbols are received by the eyes and ears and sent to the postcentral gyrus of the cortex. If the person is right-handed (and in some who are left-handed) the left cerebral hemisphere is the more developed than the right and serves a major function in the interpretation of spoken and written language. The right cerebral hemisphere may be more developed in the left-handed person. Verbal expression is achieved by association tracts from the left postcentral gyrus to the motor strip or precentral gyrus. The words are then articulated by movements of the jaw musculature, vocal chords, and tongue and coordinated respiratory movements.

A variety of tests may be used to evaluate a person's ability to receive and understand certain types of symbolic language such as letters and words. Before testing, it is important to know the patient's level of education and reading ability. Graduation from high school does not imply equivalent reading ability. How fluent is the person in the language in which he is being tested? The patient's visual acuity is assessed so that if corrective lenses are needed he is wearing them during the testing. Knowledge of the patient's hearing acuity is a significant factor because if he is hard of hearing and the examiner does not know it, it could be misinterpreted as an inability to comprehend.

Methods of Testing Language Function. The following tests will indicate whether or not the patient has basic language skills:

1. Point to common objects, such as pencil, clock, pillow, book, chair, and have the patient name each one. Use only single nouns and verbs.
2. Have the patient match printed and written words with pictures.
3. Have the patient read some simple words, both printed and written.
4. Write out some simple commands and ask the patient to read them and perform the activities, for example, "Tap right foot"; "Make a face."
5. Give simple verbal command for the patient to follow, such as, "Stand up"; "Bend your leg"; "Shake my hand."
6. Give a complex verbal command for patient to follow, such as "Look at the ceiling and raise your arm"; "Left hand on right knee"; "Right hand on head."

It should be noted that when there is impairment of the cerebral centers for comprehension, the ability of a person to deal with abstractions is impaired. To facilitate testing of such patients, concrete objects associated with present circumstances should be used as much as possible.

Tests may be used to evaluate the ability of the patient to express himself verbally and in writing. For example he might be asked to write or verbally give a description of an object or a place. The nurse examiner already will have had some indication of the expressive abilities of the patient because, when testing for reception of communication, a verbal response is sometimes required.

In eliciting verbal responses it is necessary to avoid questions that are used so often in daily life that the answer is automatic; for example, "How are you?" "Fine." Some routine questions can be answered by patients who do not understand the words or are unable to express what they really want to say simply by timing of the question. For example, "Hello, how are you?" is usually said almost immediately on meeting a person, not in the leave-taking. Some persons who cannot express their thoughts because of brain impairment use what is called automatic speech, in which they can sing familiar songs, count, answer questions that are frequently asked, and give their name and address.

The character of the speech patterns should also be appraised. Does the patient initiate conversation and ask questions spontaneously? Does he speak in a monotone? Does the voice have a nasal quality? Does he use simple, single noun and verb sentences, or are his thoughts expressed in more complex sentences?

Responsiveness

Impairment of consciousness occurs on a continuum. The descending order of the continuum is from spontaneous verbal and motor activity and attentive cooperation to complete absence of any motor or reflex responses. Deterioration or improvement of consciousness occurs within the sequence [3]. With deterioration, the alert patient becomes less able to answer questions, slower, and more difficult to arouse. First, there is a general uncooperativeness and then incapacity to cooperate.

Disorientation may follow or coincide with the loss of ability to cooperate. Disorientation is progressive and in a consistent pattern. First, the patient is disoriented in relation to time, to place, to person, from others, and then from self. The inability to follow simple commands, e.g., "Open your mouth," "Close your eyes," "Squeeze my fingers," usually occurs after disorientation to person. Beyond this level of function it is necessary to use painful rather than verbal or auditory stimuli. Pain can be induced by applying pressure over the styloid process in the neck, on the supraorbital nerve, the root of the fingernail, or the periosteal surfaces of bone or by squeezing muscle bellies or tendons. The supraorbital nerve is located in the eyelid against the supraorbital bone, just above the globe of the eye. Pinching the biceps, Achilles tendon, or the pectoralis muscle of the upper chest may be sufficiently painful to elicit a response. At first, responses to pain are somewhat purposeful; there is resistance or withdrawal and grimacing. Purposeless responses of chewing or hyperventilating are indicative of extremely depressed levels of consciousness as are decerebrate and decorticate posturing. When motor responses to pain cannot be elicited, the corneal and cough reflexes may still be present.

When monitoring a patient for signs of improvement or deterioration of consciousness, it is important to be aware of where he is on the continuum and what direction the progression is. Some examiners record the progression on the continuum by dividing the continuum into stages or levels of consciousness such as lethargy, semicoma, and coma. These terms lead to ambiguity and the need for interpretation. It is better to describe the phenomena observed or elicited from the patient and the type and amount of stimulation needed to elicit the response. This permits comparisons of the patient's responsiveness over time and between examiners and easier recognition of changes in the patient's responsiveness.

When examining an unresponsive patient one should always be looking for the cause of the altered consciousness. The breath odors, signs of trauma or of hemiparesis, previous illnesses, or drug use are clues to the possible cause.

Muscle strength, blood pressure, pulse, respiratory pattern, temperature, and pupillary light reflex are correlated with the level of responsiveness to recognize and evaluate increasing intracranial pressure. Changes in orientation, arousability, and muscle strength are likely to be the first signs of increasing intracranial pressure in the patient who is on the alert, oriented, cooperative end of the continuum. A subtle hemiparesis can be first detected by testing for ulnar drift. This is done by instructing the patient to put his arms out in front with the elbows straight and the fingers spread and then to keep his eyes closed. He holds this position for approximately a minute, and the examiner observes for flexing and internal rotation of the elbow. Normally, a person can hold the position without flexing of the elbows, but one with hemiparesis cannot do so. The patient with marked muscular weakness of an arm will not be able to hold the arm up at all, and the patient with hysterical or functional weakness will let the arm drop straight down with the elbow straight.

The effect of increasing intracranial pressure on the blood pressure, pulse, respirations, temperature, and pupillary light reflex is shown in Figure 13-1. Fixed, dilated pupils and cessation of respirations are the end states.

The patient should be roused to his fullest level of response each time he is evaluated. This is likely to be after activities are done with him or for him, or it may be achieved by a brisk massage around the mouth. The examiner should be careful to maintain the patient's dignity and be cognizant of the sequelae of the stimulation (i.e., bruising) and the need to clarify to family members the purpose of the vigorous stimulation.

If neurologic examination is needed to determine the presence of increasing intracranial pressure, it must be done thoroughly to establish a baseline for detection of deterioration or improvement and for the prescription of therapy. Delay in instituting therapy for increasing intracranial pressure may have dire consequences.

MOTOR FUNCTION EXAMINATION

For a thorough inspection of motor functioning it is important that the patient be undressed except for a loincloth. Women may also wear chest covering.

Muscle Bulk

Muscles are tested in pairs. The size, contour, and strength of the muscle on one side is immediately compared with the one on the opposite side. A general comparison of body contour is made with the average normal figure of like sex and age. A concept of normal muscle bulk is gained with experience.

The limbs are positioned symmetrically for comparison, and the muscle contours are inspected during contraction and rest. When there is suspicion of atrophy, measurements should be made of the circumferences of the limbs bilaterally at their maximum girth. Corresponding points should be accurately marked for measuring above and below the patella, the elbow, and other appropriate bony prominences. The tension applied to the tape measure must be the same for both sides. The points at which the measurements are taken, as well as the circumferences, should be recorded for evaluation of the progression of the atrophy. Differences of less than 1 cm are not significant.

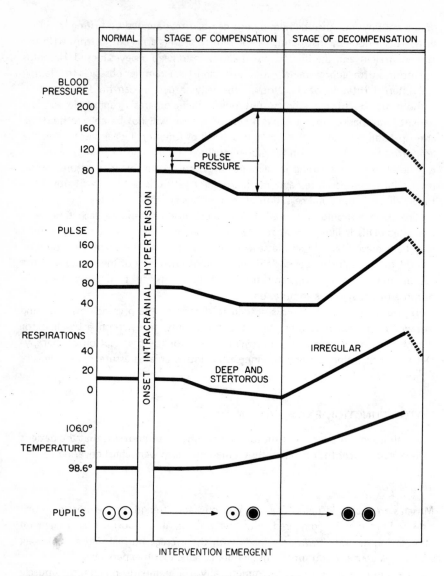

FIGURE 13-1. Increasing intracranial pressure signs.

Asymmetrical muscle wasting is not difficult to detect, but symmetrical wasting is easily missed. Hypertrophied muscle will be seen occasionally, but atrophy and weakness occur much more frequently. Wasting may be from lower motor neuron lesions, myopathy, or disuse from paralysis due to upper motor neuron lesion or joint pain, as in arthritis.

Muscle Tone

Muscle tone, or tonus, is the slight muscular resistance felt by the examiner when the relaxed limb is passively moved through its range of motion. It is the end result of all neural activity from many sources. The qualitative evaluation of tonus is difficult and largely a matter of personal experience.

The patient is instructed to relax and to let the limb being examined "hang loose." This is difficult to do, and to achieve the desired degree of relaxation it may be necessary to divert the patient's attention. Each limb in turn is palpated, passively shaken, and moved through flexion, extension, and rotation. The range of motion is done both rapidly and slowly while feeling the degree of resistance. Normal tone has a mild even resistance to movement through the entire range. It is a quality of resilience rather than complete flabbiness. The swing of extremities is determined by tonus. Swing can be tested by the examiner flipping the patient's arms out from the hips and allowing them to drop, and by raising the patient's legs and letting them drop while the patient sits on the side of the table. The duration, regularity, and pattern of the swing are observed. The normal limb swings freely with a regular motion like a pendulum, which decreases in a steady even manner.

Muscle tone may be increased (hypertonicity) or decreased (hypotonicity). The alteration may be general or focal, with tonus different in separate muscle groups. In hypertonicity the increased resistance may be predominantly in extensor muscles, in flexor muscles, or in both; there is increased flexion of joints, muscle bellies stand out more, and limbs at rest tend to remain in a fixed posture. Hypertonicity is associated with brisk reflexes and is characteristic of upper motor neuron lesions. Spasticity and rigidity are manifestations of hypertonicity. Sudden passive movements of the joints are initially met with considerable resistance, evidenced by spasms, but when overcome, the movement continues more easily. *Rigidity* is a steady contraction of flexors and extensors which causes increased resistance to passive movement throughout the full range of motion in any direction.

In hypotonicity the muscle feels soft and flabby, there is a looseness of extremities on shaking them, and the joint can be moved beyond the usual range of motion. The extremity tends to assume a position dictated by gravity. There is loss of the normal slight flexion of joints, and there is a flattened appearance of the muscle body instead of the rounded contour. Lower motor neuron lesions and muscle disease are causes of hypotonicity. The patient complains of such symptoms as slowness, dragging of the foot, and lack of arm swing in disturbances affecting muscle tone.

Muscle Strength

Ability and confidence in detecting muscular weakness, especially if minimal, can be attained only by testing a variety of patients with muscular weaknesses and normal strength. Practice is the only means of gaining a feel for what is normal range. When testing muscle strength, it is the muscle fibers and their innervation that are being tested. Knowledge of muscle innervation is essential in pinpointing neurologic lesions, and knowledge of the function of specific muscles is needed to understand abnormal gaits and muscular function deficits. The use of muscle and nerve anatomy charts can help one to determine and describe better which muscles, peripheral nerves, and spinal cord segments are involved.

Muscular strength can be tested and described with limited knowledge of specific muscles and nerves by the function performed in reference to a particular joint. The functions are flexion, extension, abduction (away from midline), adduction (toward midline), supination (face up, palm up), pronation (face down), and rotation. The muscle and joint functions are tested in a cephalocaudal (head to foot) order from the shoulders down to the elbows, wrists, hands, hips, knees, ankles, and feet (see Table 13-1).

For efficiency and assistance in localizing the lesion it is helpful to develop a scheme for examining muscle strength, tone, size, and reflexes that begins at the head and neck and moves downward to the arms and then the legs.

During the motor examination there should be unobstructed observation of the patient, so that the muscles and joints can be inspected, palpated, and tested for strength. The patient should be in the position that gives him the greatest body stability. In the routine examination, the patient should be seated. Symmetrical muscle pairs are directly compared (i.e., one arm is tested then the other) for relative strength. Proximal and distal muscle groups are tested. If the patient experiences muscular difficulty under certain conditions such as cold or exertion, these conditions should be reproduced with cold water or repeated movements of the involved muscles. The examiner generally tries to match strength with the patient, using the principles of leverage and the fact that muscles are strongest when they act from their shortest (flexed) length.

Generally, the patient is instructed to hold a position of strength and to resist with maximal effort the pressure applied by the examiner and to continue to resist until instructed to stop. The opposing pressure is applied gradually and is continuously increased to the maximum or until the patient is overpowered. The comprehending, cooperative patient, with either strong or weak muscles, will have a smooth steady counterpressure, and the joint will move as the examiner varies the pressure applied.

The patient with an hysterical type of weakness is likely to have a jerky contraction, or sudden cessation of effort, or both. This abrupt giving way and lack of following through are major clues to functional (hysterical) weakness. Functional weakness of a leg may be detected by placing one's hands under the

Table 13-1. Muscle Strength Testing

Muscle Function	Patient's Movement	Examiner's Resistant Motion
Neck		
Flexors	Chin on chest	Fingertips against forehead;
Extensors	Head backward	palm of hand against occiput
Fingers		
Flexors (C 8)	Squeezes examiner's fingers hard; makes fist	Compares grips and attempts to withdraw to straighten fingers
Extensors (C 7)	Fingers out straight	Attempts finger flexion
Adduction (C 8– T 1)	Holds paper between adjacent fingers	Pulls paper
Abduction (C 8–T 1)	Fingers straight out and spread apart	Squeezes adjacent fingers together
Wrist		
Flexors	Flexes wrists	Tries to extend wrist
Extensors	Pronates forearm and cocks up wrist	Presses dorsum of hand to push wrist down
Elbow		
Flexors (biceps, C 5–6)	Flexes elbow 90° and attempts to bend more	Prevents flexion
Supinators (palm up) Pronators	Rotates wrist in one direction then the other	Resists efforts to rotate
Extensors (triceps, C 6–8)	Flexes elbow varying degrees and attempts to straighten	Prevents straightening
Shoulder		
Abduction (deltoid C 5–6)	Holds out upper arm horizontally	Attempts to depress elbow
Adduction	Holds upper arm close to chest	Attempts to raise elbow horizontally
Ankle		
Dorsiflexors (L 4–L 5)	Walks on heels; pulls foot and toes upward	Pulls downward on foot
Plantor flexors (S 1–S 2)	Walks on toes; push down	Pushes against bottom of foot
Knee		
Flexors (hamstring L 5–S 1)	Sitting: holds knee bent at 90° angle. Prone: Partly flexes knee and tries to flex further	Resists above ankle
Extensor (quadriceps L 3–4)	Squats; arises; slight flexion of knee and resists bending	Attempts to flex knee
Hip		
Flexors (L 2–L 3)	In bed; Raises leg about 45° and holds 15–20 seconds (wobbling or drifting downward indicates weakness). Sitting: Raises knee up	Downward pressure directly above knee
Extensors (L 4–L 5)	Ascends step, rising from squatting position	
Abductors (L 4–L 5)	Holds knees apart	Tries to approximate knees
Adductors (L 2–L 3)	Holds knees together tightly	Tries to separate knees
Trunk		
Abdominal	Rises from lying to sitting	
Back	Side or prone: Elevates leg or head	

supine patient's heels while instructing him to lift the weak leg. Normally, with unilateral leg weakness, there should be pressure felt from the heel of the unaffected leg as it is used for leverage if full effort is put forth to move the contralateral leg. Much urging is required to get any muscle contraction in nonorganic weakness.

To make the patient's record meaningful for examiners and useful in determining changes in muscle strength a standardized scale is used for grading muscle power [3].

Value	Functional Level
5	Full range of motion against gravity with full resistance.
4	Full range of motion against gravity with some resistance.
3	Full range of motion against gravity.
2	Full range of motion with gravity eliminated.
1	Palpable increase in muscle tension. No joint movement.
0	No evidence of contraction.

This scale is intended for lower motor neuron lesions and is only useful in the fully cooperative person, for it is based on the ability of a person to contract a muscle group with his maximum effort against applied resistance.

Contracture, pain, involuntary movements, spasticity, rigidity, ataxia, and deformity may all interfere significantly with evaluating muscle strength.

In the unconscious or demented patient, observations are made of his performance, noting, for example whether or not there are spontaneous movements or withdrawal in response to noxious stimuli, the presence or absence of muscle tone when dropping the lifted limb of the unconscious, and equal bilateral body responses.

The motor examination begins the moment the examiner meets the patient, as she observes how the patient walks, stands, sits, and performs other spontaneous activities. In the routine physical examination, the strength of a few movements is always sampled. These include the cranial nerves, elbow, wrist, hip, knee, and ankle flexors and extensors. Depending on the patient's history and physical findings much more may be done.

The patient who has muscle weakness will tend to enumerate specific functions which give him difficulty, such as turning a doorknob, rising from a chair, stumbling, chewing, or caring for hair, rather than stating vague complaints of being weak, tired, fatigued.

When muscle weakness is detected, the involved muscles are carefully inspected for atrophy or unusual bulk, tenderness, fasciculations, and tone.

Muscle weakness is indicative of pyramidal pathway disturbance in the cerebrum, brainstem, or spinal cord; in peripheral nerves; at the neuromuscular junction; or in the muscle itself.

The systematic assessment of the muscle groups as outlined above helps the nurse examiner to define specifically which muscle functions are weak and to grade the weakness. The nurse examiner is also concerned about the functional abilities of the patient for such things as activities of daily living. This is determined by observing the patient get out of bed, brush his teeth, dress, feed himself, and so on.

Joint Function

To examine an extremity is to study the elements of it — reflexes, muscles, joints, skin, subcutaneous tissue, and related vascular and nervous structures. Joint and bone examinations are integrated into the examination of each extremity. Any bony structure or joint (s) implicated by the patient's history or the physical findings should have a detailed examination.

Bones are assessed for angulation, masses, tenderness to palpation or percussion, and structural integrity. Joints are inspected and palpated, and bilateral comparisons are made of alignment, shape, circumference, range of motion, state of joint fluid (effusion), stability, scars, draining sinuses, warmth and redness of overlying skin, presence of swelling, wasting of adjacent muscles, and tenderness.

The patient is asked to move affected or selected joints through as full a range of motion as he can. If there are limitations, passive range of motion is done by the examiner. The limb is supported above and below the joint, and the patient's face is observed for expressions of pain during the test. Joint range of motion is estimated in terms of degrees of the arc of a circle. The neutral position (no flexion, no abduction, and so on) of the extremity or trunk is used as a starting point. It is considered 0 degrees. Any flexion, abduction, or hyperextension is measured in degrees from there. *Measuring and Recording of Joint Motion,* published by the American Academy of Orthopaedic Surgeons, contains criteria by which the measurements can be obtained for specific joints. A simple instrument called a goniometer helps one make more accurate measurements.

A variety of terms is used to describe deformities of the extremities. The use of the terms *varus* (toward midline) and *valgus* (away from midline) has been frequently confused. They are correct only for describing deformities. The terms *adduction* and *abduction* are used in descriptions both of deformities and normal range of motion. Deformities resulting from fractures are described by the relationship of the distal portion to the proximal. A "posterior dislocation of the elbow" means the ulna and radius is dislocated posterior to the humerus. The angulation of bone, such as might occur with a fracture, is sometimes described by the direction in which the apex of the abnormal angle points, i.e., posterior, lateral, medial, anterior. Proximal, middle, and distal contractures should be described in specific detail, e.g., "a flexion adduction contracture of left hip." Extremity lengths should be measured for objective comparisons when the examiner is uncertain of variations. The measurement is taken between two bony prominences, with the extremities in symmetrical, extended positions. The crest of the anterior superior iliac spines to the medial malleoli of the ankle are the lower extremity landmarks, and the acromion of the shoulder to the radial styloid projection above the thumb are landmarks for the arms.

Effusion, or increased synovial joint fluid, causes a uniform swelling of the joint and obliterates the normal landmarks. A sense of fluctuation can be felt. To elicit fluctuation in the knee, it is extended, and the pouch above the patella is squeezed toward the joint with one hand. In the presence of effusion this hand will feel an expanding impulse when the lateral aspects of the knee are squeezed with the opposite hand. Effused joints are usually held in flexion and attempts to extend it cause pain.

Roughened joint surfaces or bone fractures may produce a grating (crepitus) that can be heard or felt over the moving joint or fracture. Bony overgrowths (nodules) occasionally may be felt along the margins of large joints like the knee and the elbow or the distal phalanges of the fingers.

Flexibility of the upper spine is appraised by instructing or assisting the patient to tip his head backward (hyperextension) and forward (flexion), toward each shoulder, and then to turn it from side to side (rotation). Bending over to touch the toes and rotating the shoulders from the pelvis tests the flexibility of the lower spine. The patient should be able to accomplish these movements easily in the absence of disease and changes of aging.

Backache is an affliction frequently seen in today's society. Evaluation of the complaint is difficult because objective symptoms are often not found. This does not negate the symptom, and careful evaluation of spinal function and obtaining data on occupational and other activities provide salient clues to the probable cause and severity of the problem. Appraisal of spinal motion is done in conjunction with the examination of the upper and the lower extremities.

In radiculopathies (disease of the nerve roots), flexion, extension, and rotation of the cervical lumbosacral spine may produce pain, and movement may be limited in one or more directions. In compression of lumbar or sacral nerve roots from a herniated disc, the patient's pain may be reproduced by the straight leg raising test. With the patient supine, the legs are kept straight and raised one at a time by the examiner. The degree of leg elevation from the bed at which the patient feels pain, which leg is affected, and the site of the pain should be noted. Dorsiflexion of the foot by the examiner while the leg is raised to a 45° angle will stretch the nerve even more and may reproduce the pain that straight leg raising alone did not. Sharp pain radiating down the leg is indicative of sciatic nerve irritation; whereas the discomfort from muscle tightness is not. Back pain symptoms are correlated with the muscle strength, reflex, and sensory findings of the lower extremities.

When observing a side view of an erect, well-developed person with good postural habits, one should, figuratively speaking, be able to draw a perpendicular line that begins at the lobe of the ear, goes through the shoulder, the trochanter of the femur, the center of the knee, and to the front of the ankle. The spinal silhouette should have a gentle C curve of the cervical spine with the concavity posterior, the dorsal spine with a convex curve to the posterior, and the lumbar spine curving forward and then back at the sacral spine. The head should be held back and the chin up, so that the chin is not projected beyond the same line as the chest. The abdomen should be flat.

When viewed from the back the iliac crests should be at the same level and the shoulders squared and of equal height while the arms hang easily at the sides. The scapular wings should be even and move symmetrically, and the spinous processes of the vertebrae should be in a vertical line. Deviations from a straight vertical line may be seen more readily by putting a mark on each spinous process. Lateral curvature of the spine is called *scoliosis*; round shoulders and exaggerated posterior curvature of thoracic spine is called *kyphosis* and an increased lower back (lumbar) curvature is called *lordosis.*

Muscle Stretch Reflexes

Voluntary muscles contain stretch-sensitive receptors which, when stimulated by mechanical stretching, send impulses through the afferent fibers in peripheral nerves and dorsal roots to anterior horn cells of the spinal cord. The anterior horn cells are excited at the same cord segment and send efferent impulses via the anterior root and motor nerve to the same muscle, leading to a brief contraction of the muscle. This is a simple monosynaptic reflex that may be diminished or lost with interruptions of afferent (sensory) fibers. It is also diminished with extensive destruction of efferent (motor) fibers and anterior horn cells. Release of this monosynaptic reflex from the influence of higher levels of the pyramidal tract and cerebral motor cortex produces hyperreflexia (exaggerated reflexes). Extreme hyperreflexia leads to clonus.

Only a discrete mechanical stimulation (i.e. a quick blow of the reflex hammer) will elicit muscle stretch reflex (MSR). To produce a brisk and consistent stroke with the reflex hammer, it is held loosely between the thumb and index finger, and the swing is made from the wrist, allowing the hammer to fall by gravity against the tendon. The broad head of the hammer is used to strike accessible tendons (e.g., the Achilles) and the pointed end for smaller, less accessible tendons (e.g., the biceps). Complete relaxation of the patient and a proper degree of muscle tension are the other two factors that must accompany an adequate stretch stimulus to elicit consistent muscle stretch reflexes. These two factors are basically dependent on proper positioning of the patient and the extremity. When seated, the patient should be comfortable and have both the arms and legs in a relaxed position with the forearms on the thighs and the feet on the floor or dangling freely. With too little or too much muscle stretch, a reflex cannot be elicited. Usually, positioning midway between full extension and full flexion obtains the proper degree of tension. Practice helps in determining this degree.

If these measures do not produce muscle stretch reflexes, reinforcement techniques may help. These involve instructing the patient to contract muscles other than the one being tested. For instance, have him interlock his fingers and pull while the reflexes of the lower extremities are being tested, and squeeze the knees together while the upper extremities are tested.

The biceps, triceps, brachioradialis, patellar, Achilles tendons, and jaw reflexes are the common reflexes tested in general physical examinations. Methods of testing some of these reflexes are shown in Figure 13-2.

The biceps reflex (cervical nerves [C] 5 and 6) is tested by the examiner's placing the tip of his thumb or index finger over the biceps tendon at the antecubital space, pressing firmly to produce slight tension, then striking a sharp blow on the finger with the reflex hammer. The patient's arms should be positioned symmetrically. This is achieved in the recumbent patient by placing both hands in identical position on the abdomen. When the patient is sitting, his elbow is supported by the examiner's hand and his hand is placed on the examiner's forearm or the pronated forearm is placed on the patient's thigh. The reflex response is flexion of the arm (Fig. 13-2A).

The triceps reflex (C 6, 7, and 8) is tested on the supine patient with the forearm flexed on the anterior chest and the tendon struck directly above the elbow. With the patient in the seated position the arm may be supported at the wrist to change the muscle tension if no response is obtained with the arm resting on the thigh. This tendon is short and difficult to percuss without hitting muscle fibers too. The reflex response is extension of the arm (Fig. 13-2B).

The brachioradialis reflex (C 5 and 6) is tested by striking the distal radius just above the thumb with the patient's forearm midway between pronation and supination and the elbow at a right angle. The patient's hands are on the abdomen when he is in a recumbent position but on the knees or held by the examiner when the patient is sitting. The response is flexion of the forearm on the arm and usually also flexion of the fingers and hand [1] (Fig. 13-2C).

The quadriceps reflex (knee jerk) (lumbar nerves [L] 2, 3, and 4) is elicited by striking the tendon just below the patella when the patient is seated with legs dangling. The patient should sit far enough forward so the legs swing freely and the knees are apart. To help evaluate the extent of the response, the examiner's hand may be placed on the patient's knee. When the patient is supine, the knees are bent slightly (about 20°) by lifting the thighs, to create slight muscle stretch. The reflex response is quadriceps contraction and knee extension (Fig. 13-2E).

Achilles reflex testing (ankle jerk, sacral nerves [S] 1 and 2) requires that slight stretch be placed on the tendon. Several positions can be used. In all positions, slight dorsiflexion should be induced by gentle pressure on the ball of the foot. For access to the Achilles tendon of the bedfast patient, the foot and ankle can be placed on the opposite shin by flexing the knee and externally rotating the hip. With the prone patient the knees are bent to a 90° angle; the

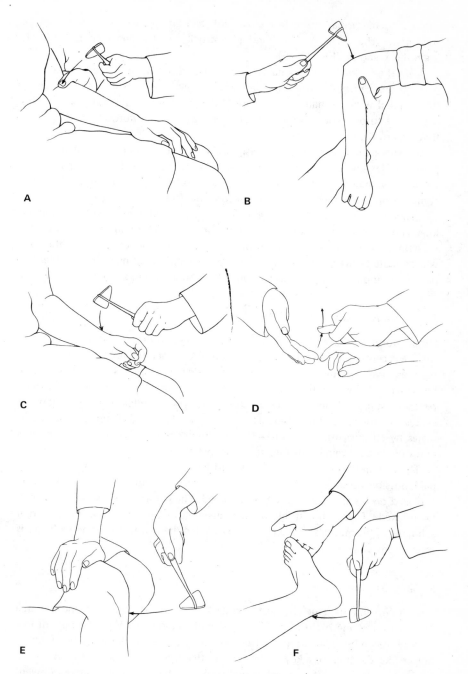

FIGURE 13-2. Technique of obtaining muscle stretch reflexes. (Figures 13-2, 13-3, 13-5, 13-6 reprinted from J. F. Simpson and K. R. Magee. *Clinical Evaluation of the Nervous System.* Boston: Little, Brown, 1973.)

ambulant patient may kneel in a chair with feet and ankles suspended over the edge of the chair. The Achilles tendon is struck directly, and plantar flexion is the reflex response (Fig. 13-2F).

Jaw reflex (pons, Vth Cranial Nerve) is elicited by having the jaw relaxed and partially opened with one finger pressing downward on the chin; the finger is then tapped with the hammer. Closure of the jaw is the response. Normally, this is difficult to obtain and so, if it is obtained without reinforcement, it is likely that hyperreflexia is present.

In general, if one receives no response when attempting to elicit a muscle stretch reflex, be sure to (1) strike the blow crisply, and (2) alter the muscle tension by adjusting the position of the extremity, changing the finger compression of the tendon or using reinforcement.

In hyperreflexic states of the legs, clonus may be elicited by slightly flexing the knee and then briskly jerking the foot upward and slightly outward and holding it. With the continued application of pressure to the sole of the foot, the foot will oscillate between flexion and extension. This will continue for as long as the pressure is applied. Only clonus sustained beyond a few jerks is pathological.

Superficial Reflexes

Other motor cortex and pyramidal tract reflexes can be elicited by stimulating surface receptors in skin. The abdominal reflex (upper and lower) is tested in all four quadrants with a brisk stroke toward the umbilicus. The response is movement of the umbilicus toward the quadrant stimulated. The supine relaxed position is used. Upper motor neuron lesions and abdominal distention are causes of absence of the reflex. The cremasteric (L 1 and 2) reflex is tested in males by stroking the inner surface of the upper thigh. The normal response is quick upward movement of the ipsilateral testicle.

The anal reflex (S 3, 4, and 5) should be evaluated when there is low back pain, possible cauda equina lesions, or sacral nerve root compression. The patient is placed on his side and the buttocks spread. The perianal area is then scratched or pricked. There should be an obvious quick contraction of the external sphincter. This may also be evaluated by feeling the contraction when a finger is inserted into the rectum.

Pathological Reflexes

Except in infants, the Babinski reflex is pathognomonic of motor area dysfunction of the brain or corticospinal pathway disease. With the patient in a relaxed, recumbent position and legs extended, a firm stroke is applied with an object like the thumb, a key, or an orange stick against the sole of the foot (Fig. 13-3). The stroke is begun at the lateral aspect of the heel, moved slowly upward toward the little toe, and then across the ball of the foot toward the large toe. The normal response is plantar flexion of the toes. The pathological Babinski

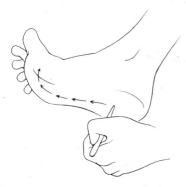

FIGURE 13-3.   Technique of eliciting the Babinski reflex. The sole is stroked firmly along the path indicated.

response consists of extension of the big toe and flexion and spreading of the small toes. Flexion of the leg may even occur. The response may be equivocal and therefore difficult to evaluate when there is voluntary withdrawal that is not pathological. The voluntary withdrawal is faster and associated with rapid withdrawal of the leg. The Babinski sign is slow and usually disappears quickly when stimulation ceases. The examiner should strive to achieve a consistent response. This may require varying the stroke pressure, speed, and length.

The Hoffmann reflex is tested by flicking the nail of the middle finger. Normally there is little if any response. In hyperreflexia there is a flexion of the thumb and finger.

Symmetrical reflexes should be compared immediately; e.g., one Achilles reflex is tested and then the other, for immediate comparison. Asymmetry and discrepancy between one part of the body and another is assessed. Any isolated reflex change, either hyporeflexia or hyperreflexia, requires consideration by the examiner and correlation with muscle bulk, strength, and sensory findings. Decrease of muscle stretch reflexes occurs when the reflex arc is interrupted. The interruption can be in the spinal cord, the sensory or motor nerves, or the muscle. Exaggerated reflexes frequently represent upper motor neuron disease located anywhere from the cerebral cortex to the appropriate anterior horn cell.

Reflexes are graded on a 0 to 4+ scale and recorded on a stick figure (Fig. 13-4).

Coordination and Equilibrium

Coordination and equilibrium are achieved by the integrative functioning of the cerebellum, posterior columns of the spinal cord, and the vestibular mechanism of the ear. Injury to the proprioceptive system, the receptors and nerve pathways for the sense of movement and position of body parts, will produce incoordination, ataxia, and imbalance.

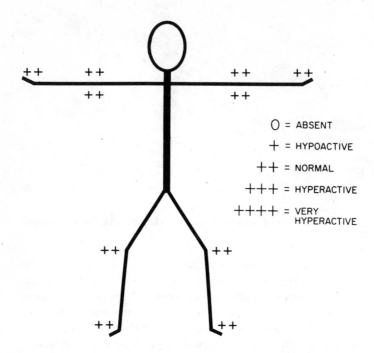

FIGURE 13-4. Stick figure for recording muscle strength reflexes.

Coordination. Coordination is the synergistic action of muscles functioning in proper sequence to produce a smooth, purposeful movement. Incoordination occurs because of improper programming of the involved muscles, which causes errors in the speed and the dexterity of movement as it is performed. These can be evaluated by the use of some simple tests.

The finger-to-nose test is performed with the patient in a sitting position with his arms extended forward; then, using alternating hands, the patient touches the nose with the forefinger and returns the arm to the extended position. This test is done first with the eyes open and then with the eyes closed. The patient should be observed for smooth movements and the maintenance of proper body posture.

Another test is forefinger approximations. The patient extends his arms out at the sides and then brings them foreward until the forefingers meet at the midline. This test is done first with the eyes open and then with the eyes closed.

Diadochokinesia, "or diametrically opposite hand movement," is evaluated using several different tests. With the patient in a sitting position, the palms of his hands are placed downward on top of the knees and he is then asked to alternate the hands rapidly from pronation to supination. The hands are compared for equality of movement. Another test is to have the patient place the heels of his hands on top of the knees and then ask him to tap his knees with his fingers, using a rapid motion. Coordination is also demonstrated by touching the tips of the forefinger and the thumb in a series of rapid approximations. While observing the performance of these tests it is important to remember that the very young and the elderly may perform less well than young and middle-aged adults.

The heel-to-knee test will demonstrate coordination of the legs. In a supine position, the heel of one foot is placed on the patella of the contralateral leg. The heel is slid down the skin toward the foot without removing the heel from the skin surface. Any deterioration in the quality of the movement should be noted.

While the tests are being performed, some specific observations should be made concerning the initiation of the movement, the direction the extremity takes toward the goal, and the manner in which the extremity is returned to the resting state or end point. Normally, the beginning of the movement should be promptly initiated and show no evidence of slowness or hesitation. The movement should be smooth, purposeful, and reach the goal directly and accurately without taking circuitous routes. The return to the original resting position should be performed smoothly, without evidence of past pointing or extraneous movements.

Equilibrium. Equilibrium is tested by asking the patient to stand erect with his feet together. This is done first with the eyes open and then with the eyes closed. With his eyes open, the patient may then be asked to walk, first naturally, and then in tandem fashion (placing the heel in front of the toe). The nurse examiner should remain near the patient and be ready to prevent injury in case the patient should begin to fall. Normally, the patient should be able to maintain his balance (even on one leg alone) and to walk tandem with the eyes open or closed. The patient who cannot stand steadily with the feet together and who has increasing difficulty with the eyes closed is said to have a positive *Romberg's sign.* This is positive only if there is actual loss of balance, causing a shifting of the feet in order to restore balance. Swaying of the trunk alone is not regarded as a positive Romberg's sign.

While the patient is performing tests of coordination, care must be taken to prevent him from injuring himself. Patients with disequilibrium may lose their balance easily. When lack of coordination is present, the muscles are not working synergistically, and they may be operating at the wrong time. To compensate for this, the movements become jerky and have increased force. Thus, in the finger-to-nose test, the patient, when attempting to touch his nose, may hit his face.

Abnormal Movements

Ordinarily, movements of the musculoskeletal system are under voluntary control. However, certain pathological conditions of the extrapyramidal tracts will produce muscle movements over which voluntary control is inhibited or ineffective. These involuntary movements may involve only a single muscle fiber or may extend to include multiple muscles in the limbs, trunk, and head. Some of the more common abnormal movements are fasciculations, tremors, chorea, and tics.

Certain types of abnormal movements occur at complete rest, with increased muscle tonus, or at the completion of a movement. Description of the involuntary movement in relation to these three phases is most helpful in properly identifying the movement. Movements occurring at complete rest can best be observed with the patient in a supine position during maximum muscle relaxation. To initiate movements produced by increased muscle tension, the extremities may be actively held in a stationary position of extension and adduction. The extremity may also be flexed and gently tapped with a percussion hammer. Abnormal movements occurring at the termination of an activity can be observed by having the patient drink from a cup, reach for an object, or do any of the coordination tests.

Characteristics of the abnormal movement pattern should be assessed in a systematic way. Identify the location and degree of muscle involvement. Some movements, such as tics and fasciculations, will begin in the region of the head and shoulders and involve only parts of muscles. Other involuntary movements frequently begin in distal extremities, gradually progressing toward the trunk and including more muscle to produce more extensive movement. The onset of the involuntary movement may be slow or so abrupt as to endanger equilibrium. The amplitude of the movement can be grossly visible or so fine that it is barely detectable. Fasciculation is an example of a movement of such a low amplitude that it appears wormlike. Movements of very low amplitude are more difficult to observe in an obese or muscular person. Fascicular reflections on wet skin from a good light can help make them more clearly visible, but care should be taken to keep the patient warm. Shivering caused by cold can resemble and be mistaken for fasciculations. Fasciculations can be palpated and auscultated. A light tap on the muscle mass with a percussion hammer can initiate fasicular muscle movements.

Involuntary movements may have a rhythmic quality, as is characteristic of tremor, or may be jerky, like chorea. Some movements are repetitive, like the pill-rolling tremor in parkinsonism, while other involuntary movements are dissimilar one to another.

SENSORY FUNCTION EXAMINATION

The function of three areas of the central nervous system is appraised by testing sensory discrimination. These areas are the posterior columns and the spino-thalamic tract of the spinal cord and the sensory cortex of the parietal lobe.

The posterior columns transmit deep-structure sensitivities, which consist of vibration, position sense, and deep-pressure pain. The fibers enter the spinal cord through the dorsal roots and ascend on the same side of the posterior columns to the medulla. In the medulla the fibers cross and ascend through the thalamus to the sensory cortex on the side of the brain opposite to the area stimulated.

The pathways for superficial cutaneous sensations of light touch, superficial pain, and sensitivity to temperature enter the spinal cord through the dorsal roots and cross over to the ventral surface of the opposite side of the cord. After crossing, the impulses travel upward in the lateral spinothalamic tract to the thalamus and from the thalamus to the sensory cortex of the parietal lobe.

Vibratory and position sense, deep and superficial pain, and tactile and thermal sensitivity are thus dependent on intact receptors, peripheral nerves, spinal cord pathways, and thalamic and sensory cortex function. Fine discrimination of sensory stimuli is the function of the sensory cortex. When cortical sensitivity is lost, the basic sensation is recognized, but there is little discrimination of its qualities.

The sensory part of routine physical examinations is a head-to-toe survey of the patient's ability to perceive superficial and deep sensations and to make fine sensory discriminations. All are checked in a brief fashion to exclude the presence of a sensory deficit. A pin and cotton are used to test for pain and touch on the face, trunk, forearms, upper arms, thighs, and lower legs. The hands and feet are tested for vibration sensitivity with the tuning fork, and also for position sense. The examination may be limited to these tests when the patient's history has aroused no suspicion of sensory involvement of any kind. A painstaking assessment is done of any areas expected to show impairment from the history related by the patient.

Both sides of the body and the proximal and distal parts are compared for equality of reaction by testing back and forth between the areas with each sensory stimulus and comparing thresholds and responses.

Under normal conditions, a person has sensory responses to all stimuli, and sensations over the body surface are felt equally on both sides of the trunk, extremities, and face. Abnormal reactions that follow anatomic divisions indicate a disruption somewhere along the pathways from the receptors to the sensory cortex of the cerebrum.

The sensory examination is likely to be difficult when the examiner is attempting to map out the margins of the areas of sensory loss and to compare thresholds to stimuli, because this procedure involves a subjective reaction from the patient, and the patient is suggestible to a significant degree. This suggestibility stems from clues that inadvertently are given with the application of the sensory stimulus; for example, the way questions are phrased or the visual clues received by the patient. All sensory testing should be carried out with the patient's eyes closed or his face screened so he cannot see the body part being tested or the examiner's movements or facial expression. The application of each stimulus should be in a random, unpredictable order, purposefully designed to prevent the patient from anticipating any particular site sequences or intervals between applications of the stimulus. The intervals between stimulus administration should be varied slightly so that stimulation is not rhythmic. This will help to maintain the patient's attention and prevent predictability.

Reasonably definitive results can be gained provided the patient is clearly told what is going to be done and how he is to answer. A brief practice demonstration with the patient's eyes open will facilitate comprehension and avoid unclear results. Only consistent, demonstrable sensory abnormalities on several examinations are acceptable. It may be necessary to check and recheck to map out margins and to compare thresholds. Diminutions in sensation occur more than does total loss, so watch for gradual as well as abrupt changes. The sensory section of the examination may be repeated later if there are questionable changes. It should not be done when the patient is fatigued because it requires that he be alert, attentive, and cooperative. The above applies to sensory testing in general, as do these:

1. Test from the decreased area to the normal areas.
2. Test across dermatomes, i.e., up the trunk, across the midline, and across the dorsa of hands and feet (Fig. 13-5).
3. Test the length of the body, both sides, and all four extremities.
4. Test the saddle area (the buttocks and genitalia).

Vibration

Vibratory perception is tested by applying a vibrating tuning fork (128 cps) to bony points such as the ankle, knee, hip, wrist, elbow, and shoulder on both sides of the body. Begin at the periphery and work toward the center. If the response is normal in the distal site, it will be normal in the proximal areas. Ask, "Do you feel the buzz," as the tuning fork buzz is demonstrated. Then test by instructing the patient to report each time he feels the buzzing and when it stops. Strike and apply the fork with a consistent degree of force and firmness. Since the patient hears the tuning fork being struck to set it vibrating, strike the fork before each application, but vary the stimulation as follows: (1) sometimes stop the vibration of the fork with the hand before applying it, (2) sometimes after applying it for varied intervals, and (3) sometimes let it run down. Squeeze the vibrating ends to stop it. Compare thresholds in various areas by the length of time the vibrations are discernible to the patient while the fork runs down.

Normal function is recognition of the vibration and awareness of its cessation. Persons over 60 may have diminished vibratory sensation in their feet and lower legs. The level of bone sensory perception corresponds with sensory level in the overlying skin.

Proprioception

Proprioception, the sense of movement and of position of body parts, is tested in all four extremities. First, the patient is instructed to say "Up," or "Down,"

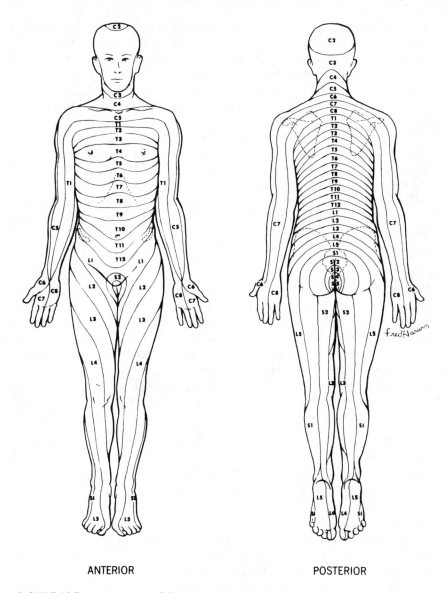

ANTERIOR   POSTERIOR

FIGURE 13-5.   Arrangement of dermatomes.

as digits are passively extended or flexed. One hand supports the patient's completely relaxed foot or hand, while the other hand grasps a digit by its sides and wiggles it up and down. Then movement is stopped in one direction or the other randomly. Do the exercise five times, as the probability of success by chance is 50 percent [2]. Take care not to use a different tone of voice or to ask a question between the up and down positions or to apply different pressures. The patient may respond to these associated stimuli.

Once the patient understands the test he should easily detect movements of a few millimeters and be able to identify which toe is being manipulated and the direction of the position at the end of the movement. Recognition of position and direction of movement permits coordinated movements.

The novice examiner usually uses the great toe and thumb. The third and fourth digits are the greatest challenge because the first, second and fifth digits have the richest innervation [2].

Deep Pain

Deep pain is pain from deep-lying muscle, fascia, bone, and ligaments. Firm squeezing of the structures causes an unpleasant pain. The areas squeezed are usually the Achilles tendon and the muscle at the junction of the thumb and first finger. Other areas are the calf and forearm muscles, the trapezius at the sides of the neck, the testicles, and the supraorbital notch. Note the amount of pressure required to elicit pain. Normally, these parts are tender to pressure, and as the patient becomes conscious of firm and prolonged pressure, he will rise slightly in protest, grimace, withdraw, or resist. This may be the only sensory testing that can be done in the obtunded patient.

Light Touch

Light touch (superficial tactile sense) of the skin surfaces is tested by stroking them with a wisp of cotton or with the fingers; cotton tests a finer response. The patient is instructed to say "Now" and "Right" or "Left" each time he is touched. Avoid asking, "Do you feel this?" as this is too suggestive. Sometimes, do not touch him when he expects you to. Periodically, ask him to point with a finger to the exact site of the stimulation. Normal skin has various areas with different thresholds to touch. Hairy and thin skin is more sensitive than horny skin. Lines are drawn on the skin to map out the regions of the loss. Diminished sensation is called *hypesthesia;* increased sensations, *hyperesthesia;* complete loss of sensation, *anesthesia.* Record the specific stimulus and the elicited sensation exactly.

Superficial Pain and Temperature

Superficial pain is elicited by pricking the skin with a pin hard enough to cause an unpleasant sensation. This can be determined on your own hand. Demonstrate "sharp" and "dull" respectively with the point and head of a safety pin.

Then apply the sharp and blunt ends in random order, and ask the patient to stipulate whether the stimulus is sharp or dull. Again, avoid asking, "Is this sharper than that?" Rather ask, "Is there a difference between this and that?" If the response is affirmative, ask, "What is the difference?" You may sometimes state the opposite of the actual situation to test suggestibility; for example, "Is this sharper than this?" When it is actually duller.

Pain thresholds vary over different body surfaces but pain can be perceived on all surfaces. Complete loss of pain sensation is called *analgesia. Hyperalgesia* and *hypalgesia* are the terms for increased and diminished pain respectively. In hyperalgesic states the patient winces the moment the area is touched with the pin.

Superficial pain and temperature pathways are so close anatomically that testing one evaluates the pathways of the other. Pain sensation is tested in the routine physical examination, and, if it is altered, sensory response to temperature is assessed. Sensitivity to temperature is effectively tested by the random application and alternation of two test tubes, one filled with hot water and the other with ice water. The tuning fork may be used instead by heating one prong with hot tap water. The temperatures used for testing must differ from skin temperature and the temperature of the environment. Excessive heat or cold causes a painful, not a thermal, response. The patient is instructed to state "Hot" or "Cold" each time he is tested. The skin should be observed for signs of loss of sensation such as trauma and cigarette burns on the fingers and irritation of the feet by the shoes.

Mapping The Area of Loss

Mapping the exact distribution of sensory loss is done in order to determine whether it is confined to a peripheral nerve, has a dermatomal distribution, or involves one entire side of the body.

In organic lesions the margins can be defined with reasonable reproducibility and are compatible with the anatomy of the nervous system. Bizarre, nonanatomic distributions occur with functional disturbances. These may be most quickly seen by having the patient draw on his own skin the area of numbness.

To delineate the margins of sensory changes, the area of sensory loss is marked on the skin with a ball-point pen during the testing of each type of stimulus. A different-colored line is used for the different stimuli. A sketch of the affected areas or a sensory dermatome chart may be a helpful way of recording the involved arrangement. The overall picture of the patient will conform to the sensory dermatome chart or sketch, but he may have certain minor variations in distribution.

Stereognosis

Stereognosis is the use of tactile sensation to identify objects in the hand. With the patient's eyes closed, the examiner places a series of small objects in the patient's hand one at a time, and the patient is asked to identify each one. The objects can be anything from the examiner's pockets, such as scissors, coins, pen, pencil, paper clips, or safety pin. Usually, most of the work of identification will be done not with the palm but with the fingers, which will hold the object and feel and manipulate it. If the patient demonstrates inability to handle the object well with the fingers and instead holds it in the palm of his hand, he frequently may be unable to name the object correctly. This may be due to peripheral neuropathy, posterior column disease, or parietal involvement.

Graphesthesia

Graphesthesia tests the patient's ability to identify numbers or letters traced on the skin. It is especially helpful in identifying sensory loss when the patient has poor coordination or cannot make fine movements of the hand for stereognosis sensory tests. Although the test is most often performed on the hands, other body parts such as the sole of the foot and the truncal area also can be used. The patient is instructed to close his eyes; then, one at a time, single digits or letters are written on the skin. On the hand, the characters should initially be drawn 0.5 cm high; on the arm, 1.5 cm high; and on the trunk, 2 cm high. If the patient cannot identify what was written, the height is increased with each subsequent trial. Normally, the letters or numbers should be identified as rapidly as when written on paper.

Two-point Discrimination

Two-point discrimination is a more precise evaluation of tactile sensation than the tests previously described. The patient should be able to differentiate between being touched with one point or two points. If touched with two points simultaneously, the distance between the two points is important to quantify. With the fingers and toes, a distance of 5 mm between the two points is normally sufficient to distinguish two points. If a greater distance is needed, a sensory defect is present. If the dorsum of the lower leg (shin) is used, the normal distance at which two-point discrimination is made is 10 cm [4].

The test is conducted using either a pair of calipers or two pins held to simulate a compass. The procedure is explained to the patient, and the one- and two-point stimuli are demonstrated. With eyes closed, the patient is then asked to tell whether the stimulus has one or two points. The stimuli are applied in random fashion, sometimes touching the skin with one point and at other times with both points. When applying two-point stimulation, the examiner should make sure that both points make skin contact at the same time; otherwise, each point will be experienced as a separate stimulus. If, when using two points, the stimuli are not recognized as being two, the distance between the points should be increased until the patient makes the discrimination. This distance is then recorded. If the shin is used, the examiner can use his fingers. The normal distance between which the two points are felt simultaneously will vary, depending on which part of the body is being tested. A general rule of thumb is that the trunk, arms, and legs do not have so fine a touch discrimination as do the hands and feet.

Since sensory abnormalities are related to disturbances in the nerve supply to the different parts of the body, some knowledge of peripheral and central pathways is indispensable in interpreting the abnormalities. Considering the sensory findings along with the patient's complaints, reflex changes, and motor weakness may make apparent a pattern that will enable localization of the defect. As previously mentioned, the objective of this chapter is merely to help the nurse examiner distinguish normal from abnormal findings. She will need other resources to enable her to localize lesions.

CRANIAL NERVE FUNCTION EXAMINATION

The testing of the twelve pairs of cranial nerves is done in order of their numbers, so that none is omitted. A device for remembering the order of the cranial nerves is "*O*n *o*ld *O*lympus' *t*owering *t*op *a Finn a*nd *G*erman *v*iewed *s*ome *h*ops." The first letter of each of the 12 words is the same as the first letter of the names of the cranial nerves.

Olfactory Nerve (Cranial Nerve I)

Cranial nerve I subserves smell, and to test its function, the patient is instructed as follows: "Close your eyes and tell me when you first smell this, then try to identify the odor." One nostril is occluded by finger compression and an odoriferous substance like tobacco, coffee, or peppermint is sniffed through the other nostril. The substance is first held away from the nose and gradually brought closer for the patient to identify. The other nostril is then occluded, and this time the substance is not presented. This assesses the patient's suggestibility and attention. In every sensory test such safeguards must be built in to assure objective results. Finally, a substance is presented to the untested nostril. Appreciation of an odor without precise identification of the substance is sufficient to rule out *anosmia* (loss of the sense of smell).

Anosmia may be caused by a number of factors. The common cold and allergic rhinitis are the most common causes; therefore, before testing the function of smell, possible obstructions of the nasal passages should be ruled out. The patient usually notices loss of taste rather than smell, since taste is influenced by smell.

The olfactory nerve need not be tested in routine examinations. It is pertinent in head trauma and tumors at the base of the frontal lobe, which may cause olfactory tract damage.

Optic, Oculomotor, Trochlear, and Abduceus Nerves (Cranial Nerves II, III, IV, and VI)

Methods of appraising functions of these nerves and appraisal methods are detailed in Chapter 7, on vision. Evaluating visual acuity, visual fields, and motor function of the eye is an integral part of the neurologic examination.

Trigeminal Nerve (Cranial Nerve V)

The trigeminal nerve supplies sensation to the face and motor innervation to the muscles of mastication (Fig. 13-6). It consists of three peripheral branches from the gasserian ganglion outward: the ophthalmic branch (first division); the maxillary branch (second division); and the mandibular branch (third division). Sensations from the cornea and the forehead are transmitted via the ophthalmic branch. The maxillary branch is the sensory supply for the lateral aspect of the nose, the skin of the cheek, the upper teeth and jaw, and the mucosa of the uvula, hard palate, and nasopharynx. The mandibular branch is the only branch that has both motor and sensory fibers. It carries sensory stimuli from the ipsilateral side of the tongue, pinna of the ear, lower teeth, gums, jaw, floor of the mouth, and the buccal surfaces of the cheeks. The motor fibers innervate the temporal, pterygoid, and masseter muscles (the muscles of mastication).

The technique for testing sensations is as described in the section on sensory function examination. The patient is instructed to keep his eyes closed for facial testing to avoid responses based on visual rather than cutaneous clues. The skin

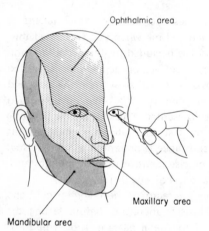

Ophthalmic area

Maxillary area

Mandibular area

FIGURE 13-6.   Distribution of trigeminal nerve innervation to the face, and technique of eliciting corneal reflex. Note sparing of angle of the jaw.

of the forehead, cheek, and jaw should each be tested for pain, touch, and temperature and on both sides of the face, so that all three branches of both the trigeminal nerves are evaluated. Start with a normal area, rather than a numb area, to establish that the patient understands the directions. Then alternate areas and sides randomly. Assess for decreased or increased sensitivity and equality of response of the two sides.

The afferent pathways of the corneal reflex are the trigeminal nerves; the efferent pathways are the facial nuclei. To test the right cornea reflex the patient looks to the left, and a cotton tip is introduced from the right, out of the patient's visual field in order to minimize visually stimulated blinking. The cornea is touched lightly with the cotton. The cornea, not just the sclera, must be touched. Care should be taken to stimulate but not scratch the cornea. The normal response is rapid closure of the eyelids, similar to that occurring when a foreign body enters the eye. It is common for both eyes to blink. If there is no ipsilateral blink, ask if the stimulus was felt and observe for a consensual blink. Each corneal afferent tract goes to both facial nerve (efferent) nuclei to close both eyes. If the facial nerve on the side tested is destroyed, the patient will feel the stimulus, and there will be a consensual blink but no ipsilateral blink. On the opposite eye there will be an ipsilateral blink but no consensual blink.

The mastication muscles are tested by having the patient clench his teeth and palpating the muscles of the side of the face (masseter and temporal) for force of muscle contraction and bulk. Normally, they are firmly contracted, and attempts to open the jaw by downward pressure on the chin are resisted. The pterygoid muscle is tested by pressing laterally on the jaw while the patient's mouth is partly open. With one-sided pterygoid weakness, the jaw deviates toward the weak side. The deviation may be seen as the mouth is opened slowly. Look at the relative positions of the upper and lower teeth for jaw deviation when the mouth is opened.

Facial Nerve (Cranial Nerve VII)

Motor innervation to muscles of facial expression, taste on the anterior two-thirds of the tongue, and general sensation to portions of the external ear are mediated by the facial nerves. Their function is determined by asking the patient to wrinkle his forehead by frowning and raising his eyebrows (frontalis muscle), closing his eyes tightly (orbicularis oculi muscle), pursing the lips by whistling (orbicularis oris muscle), retracting the angles of the mouth by smiling (lower facial muscles), and drawing his lower lips downward and laterally by vigorous effort to show teeth (platysma and triangularis muscles).

There should be equality of function and strength between the two sides of the face. Some degree of facial asymmetry is common, especially of the mouth with smiling and talking, and must be distinguished from muscle weakness. Gross weakness is apparent from marked asymmetry, but lesser degrees of weakness can be detected only when deliberately sought by testing the various muscles of facial expression.

Two types of facial nerve paralysis may be observed, depending on the site of the disruptive lesion. Lower motor neuron lesions in the facial nucleus of the facial nerve cause complete paralysis of one-half of the entire face. The muscles of that side of the face sag, and the normal lines around the lips, nose, and forehead are less pronounced. The mouth is drawn to the strong side with smiling; there is inability to close the eye; the patient may drool; and the cheek on the affected side may puff out with expiration. The central type of facial paralysis is due to a lesion above the facial nucleus, such as in the motor area of the cortex. The forehead function is intact because the primary motor neurons of the brainstem supplying the forehead muscles are innervated by both sides of the motor cortex. The lower facial muscles are paralyzed for voluntary movements but an involuntary grin is still possible, with innervation from extrapyramidal circuits. There may be slight weakness of eyelid closing and palpebral fissure widening.

The muscles of facial expression are tested in the patient with a depressed level of consciousness by observing wincing in response to noxious stimulation, for example, applying pressure to the supraorbital nerve.

Taste on the anterior tongue is not routinely tested unless the examiner wishes to determine if the taste fibers of the facial nerve are also involved. The technique for testing taste is described in the section on the hypoglossal nerve.

Auditory Nerve (Cranial Nerve VIII)

Auditory nerve testing is discussed in Chapter 8.

Glossopharyngeal and Vagus Nerves (Cranial Nerves IX and X)

The glossopharyngeal and vagus nerves run close together, and because their functions are so similar they are tested together.

The glossopharyngeal is a mixed nerve. The motor portion produces elevation and construction of the pharynx. It is the sensory nerve to the posterior third of the tongue, soft palate, tonsillar pillars, and pharynx. The vagus is also a mixed nerve innervating the larynx. In addition, it has visceral innervation functions, with implications for the cardiovascular and gastrointestinal examinations.

The taste function of the glossopharyngeal nerve can be evaluated by having the patient first rinse his mouth with clear water to remove any existing substances that could affect taste. The tongue is then protruded. Sweet, sour, salt and bitter substances are separately applied to the anterior two-thirds (innervated by the facial nerve) and posterior third (innervated by the glossopharyngeal nerve) of the tongue. The mouth is rinsed with water after the application of each substance. The patient is asked to identify each substance by pointing to or selecting a card on which is written the word describing the substance. Sugar crystals or glucose solution will produce sweetness. Unsweetened lemon juice or vinegar will give a sour sensation; table salt gives a salty sensation; quinine will elicit a bitter taste and should be used last. The substances in crystalline form can be applied directly with an applicator. Those in solution can be applied with a medicine dropper. Taste sensation is frequently diminished or absent in the aged and also following head injuries. If olfactory acuity is diminished, there is a direct effect on the gustatory sense, and taste may then be simultaneously decreased.

The lesions of the vagal system affect the patient's ability to swallow and can be determined by having him drink some water. This is best performed with the patient's head elevated. Nasal regurgitation or coughing indicates palatal weakness. Care should be taken to prevent aspiration of the liquid.

The gag reflex is stimulated by touching each side of the pharyngeal wall with a tongue blade. The glossopharyngeal nerve is the sensory component of the gag reflex and the vagus the motor component.

The presence of hoarseness or diminishing strength of coughing may indicate laryngeal weakness.

For good visualization of the back of the mouth, the tongue is depressed with a tongue blade and the oropharynx illuminated by a light directed from behind or to the side of the examiner. The pharyngeal walls and soft palate are observed for symmetry and their relationship to the midline position. As the patient says "Ah," the soft palate should elevate equally on both sides. The pharyngeal muscles will contract during the "ah," moving toward the midline. Weakness on one side will produce deviation to the unaffected side and distort the midline position. If there is weakness of the soft palate, the voice will have a nasal quality.

The Spinal Accessory Nerve (Cranial Nerve XI)

The spinal accessory nerve innervates the sternocleidomastoid and trapezius muscles. The sternocleidomastoid muscle originates behind the ear and inserts into the clavicular area. When the head is turned to the side, this muscle can be observed as the longitudinal ridge which becomes prominent on the contralateral side of the neck. The sternocleidomastoid muscle is observed bilaterally for muscle mass, symmetry, and contour from the neck to the shoulders. Ordinarily, its shape is readily identified, but atrophy of this muscle could make it difficult to observe. In athletes, the muscle contour will be prominent but symmetrical. In the presence of abnormal head movements the sternocleidomastoid muscle would be likely to show more hypertrophy on one side.

Because of the origin and insertion of the sternocleidomastoid muscle, contraction of this muscle on one side will cause a downward movement of the head, with rotation of the chin to the opposite side. Muscle strength is tested by the examiner's placing one hand on the side of the patient's face and resisting movement as the patient turns his head forcibly in that direction. The examiner's other hand is placed on the firm longitudinal ridge that becomes prominent in the opposite side of the neck. The other sternocleidomastoid muscle is tested by reversing the process.

The trapezius muscles move the shoulders up and down. The patient in the upright position is observed both from the back and front to assess symmetry of the neck and shoulder junction. The shoulders should be at the same level. The scapulae should be at the same level, both with the arms down at the sides and when outstretched in front. If there is weakness in the trapezius muscle, one scapula may be lower and become more prominent than the other when the arms are extended in an anterior position.

Muscle strength can be assessed by having the patient shrug his shoulders and hold the position. The examiner places one hand on each shoulder and tries to push the shoulders down as the patient tries to maintain the shrug. Weakness is indicated by inability of the patient to maintain the position.

Hypoglossal Nerve (Cranial Nerve XII)

The hypoglossal nerve is a motor nerve, responsible for movements of the tongue. While at rest on the floor of the mouth, the tongue is observed for the amount of space it occupies, its contour, muscle mass, and the presence of any movements. The tongue should fill the entire space bordered by the lower teeth. No movements should be visible when the tongue is at rest. Normally, movements occur only when the tongue is under tension, e.g., in protrusion.

The strength of the tongue can be tested by having the patient push the tongue against the inner aspect of the cheek. As the examiner externally compresses the cheek at the point the tongue protrudes, the tongue should be able to maintain its position if no weakness is present. Both sides are tested.

The tongue is then extended out of the mouth. The tip of the tongue should be in a midline position between the two front teeth. If the tongue consistently deviates to one side, weakness of the nerve may be indicated. (The tongue will deviate toward the side of the weakness because it is a thrusting muscle.) The tongue is again observed for symmetry and muscle mass. Any decrease in size or the presence of deep lengthwise ridges may be indicative of atrophy. The patient should be requested to make rapid, repetitive movements of the tongue into and out of the mouth. The movements should be quick and strong, improving during the testing.

SYMPTOMS ASSOCIATED WITH CENTRAL NERVOUS SYSTEM DISORDERS

Headache

Headache (cephalagia) is one of the commonest symptoms encountered in routine as well as neurologic examinations. In many cases the source of headache can be suspected from the patient's history. All types of pain of the head and face are described by patients as headache regardless of the cause. The pain may be from the teeth, sinuses, nose, or throat. The guidelines that follow are primarily for headaches in the conventional sense, but they will be helpful in evaluating other types of head pain. Headaches in the conventional sense are caused by cerebrovascular dilatation (migraine), sustained tension of the muscles of the head and neck, disturbances of the cervical spine, trauma to the head, low cerebral spinal fluid pressure, and psychogenic factors.

As a screening question, in a routine examination, it is best to ask the patient if he has severe or frequent headaches, not if he has headaches. Everyone has occasional, mild, short-lived headaches which are of little consequence. What is significant is the chronic, recurring headache.

The first step is to obtain from the patient a general outline of the history of the headache in regard to onset, duration, progression of severity, frequency, location, extent, and its episodic or constant nature. This is followed by assessment of the following: possible relationships to the time of day, season, emotional status, or bodily positions; the nature of the pain, e.g. "throbbing," "bandlike," or "viselike"; the presence of associated symptoms of nausea, vomiting, scotoma, aura (such as mood changes), effect on sleep, allergies, vertigo, lightheadedness, tinnitus, family history, emotional instability, and impaired memory. The muscles of the head and neck are palpated for the presence of tenseness.

If the reason for the examination is the complaint of headache, asking the person why he sought help for the headache at this particular time may bring out important recent changes in symptoms that the person has forgotten to mention in the barrage of questions. A willingness to let the patient talk about other aspects of himself, his lifestyle, and activities of daily living as well as his immediate symptoms might help in relating these to his symptoms and providing data for estimating the emotional and physical demands confronting him.

If the assessment of a headache is approached with a preconceived idea about the patient or the diagnosis, there may be subconscious rejection of symptoms that do not fit this diagnosis. The absence of organic findings does not rule out serious disease.

Pain

Pain of neurologic origin may originate from irritation of a peripheral nerve, a spinal nerve root, the thalamus, or a sensory tract. Mechanical compression or inflammation of a peripheral nerve or of a dorsal (spinal) nerve root irritates pain and other sensory fibers. The pain and paresthesia from these lesions are perceived by the patient as occurring along the anatomic distribution of the affected nerve. The area of skin supplied by one dorsal nerve root is a dermatome, and pain of a dermatome distribution is known as radicular pain. Charts depicting dermatomes such as that appearing in Figure 13-5 help in determining which dermatomes are involved. Charts of cutaneous fields of the principle peripheral nerves are used for lesions of peripheral nerves.

If the pain has a radicular distribution, it should be determined if it is aggravated by coughing, sneezing, straining (as with defecation), or the straight leg raising test previously described.

Thalamic and sensory tract pain distribution depends on the level at which the pathway is affected. It can be over the whole side of the body or limited to large contiguous portions of the body.

The profile of the patient's pain includes many aspects — topographic, quantitative, temporal, qualitative, and the associated physiologic and behavioral and psychological processes. The evaluation is much the same as for headache pain.

Meningeal Irritation

Meningeal irritation causes a stiff neck from the muscle contraction of the extensor muscles of the neck. The degree of irritation and defensive muscle spasm is determined with the patient in the recumbent position and the examiner passively flexing the neck so that the chin rests on the chest. Little resistance will be met in the patient free of musculoskeletal defects and meningeal irritation. Marked resistance is encountered (nuchal rigidity) in meningeal irritation; at times, it may be so powerful that the back is arched (opisthotonos), and the patient can be raised off the bed like a board by lifting his head. Blood or bacteria in the cerebrospinal fluid can cause meningeal irritation.

Seizures

Brain cells that have sustained some type of injury, or have a constitutional predisposition for alterations in electrical activity, are capable of producing seizures. The repetitive dysrhythmic bursts of electrical activity from the brain cells may be localized to a specific area of the cerebral cortex or may spread to involve more cerebral and subcortical areas, manifested by loss of consciousness and generalized involvement of the whole body.

A generalized seizure often progresses in the following way: A premonitory sign or aura foretelling the advent of the impending seizure may occur seconds, minutes, or hours prior to the onset of the convulsion. The tonic phase of the convulsion begins with an audible involuntary cry, falling to the ground, loss of consciousness, stiffening of the body and extremities, and temporary cessation of respiration. The clonic phase is characterized by severe jerking movements of the extremities and labored respirations which may last for minutes. When a seizure is occurring, bed covering should be thrown off so that the patient's entire body can be observed for the extent of the involvement.

The tongue may be bitten, and urinary incontinence may occur. During the postictal period (time immediately following the seizure) the patient may be drowsy or confused and experience aphasia, temporary paralysis, headache, and fatigue. The period of time required to recover from the seizure is dependent on its severity, the areas of the brain involved, medications administered during the seizure, and the general physical condition of the patient.

To obtain an accurate and detailed history that will provide necessary information about the seizures, the examiner may need to question not only the patient but also friends, relatives, and others who can provide firsthand observations. Because of the stigma surrounding convulsive disorders and the nature of the seizure itself, the patient may be hesitant to provide information or actually may not know the details of the seizure if he has been rendered unconscious at the onset.

In eliciting the characteristics of the convulsions, the examiner must not accept ambiguous words and phrases used by the patient and must obtain a precise interpretation and clarification of the meaning with him.

The patient can be asked directly about the frequency of seizures, the time of day they occur, and precipitating factors. Note the date and time of the last seizure. Seizures frequently occur during the day, usually shortly after arising. About one-third of the patients will have a convulsion during the night, frequently in the early hours of the morning. Some patients have seizures both day and night, in this case, most occur during the daytime. Precipitating factors initiating seizures vary widely and may include sudden loud noises, music, flickering light, fatigue, worry and premenstrual changes, to name just a few.

The presence of an aura and its characteristics should be determined. The time relationship of the aura to the initiation of the seizure should be known. The type of seizure may help to locate the epileptogenic focus in the brain. The aura may be a visual, auditory, gustatory, or olfactory hallucination.

When evaluating the patient's functional return during the postictal period, it is necessary to remember that any medications given him during the seizure may be influencing his recovery, that is, his level of consciousness and ability to move around.

Medications being taken for seizure control and the frequency and times of their administration are important for the examiner to ascertain. Asking the patient the name of each medication, its action, side effects, dosage, and time and method of administration provides background information on how well the patient understands his medications and adheres to the regimen prescribed.

In talking to the patient and significant others about his seizures it is helpful to use whatever terminology for the seizures the patient uses; it may not be understood, for example, that "convulsion" and "seizures" are synonymous.

Vertigo

Vertigo is a condition in which the person is aware of an altered spatial relationship between his body and the surrounding environment. This may be manifested as a sensation that the environment is rotating around him, or that he is whirling around and the environment is stationary. Movements and positioning of arms and legs may also be somewhat unsteady. The patient with vertigo will talk about being "dizzy," "spinning," or "the room spinning around him."

The onset of vertigo may be sudden and unrelated to movement, or it may be precipitated by a change of head position. Body movement and changes in the position of the head will affect existing vertigo as well as precipitate its occurrence. Such movements and positions and their effects should be identified. The patient should flex and extend his head and rotate it in the horizontal plane.

The eyes should be checked for nystagmus during episodes of vertigo. The patient should be questioned as to the occurrence of diaphoresis, nausea, and vomiting. To help differentiate labyrinthine dysfunction from brain center impairment, tinnitus and impaired hearing, if present, should be evaluated to determine whether they are unilateral or bilateral.

REFERENCES

1. Alpers, and Mancall, E. *Clinical Neurology* (6th ed.). Philadelphia: Davis, 1971.
2. DeMyer, W. *Technique of the Neurologic Examination.* New York: McGraw-Hill, 1969.
3. Judge, R. D., and Zuidema, G. D. (Eds.). *Methods of Clinical Examination: A Physiologic Approach* (3rd ed.). Boston: Little, Brown, 1974.
4. Van Allen, M. W. *Pictorial Manual of Neurologic Tests.* New York: McGraw-Hill, 1969.

SUGGESTED READINGS

Beetham, W. P. *Physical Examination of the Joints.* Philadelphia: Saunders, 1965.
Brain, W. R. *Brain's Clinical Neurology* (3rd ed.) (rev. by Roger Bannister). New York: Oxford Medical Publications, 1969.
Daniels, L., et al. *Muscle Testing: Techniques of Manual Examination* (3rd ed.). Philadelphia: Saunders, 1972.
Debrunner, H. *Orthopedic Diagnosis.* Edinburgh: Livingstone, 1970.
De Jong, R. *The Neurologic Examination.* New York: Harper & Row, 1967.
Plum, F., and Posner, J. *Diagnosis of Stupor and Coma* (2nd ed.). Philadelphia: Davis, 1972.
Renfrew, S. *An Introduction to Diagnostic Neurology* (vols. I and II). Edinburgh: Livingstone, 1964.
Salibi, B. Levels of consciousness in acute head injuries. *Wis. Med. J.* 62:375, 1963.

AGE GROUP CONSIDERATIONS IN PHYSICAL APPRAISAL

III

THE NEWBORN   14

Judy M. Judd

GLOSSARY

acrocyanosis   Cyanosis of the hands and feet.

brown fat   Mass of tissue in neck and scalp region of the newborn and capable of greater thermogenic activity than ordinary fat, especially in periods of cold stress; also called *interscapular gland.*

congenital choanal atresia   Congenital obstruction between the posterior nares (choana) and the pharynx.

cretinism   Condition produced by the complete absence of thyroid secretion from birth.

gestational age   Number of completed weeks from the first day of the last menstrual period.

glabella   Smooth depressed area between the two superciliary arches (point between the top of the bony orbit).

harlequin color change   Vasomotor phenomenon of unknown origin and lasting only a few minutes in which, with infant on its side, the upper half is pale and the lower half is pink and red, with a clear line of demarcation; if the infant is turned, changes occur in 1 to 2 minutes. It appears more frequently in the immature.

hypospadias   Anomalous position of the urethral meatus on the ventral portion of the glans penis, rather than in its center.

kernicterus   Deposit of unconjugated and unbound bilirubin in brain cells, the most serious complication of neonatal hyperbilirubinemia.

Klippel-Feil syndrome   Shortness of the neck resulting from reduction in the number of cervical vertebrae or fusion of their spinal processes

perinatal   Period between 28 weeks gestation and 4 weeks after delivery.

supraorbital ridges   Anterior limit of the frontal bone that forms the top of the orbit.

torticollis (wryneck)   Spasmodic contraction of the neck muscles, drawing the head to one side with the chin pointing to the other side.

tracheoesophageal fistula (TEF)   Congenital anomaly which usually takes one of three forms: (1) esophageal atresia with fistulous connection between the lower esophageal segment and the trachea; (2) esophageal atresia with normal respiratory tract; (3) normal esophagus and trachea connected by a fistula.

Turner's syndrome   Retarded growth and sexual development associated with absence of one sex chromosome.

vascular rings   Congenital anomalies of the aortic arch and its tributaries, forming a ring about the trachea and esophagus and causing various degrees of compression of these passages.

HISTORY

The history of a newborn is that of past generations, especially of his parents. Since a newborn cannot be interviewed, past information will be gained mainly from his mother and from her and his medical record. It is of utmost importance that this information be accurate. If any pertinent data appear invalid or missing, another source should be sought when possible.

There are four major areas to be considered in the history of this new person: the family history, mother's obstetric history, and prenatal and perinatal events. Positive and negative findings anywhere within this history may affect the outcome of this newborn's life.

Family History

The family history covers the same areas as in the adult. Therefore only a few of the most significant influences will be indicated here. A family history of diabetes, congenital heart disease, hypertensive cardiovascular disease, sickle cell anemia, thyroid disorders, renal disease, chromosomal defects, or hereditary central nervous system disorders may have profound consequences for the infant. The economic status, race, national origin or height and weight of his parents may create special problems. The mother's general health, nutritional status, smoking and drug habits, or marital status will also influence the neonate's well-being [6] .

Obstetric History

The general obstetric history should include the number of pregnancies, the number and type of deliveries, length of labors, and size of the infants. The *high-risk areas* that should be investigated include: premature labor, prolonged labor, fetal loss before and after 28 weeks, infertility, maternal age of less than 16 or more than 40 years, previous Rh sensitization, toxemia, bleeding during a pregnancy, multiple pregnancy, hydramnios, and obesity.

Prenatal Data

The amount and quality of prenatal care and other specific prenatal conditions and events have a direct bearing on the health of the infant. Some of the facts that will affect the outcome are: last menstrual period; first visit to the physician and number of visits; laboratory finding (e.g., blood type, VDRL[*]); vital signs (blood pressure, weight gain, fetal heart tones [FHT]); type of pelvis; drugs taken; exposures to or illnesses during pregnancy (rubella, influenza, syphilis, streptococcal or staphylococcal infection, radiation); nutrition (good, poor, pica, starch). The *high-risk areas* are similar to those under Obstetric History but include, in addition, hospitalization of the mother and special tests (e.g., amniocentesis, estriols).

---

[*]Venereal Disease Research Laboratory blood test.

Labor and Delivery

Events during labor and delivery have a direct influence on the fetus. Basic information related to these events should always be readily available in a nursery area. These facts include the following:

1. How labor started (spontaneously, induced).
2. Length of labor (less than 3 hours, average, prolonged).
3. Length of time membranes were ruptured (less or more than 24 hours).
4. Color of amniotic fluid (clear, cloudy, meconium-stained).
5. Drugs taken during labor and how close to delivery.
6. Status of fetus during labor (FHT patterns, activity).
7. Presentation (cephalic, breech, transverse).
8. Anesthesia (general, local, pudendal, paracervical, caudal, spinal).
9. Type of delivery (normal spontaneous delivery [NSD], low forceps delivery [LFD], midforceps delivery [MFD], cesarean section).
10. Complications (toxemia, abruptio placentae, placenta praevia, shoulder dystocia, hemorrhage, pneumonia, nuchal cord, multiple birth, major anomaly or injury).
11. Resuscitation needed (time before first breath, oxygen, drugs, ear bulb, De Lee suction trap, laryngoscope).
12. Routine drugs (silver nitrate 1% in eyes, intramuscular vitamin K).
13. Number of vessels in cord (three is normal).
14. Elimination (time of first stool and voiding).
15. Apgar score (see Table 14-1).

General Appraisal at Birth

The major factors in success of adjustment of a newborn to extrauterine life are inherent vitality, his state of maturity, and the degree of any pathological condition which interferes with normal events. Before the infant leaves the delivery room, a gross appraisal should be done. Choanal atresia should be ruled

Table 14-1. Apgar Score for Reactions of the Newborn[*]

Score	0	1	2
Heart rate	Absent	100	100
Respiratory effort	Absent	Weak cry, hypoventilation	Good strong cry
Muscle tone	Limp	Some flexion of extremities	Well flexed
Reflex irritability (response of skin stimulation to feet)	No response	Some motion	Cry
Color	Blue or pale	Body pink, extremities blue	Completely pink

*The score is computed at 1 and 5 minutes after delivery by assigning a value (0, 1, or 2) for each aspect and totaling them. Thus a score of 0 indicates a moribund or dead infant; a score of 10 indicates optimum condition. (Adapted from Apgar, V., et al. Evaluation of the newborn infant—second report. *J.A.M.A.* 168: 1935, 1958. By permission of the authors and publisher.)

out by observing breathing while holding the infant's mouth closed. A catheter should never be routinely passed. Some authorities feel a stomach tube should be passed and the contents measured to rule out tracheoesophageal fistula and obstructions and that this catheter should also be used to test for a patent anus. Certainly, the infant should be observed for any signs of distress or anomalies which will require special care.

When the newborn's appraisal is done in the hospital, records are readily available. However, an appraisal may happen to be done in the home or elsewhere in the community, and in these situations, information sources may be nonexistent or limited to an interview with the parent or parents or to material from a public health agency referral.

CONDITIONS FOR EXAMINATION

After collection of the pertinent data in the history of a newborn, the physical appraisal can take place. The appraiser should be properly attired according to the nursery rules and should follow the accepted handwashing technique. All equipment used should be clean or sterile, and the examining room should be properly lighted and adequately warm. A detailed examination should *not* be done on a newborn immediately after birth, when he is in distress, or immediately before or after a feeding. Proper precautions for safety would include having at least an ear bulb available, closing of safety pins, and never leaving or turning from the newborn while he is on an open surface. Needed equipment should be collected before starting (if not routinely in the crib) and should include the following:

1. Ear bulb
2. Stethoscope with small diaphragm
3. Penlight or ophthalmoscope and otoscope
4. Infant tongue blade
5. Tape measure
6. Bell (or appropriate substitute)
7. Pacifier or bottle of water
8. Finger cot or catheter

The examination of a newborn requires patience, gentleness, and flexibility in routines of procedure. First, observe the neonate undisturbed. Quickly note the infant's position, color, facial expression, breathing pattern, depth of sleep, and spontaneous activity. One should now note such gross characteristics as an enlarged head, prominent abdomen, or short extremities. If the infant is relaxed, you may wish to listen to the heart or palpate the abdomen first.

Parents may or may not be present during the examination. They should, however, always be kept informed about the findings, whether normal or abnormal. If the findings are questionable, the nurse may plan to reexamine the newborn at some later time or to consult with another colleague. If a more serious problem is suspected or apparent, medical consultation, referral, or both is mandatory. Follow-up public health nurse referral should also be considered. All findings warrant careful recording for use in making later comparisons. Finally, when the examination is completed, the newborn is replaced safely and comfortably in his crib.

MAJOR CONCEPTS OF GROWTH AND DEVELOPMENT

Body Proportions

The newborn's head-to-body proportion is 1 to 4. Several measurements should be made to rule out anomalies, to provide baseline data for future comparisons should complications arise, or to demonstrate normal growth. These measurements will vary with the general size of the baby.

The head circumference average is 13½ in. (34.3 cm) and is measured by placing a metal, paper, or cloth tape firmly over the glabellar and supraorbital ridges anteriorly and, posteriorly, over the part of the occiput which gives the maximum circumference. The chest circumference averages about one inch less than the head (12½ in., 31.7 cm) and is measured at the level of the xiphoid cartilage or substernal notch in a plane at right angles to the vertebral column. The chest should be measured when the neonate is in a recumbent position and at mid-respiration. The neonate's length varies from 18 to 21 in. (45.7 to 53.3 cm). The easiest approach to measuring length is to have the infant supine. Lay the tape measure next to the baby. First measure crown to rump. This measurement is usually comparable to the circumference of the head. Then extend the neonate's leg and continue the measurement to the heel.

Estimate of Gestational Age

Since many menstrual histories are inaccurate, it is important to make an objective estimate of gestational age (Figs. 14-1 to 14-3). Some specific observations that will aid in making this estimate are shown in Table 14-2. It should be noted that new research appears to show that sole creases may not be a good criterion for gestational age in the black neonate [4]. A scoring system for external criteria is cited by Dubowitz, Dubowitz, and Goldberg [5]. It includes skin texture, color and opacity, lanugo, edema, and labia majora development.

The absence of vernix caseosa means either a very immature infant or a postmature infant. The presence and completeness of reflexes will also help one judge the gestational age (see section on reflexes). The size of newborns is variable. However, size may be related to specific complications in the mother;

Table 14-2.   Estimation of Gestational Age*

Characteristic	Below 37 weeks	37 to 38 weeks	Above 38 weeks
Sole creases	Anterior transverse crease only	Occasional creases in anterior two-thirds	Sole covered with creases
Diameter of breast nodule	2 mm	4 mm	7 mm
Scalp hair	Fine and fuzzy	Fine and fuzzy	Coarse and silky
External ear	Pliable, no cartilage	Some cartilage	Stiffened with thick cartilage
Testes and scrotum	Testes in lower canal, scrotum small, few rugae	Intermediate	Testes pendulous, scrotum full, extensive rugae

*Adapted from Usher, R., McLean, F. and Scott, K.E.   Judgment of fetal age. II. Clinical significance of gestational age and objective method for its assessment. *Pediatr. Clin. North Am.* 13:835, 1966; by Avery, Kraybill, and Mullick [2].

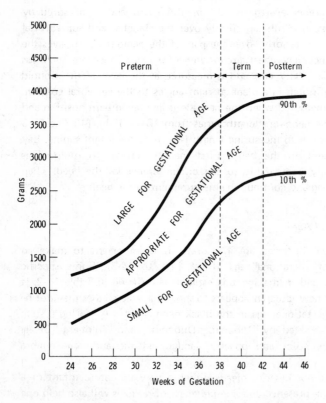

FIGURE 14-1.   Intrauterine growth status by birth weight at various gestational ages. (From Battaglia, F. C., and Lubchenco, L. O.: *J. Pediat.* 71:159, 1967. By permission.)

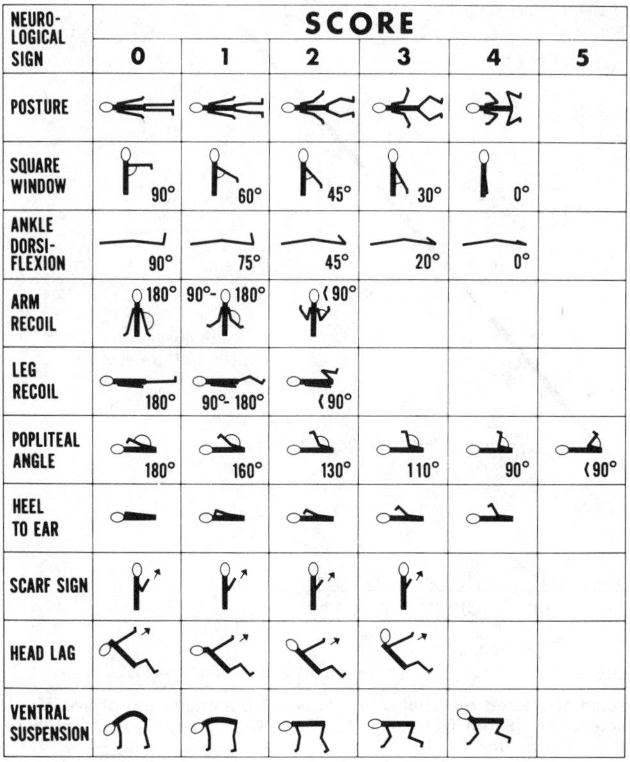

NEURO-LOGICAL SIGN	SCORE					
	0	1	2	3	4	5
POSTURE						
SQUARE WINDOW	90°	60°	45°	30°	0°	
ANKLE DORSI-FLEXION	90°	75°	45°	20°	0°	
ARM RECOIL	180°	90°- 180°	(90°			
LEG RECOIL	180°	90°- 180°	(90°			
POPLITEAL ANGLE	180°	160°	130°	110°	90°	(90°
HEEL TO EAR						
SCARF SIGN						
HEAD LAG						
VENTRAL SUSPENSION						

FIGURE 14-2.   Testing of neurologic signs related to maturity guides another important series of observations. [5]

for example, a large infant in a diabetic mother or a small infant (in relation to term) in a mother who has toxemia or smokes.

It is important to remember that any position or posture which is not characteristic may be the result of an inherent problem, such as fracture, dislocation, nerve damage, narcosis, or asphyxia. A full range of motion can be observed as the newborn moves spontaneously during the appraisal. Total flaccidity is considered abnormal and needs further investigation.

The concept of symmetry can be applied throughout the appraisal where appropriate (e.g., to movements, reflexes, observations of the face and extremities).

SENSORIMOTOR RESPONSES

The neurologic examination of the newborn requires skilled observation. It should never be attempted when the infant is hungry or sound asleep. The

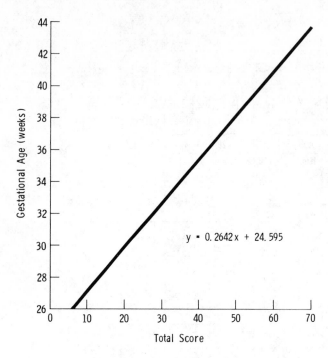

FIGURE 14-3. Gestational age based on total score derived from evaluation of neurologic signs and external characteristics. (From Dubowitz, L. M. S., Dubowitz, V., and Goldberg, C.: *J. Pediat.* 77:1, 1970. By permission.) [5]

quality of nervous system functioning is revealed by the neonate's activity, readiness of response to stimuli, spontaneous alertness, strength and character of cry, comparative use of all four extremities, vigor of feeding, and degree of postural muscle tone. You may observe some fine rapid tremors during the first few days after birth, especially on stimulation, but these usually disappear. Athetoid movements, coarse tremors even at rest, generalized stiffening, or opisthotonus are considered pathological.

Reflexes

Reflexes may be elicited all at one time, or, more ideally, in a head-to-toe sequence as the general appraisal is completed. Specific reflexes to test for are:

1. *Rooting.* Stroke the cheek, lips, or place a finger right above the upper lip. The infant should search for the finger.

2. *Sucking.* Place a nipple or clean finger into the baby's mouth, being sure to touch the palate. The infant will suck. (If sucking is present, the swallow and gag reflexes are also functional.)

3. *Ciliary.* Touch the eyelashes lightly while the infant is in a supine position. He should close one or both eyes.

4. *Doll's eyes.* Turn the infant's head from side to side. You should expect to see the eyeballs move in the opposite direction. (This reflex is difficult to test and disappears after 10 days of age.)

5. *Setting-sun sign.* If the trunk is raised and then quickly lowered to a supine position, the eyes slowly drift downward. You would *not* expect to see this sign except with cerebral damage (e.g., in kernicterus).

6. *Moro.* With the infant in a supine position, support the head and shoulders a few inches off the mattress. Then suddenly let the head drop. The reaction should be a symmetrical extending then abducting of both the arms and legs with the fingers spread (embrace). The infant may or may not cry out. This should not be confused with a startle reflex or elicited by simple banging of the crib. Absence or asymmetry of this reflex is abnormal, and the possibility of fractures, a dislocation, paralysis or central nervous system damage should be investigated. (However, be sure to repeat this reflex test at another time for verification.)

7. *Tonic neck.* The infant, when placed in a supine position, will spontaneously assume a "fencing position." As a demonstration of an immature nervous system his head will turn to one side with the arm and leg on that side extended. The opposite arm and leg will be flexed. If the infant's head is passively turned, the reversal of extremity positions will occur. This reflex may normally be absent or incomplete, but if it is still present by the second or third year, this is pathological.

8. *Grasp (palmar).* Place small objects (e.g., fingers) into the neonate's palms. He should hold on with enough force to be gently pulled to a sitting position. (Pressure on the balls of the feet will elicit a grasping attempt with the toes.) The responses should be symmetrical, with definite flexion tone in the arms.

9. *Deep tendon.* Gently tap the patellar tendon with your fingers. This reflex may be difficult to obtain or may create a more generalized response (i.e., whole leg jerks, both legs jerk). Mass responses are attributed to immaturity. (Only the knee jerk is important to test routinely in the neonate.)

10. *Babinski (plantar).* Stroke the lateral plantar surface (bottom of the foot on the side of the small toe), not the ball of the foot. The neonate should respond with an upward fanning of the toes (positive response). There is, however, no clinical significance to its presence or absence in early infancy, but it should disappear about the ninth month. Its presence thereafter is a sign of abnormality.

11. *Dancing.* If the infant is held upright with his feet touching a surface, he will usually make stepping or dancing movements.

12. Other normal reflexes observed for are blinking, yawning, sneezing, and hiccups.

Table 14-3 serves as a helpful guide for added information about some of the reflexes.

Table 14-3. Some Infant Reflexes

Reflex	Age Present (weeks)	Age When Disappears (month)
Rooting	Good at 32	9
Sucking	Strong at 34	9–12
Moro	Complete at 28	2–3
Tonic neck	? at 32	2–3
Grasp	Solid at 32	6
Dancing	Weak at 34	2–3

Tactile Sensations

The skin sensations of touch, pressure, temperature, and pain are all present at birth or shortly afterward. The lips are hypersensitive, while the skin of the trunk, thigh, and forearms tends to be hyposensitive. Cold appears to elicit a more pronounced and prompter reaction than does a heat stimulus. During the first few days of a neonate's life he is only weakly sensitive to pain. However, the soles of the feet or the lips will react much more positively to pain than do the body, hands, or feet. The presence or absence of pain should be observed for, not tested, during the appraisal. Its presence may indicate a pathological condition.

Temperature Regulation

The neonate's temperature regulation system is in poor equilibrium due to an immature hypothalamus. Heat loss is extreme and heat production low because of wetness in the delivery room, large body surface, inactivity during the first few days of life, and a low rate of metabolism. Heat is lost from the body surface by radiation, evaporation, convection and conduction. The neonate does not appear capable of shivering or perspiring. If the environment is conducive to the neonate ($70°$ to $75°$ F), his temperature will usually stabilize between $97°$ and $99°$ F, and his supply of brown fat is helpful in this process. The more immature the infant, the less stable his temperature. A cool environment is biochemically detrimental to the neonate and may result in metabolic acidosis, hypoglycemia, and increased mortality.

A rectal or axillary temperature may be taken as a part of the appraisal, but the pattern of temperature recorded on a chart, if available, would probably be more helpful.

GENERAL APPRAISAL

Head

The head is examined for size (see Body Proportions), shape, symmetry, and character of the fontanelles. Any molding usually returns to its normal shape within a few days. Soon after delivery the presentation or type of delivery may be evident from the molding: cephalic — sloping upward from the forehead; breech — flat top of head, cesarean section — round. The sutures may be felt to overlap.

If there is any extreme displacement of the cranial bones, the examiner should look for signs of intercranial hemorrhage. These signs are variable. Apneic episodes and other signs of respiratory distress are common. The commonest neurologic signs are hypotonia, diminished spontaneous movement, convulsions, coma, and lethargy. If the head is abnormally large or asymmetrical, it should be transilluminated. Transillumination is performed as follows: The neonate is taken to a completely dark room. A bright flashlight (fitted with a rubber cuff) is held tightly against the infant's head, moving it to various spots on the head. Normally, a faint halo of light, 1 to 2 cm wide, is seen in the scalp just around the cuff. If the halo is large and irregular, or if light can be transmitted from one side of the head to the other, the diagnostic possibilities include hydranencephaly, severe hydrocephalus, or a large porencephalic cyst.

The anterior and posterior fontanelles should be palpated. When the appraiser passes her fingers over the fontanelles, they should feel soft but neither bulging nor depressed. The anterior fontanelle should be *at least* as large as the tip of the little finger and is diamond-shaped and located between the parietal and frontal bones. The posterior fontanelle is located between the parietal and occipital bones, is triangular in shape, and may be almost closed at birth.

While inspecting the head, any lacerations, abrasions or skin defects of the scalp should be noted. While palpating along the sagittal suture, especially the posterior portion of the parietal bones, it is possible on some infants to be able to indent the bone easily with light pressure. You will have the sensation of pressure on a Ping-Pong ball. The shape is resumed when the pressure is removed. This indicates the presence of craniotabes, which is probably due to mechanical factors, along with a generalized deficiency in calcium metabolism. It never occurs in breech presentations and is more common in nonwhite infants.

If the neonate is 24 hours old or less, he may have *caput succedaneum,* a local area of edema, congestion, and petechiae on the scalp (presenting part); this crosses suture lines. A *cephalhematoma,* which is a hematoma under the periosteum and usually over the parietal bone, does not cross suture lines. It tends to appear on the second or third day, to be firmer to the touch than an edematous area (like touching a water-filled balloon), and disappears over a period of weeks or months.

The amount of hair may be noted but is of little consequence except to the mother. The hairline is low over the forehead, and lanugo may be present on the ears and shoulders.

Face

The face is small and round, and the lower jaw appears to recede. The face should be observed for symmetry (eye creases equal), and to see that the mouth remains on a level plane when the infant sucks or cries and that neither side of the face is motionless; if these are not observed, facial paralysis is suspected. Note the facial expression, which may indicate distress or serenity. Down's syndrome, as well as some other chromosomal and genetic disorders, may be identified by characteristic facial features.

Eyes

The neonate has almost no eyebrows but may have long eyelashes. Eye color is usually blue or gray in the Caucasian baby but may be darker in the nonwhite infant. The newborn has no protective blink. As a result of the instillation of silver nitrate 1% as a preventive against gonococcal conjunctivitis, the eyes may appear swollen (puffy) and red, with some purulent-appearing drainage. The drainage may be considerable but it is important to differentiate an infection from this normal reaction. Tears are seldom seen before the 13th to 16th day of life.

Subconjunctival hemorrhages due to labor and delivery pressures are common and not significant. Pupils should react equally to light. Eye motion is generally random and lacking in coordination. The eyes of the neonate appear able to converge for short periods of time and are especially drawn to contours. If he is shown a black triangle on a white field, his eyes will hover near the sides of the triangle, where the contrast between black and white is maximal. The infant may react to the examiner's eyes because of a like dark-light contrast. He probably has binocular vision and can see in color, seeing best at about 8 in. (20 cm). If the eyes oscillate back and forth and rotate in a peculiar searching manner, the nurse should suspect partial or total blindness.

The following observations can be made with the naked eye but are more satisfactorily made with an ophthalmoscope. The cornea and anterior chamber should be crystal-clear; otherwise, a cataract is suspected. If the cornea is enlarged or steamy in appearance, congenital glaucoma is suspected. Retinal hemorrhage may only be seen with an ophthalmoscope and is a sign of severe birth trauma. The neonate is not too cooperative in opening his eyes, so patience is required. It may be helpful to place the baby in a supine position, raising his head slightly and shading his eyes from a bright light. Another maneuver that may work is to rock the whole body from an upright to a horizontal position several times.

Nose

The most pertinent observation related to the nasal passages is congenital choanal atresia (see the section on appraisal at birth). Dried mucus or lint in the nose may cause sneezing, noisy breathing, or both. The nose may be flattened due to delivery. This will correct itself in a few days. Milia, small white nodules which are clogged sebaceous glands, are usually found over the surface of the nose and sometimes elsewhere on the face. A severely stuffy nose or saddle nose are indications of congenital syphilis.

The sense of smell is well developed in the newborn. Some reactions of the neonate when exposed to strong odors (e.g., ammonia, acetic acid) are crying, squirming, grimacing, sucking, and a changing respiratory rate. However, there is a wide range of individual differences in these reactions, as well as varying reactions in the same infant.

Mouth

The lips may appear dry but pink. A harelip should be noted. By the end of the first week of life a sucking blister will be developing. The mouth can be forcefully opened but is best examined when the infant is crying. A tongue blade may be useful. The gums should appear a healthy pink; tooth buds should be visible. Rarely, erupted teeth are seen. If present, it is better to remove them to avoid trauma, or aspiration or both, since they are usually loose. There should be no cysts or tumors of the mouth. The tongue should not appear too large for the mouth. A continued rhythmic protrusion of a normal-sized tongue suggests increased intercranial pressure. The frenulum linguae should be of adequate length. The palate should be visualized and palpated with a clean finger or finger cot, to be sure it is intact. Epstein's (epithelial) pearls, small shiny whitish-yellow nodules, may be seen at the junction of the soft and hard palate. These should not be mistaken for thrush, which is a yeastlike fungus (*Candida albicans*) infection of white patchy exudate on the tongue, palate, and other mucous surfaces of the mouth and pharynx.

The newborn appears to have a more developed sense of taste than of sight or hearing. He reacts to a sweet taste with contented sucking. If offered fluid with a salty, sour, or bitter taste his reactions will be mainly negative, that is, he will appear to show discomfort. However, the newborn probably would not refuse harmful fluids because of the taste, so care that nothing toxic is given to the infant is essential.

Infant Cries

The neonate will probably cry spontaneously during the examination. If not, he may be stimulated to cry by slapping the bottom of his foot. Crying is the beginning of vocalization. When a neonate cries, he holds his head in the midline position, and there is mass activity. The cry should be observed for its nature, pitch, intensity, frequency, and effort.[†] Listening carefully, the nurse can distinguish a normal from an abnormal cry.

[†]Feingold, M. *Baby Cries: The Differential Diagnosis* (audio production tape). Medcom, Inc., New York, N.Y.

Normal Cries. The normal cry has a normal pitch; loudness varies with breathing and can increase when the baby wants it to do so. A normal cry of discomfort at first is monotonous in pitch, staccato-like, and intermittent. It will increase in its incessantness. A cry of pain rises in pitch. A cry of rage is longer, the breath is held and the face often becomes purplish. Gasping sounds usually accompany the rage cry.

Abnormal Cries. A cry indicating illness goes from strong to weak. The cry in central nervous system damage is a high-pitched, shrill shriek. A normal but extra sound at the end of a cry or hoarse, high-pitched inspiratory crow indicates a larynx problem. The cry in creatinism is hoarse, not loud or frequent, of low intensity, and sluggish. The cri-du-chat cry, like the mewing of a cat, is indicative of a chromosomal abnormality. The infant whose mother is drug-addicted has a high-pitched cry.

Ears

The ears may temporarily be misshapen by intrauterine positioning but rapidly assume their normal configuration. In the full-term infant, cartilage formation gives firmness and support to the structure. If the ears appear low in placement, or if some malformation is present, renal anomalies or chromosomal disorders should be suspected. Preauricular fistulas or tubercles may be present. Visualization of the canal and drum may be difficult because of the angle of the canal and the presence of vernix caseosa. However, an attempt to examine the canal and drum with an otoscope should be made to rule out infection and anomalies.

Hearing is possible for the neonate after the eustachian tubes become aerated, which occurs about 24 hours after birth. If a bell is rung or an electric device sounded, the infant may react by cessation of activity, increased movement of the body, limbs, or eyes, and blinking [8]. However, deafness can not be diagnosed with certainty in the newborn.

Neck

The neck is short and weak (see the section on neuromuscular development). Because of this, skin folds are deep and moist and a common site of pustules. The neck should be inspected and palpated for masses or a goiter. Although an immature infant's head can be rotated so that the chin goes well beyond the acromial tip, the normal newborn's chin stops at the acromial tip. Abnormally decreased mobility of the neck may occur if there is an anomaly of the vertebrae (e.g., Kleppel-Feil syndrome). Webbing of the neck is a feature of Turner's syndrome. Congenital torticollis may be due to a maldevelopment or to hematoma of the sternocleidomastoid muscle. It is most commonly seen in breech or difficult cephalic deliveries. Diagnosis is seldom possible in the newborn period. A firm, circumscribed noninflamed or discolored mass felt on the sternocleidomastoid muscle of an infant at about 2 weeks of age would be a hematoma.

Skin

The skin should be inspected in its entirety. There is a loose attachment of the epidermis to the underlying dermis. Turgor and elasticity are to be expected. Depression of the fontanelles may be one sign of dehydration.

At birth the skin is a purplish red, and acrocyanosis is present. Within hours, only the palms and soles still appear cyanotic. To differentiate poor peripheral circulation from true cyanosis, vigorously rub the palm or sole. Normally, it will quickly turn pink. Generalized cyanosis is abnormal (see Chaps. 9 and 10). An ashen-gray cyanosis may indicate septic shock. Within 24 hours, some babies have a "boiled-lobster" look. This very red appearance is a normal reflection of a high hematocrit and thin subcutaneous fat layers. Pallor may indicate blood loss, erythroblastosis, or cutaneous vasoconstriction (shock, heart failure), and the medical staff should be alerted.

Jaundice that appears during the first 24 hours is abnormal and usually indicates hemolysis or sepsis. If physiologic jaundice, which appears after 24 to 36 hours, is severe, further investigation is also indicated (i.e., bilirubin level). Jaundice can best be observed in daylight. Press your finger against the infant's nose or abdomen. On release, the skin will appear yellow, not white, if jaundice is present. On nonwhite babies' skin, jaundice can be more easily detected by observing the color of the palate and sclera.

Pigmentation is variable and usually dependent on racial origin. Mongolian spots, which are blue or blue-black spots of varying size, are found especially in the sacral area. The majority are in Oriental or black infants but, rarely, may appear in the Caucasian infant also. In the black infant, pigmentation is most prominent in the nail beds and genitalia. Generally, these babies may not reach their regular pigmentation for several weeks. A harlequin color change may be observed but is more apt to occur in an immature infant.

The newborn has many skin "markings" that are normal but peculiar to him. These are as follows:

1. *Milia* (clogged sebaceous glands) are usually present on the nose and maybe the cheeks for several weeks and appear as "whiteheads."
2. *Lanugo* is fine downy hair found on the forehead, ears, and shoulders. While it is more noticeable in the premature, it is not necessarily a sign of prematurity.
3. *Erythema toxicum* is a transient maculopapular rash which appears to be urticarial with a blanched, wheal-like appearance. At times, the center has vesicles of clear fluid which should not be mistaken for impetigo, which is purulent.
4. *Petechiae* may be found and usually relate to a long labor or rapid delivery. They may indicate intrauterine infection or thrombocytopenia. (Any increase in bruising should be noted.) Generally, a routine injection of vitamin K will help control any bleeding

tendency of the young neonate before the coagulation processes become established on about the fifth day.)

5. *Superficial telangiectasia,* reddened, vascular unraised areas, are found in the nape of the neck (stork bites), or on the upper eyelids or upper lip (flame nevi). These disappear within the first year and should be differentiated from larger, bright red or dark purple, often elevated hemangiomas which often persist. (Examples of these are the port-wine stain and strawberry and cavernous hemagiomas.)

Vernix caseosa, the whitish, cheesy, greasy protective material found on the skin at birth, will be absorbed but may still be seen after several days in skin folds, especially the labia. A yellow discoloration of the vernix is abnormal and some fetal pathological process can be assumed (e.g., erythro-blastosis, anoxia, postmaturity). The skin usually becomes dry in the first weeks, but the dryness is more extreme in the postmature neonate or one who was malnourished in utero. These infants need to be watched for signs of hypoglycemia (low blood sugar), manifested by apnea, cyanosis, rapid and irregular respirations, tachypnea, jitters, tremors, twitches, lethargy, convulsions, coma, abrupt pallor, upward rolling of the eyes, sweating, weak cry, and refusal to eat. Extensive desquamation of the palms and soles, together with radiation fissures around the mouth, pustular rash, and nasal discharge, is an early sign of congenital syphilis.

Localized edematous areas (e.g., caput succedaneum) are normal. Generalized edema is abnormal and might indicate hydrops fetalis, hyaline membrane disease, or congestive heart failure. Localized edema of the dorsa of the hands and feet may be the only clue to Turner's syndrome during the newborn period.

Back

Turn the neonate on his abdomen and inspect the back. The ribs and vertebrae can easily be palpated for anomalies. Large openings in the vertebral body cause herniation of the contents of the canal. These are cystic masses and must be differentiated from a more solid tumor. Look for tufts of hair along an intact spinal column; these may indicate a pathological condition beneath. Inspect a deep coccygeal dimple for a dermal sinus with perhaps a dermoid cyst at the end of the sinus.

Extremities

With the neonate lying on his back, evaluate all four extremities for gross deformities and activity. Observe and test the range of motion at all joints (see Reflexes). Intrauterine positions may influence the "position of comfort" assumed but should be distinguished from a pathological condition. The lower extremities in a breech presentation may take several weeks to assume a normal position. Injury to the brachial plexus causes the arm to assume a characteristic position of extension, adduction, internal rotation, and pronation. All newborns are bowlegged, flat-footed, and have cold extremities. The active infant may have abrasions on his knees, ankles, or toes.

Polydactyly (extra digits) should be checked for on both hands and feet. Polydactyly, especially of the hands, is relatively common in the black population. It should be established by x-ray if there is bone involvement. The presence or absence of webbing should also be determined.

It is important to find a dysplasia of the hip or a dislocated hip as early as possible. With the baby still on his back, flex his thighs, one at a time, outward and downward to the table or mattress. If one thigh does not easily abduct, suspect the diagnosis. Also listen for a consistent sharp click heard on the affected side during abduction and high or extra creases in the affected thigh. Dysplasia may be diagnosed by Ortolini's sign, as follows: Active attempts are made to subluxate the femoral head in and out of the acetabulum by a firm anteroposterior pushing and pulling with the pelvis fixed with the other hand. If dysplasia is present, one can feel and often see the head slipping in and out of the acetabulum, and triple diapering should be used to keep the hips in a partially flexed and abducted position.

Thorax

The thorax is cylindrical, having equal anteroposterior and lateral diameters (see Body Proportions). Hypertrophy of the breasts may be present in both females and males as a result of estrogen from the mother crossing the placenta. Signs of inflammation should not be present. Supernumerary nipples may be present. The ribs are flexible. The xyphoid cartilage may be felt and often can be seen below the sternum in the epigastrium. The fingers should be passed over the clavicles to rule out the most commonly seen fracture in the newborn. It will feel like a "knot" but may not be felt until the third or fourth day of life. One should also observe for evidence of pain on pressure, asymmetry of angulation, and a complete Moro reflex (see Reflexes). Common congenital deformities of the chest include: (1) funnel chest, in which the lower portion of the sternum is depressed and (2) pigeon breast, in which the sternum, together with the costal cartilages, is prominent, and the lateral walls of the thorax are correspondingly depressed.

Respiration

The respiratory pattern should be observed before the infant is disturbed. In the normal neonate, respiratory movements are predominantly diaphragmatic. The abdomen rises and falls with inspiration and expiration, while the thoracic cage remains relatively immobile. If intercostal muscles are being used to any extent, a pathological condition should be suspected. Normal breathing rate varies between 30 to 60 respirations per minute but tends to be more rapid during the first hours after birth and with activity. The normal respiratory pattern varies considerably. Irregular, shallow respirations, short periods of apnea, breathing of the Cheyne-Stokes type, followed by several deep breaths, are all common in the neonate. Transient tachypnea may normally occur, especially in an infant born by cesarean section or in a breech presentation. If tachypnea (over 60 respirations per minute) is at a sustained rate, it is abnormal.

Other signs of distress include generalized cyanosis, respiratory grunt, retractions of the chest on inspiration and flaring of the nostrils on inspiration. Inability to handle mucus will cause a problem to the neonate, especially in his "second period of reactivity" after birth [1].

Gentle percussion gives a resonant note over the lung fields. If done heavily, data will be inaccurate. It is difficult, especially for the inexperienced, to learn much about the lungs by percussion. Although the lungs and heart should be examined simultaneously, they are discussed in separate sections for clarity of understanding.

Proper stethoscope technique is vital if accurate data are to be obtained (see Chaps. 9 and 10.) For example, rapid respirations may produce a sound which on auscultation may be confused with a heart murmur. An adult-size diaphragm is not ideal for auscultation because it will cover too large an area of the baby's chest wall and fail to conform to the curvature of his chest.

Ausculatory signs in the lungs are of less value in the neonate than in other pediatric age groups. . . . Diminished breath sounds occur in hyaline membrane disease, atelectasis, emphysema. . . . Fine rales are produced in terminal bronchioles and alveoli by the rush of air through fluid within them. These rales are classically described as crackling in character . . . . Rales are heard in some infants with hyaline membrane disease, pneumonia, pulmonary edema and occasionally in normal babies. They are sometimes only audible after deep inspiration, which must be induced by stimulating a cry [6, pp. 100–101].

If labored breathing is noted, it may be due to abnormalities of the respiratory system or other systems of the body. Choanal atresia, anomalies of the epiglottis and larynx, or vascular rings should be suspected if there are signs of upper airway obstruction.

Circulation

The methods used in examining the cardiovascular system of the newborn are observation, palpation, percussion, and auscultation (see chap. 10 for techniques).

Inspection.   Inspect the chest wall at about the fifth intercostal space in the midclavicular line for local pulsations on the chest wall. Pulsations are more prominent in small babies. If pulsations are prominent in the epigastrium, the heart is probably considerably enlarged.

Palpation.   To identify the normal apical impulse, feel at the fifth intercostal space. Detection of an abnormal heart position early in the examination is an important initial step in establishing a correct diagnosis and of particular importance with a dyspneic infant. In *pneumothorax,* the apical impulse moves away from the affected side due to the shift of the mediostinum. In *diaphragmatic hernia,* the apical impulse is displaced to one side of the chest. In *dextrocardia,* the apical impulse is in the right chest. (Compare the right and left chest.)

Percussion. The size and configuration of the heart may be judged by percussion but in the neonate they are difficult to estimate by this method.

Auscultation. Auscultation is the most informative component of the physical examination of the heart when done by a skilled nurse practitioner. In the neonate the first and second heart sounds resemble the syllables "toc-tic" and are normally well defined and clear. The second sound is somewhat sharper and higher-pitched than the first. Murmur at birth does not necessarily mean heart disease. It may be a late-closing ductus arteriosus. Only after several weeks will a murmur assume its normal intensity. Therefore only the ones that persist and increase in intensity are most likely to be significant. If present, these require medical follow-up, together with x-rays of the chest and an electrocardiogram. Localization of a murmur in the newborn may be difficult. Most murmurs are systolic and occur after the first sound and at or before the second sound. Continuous murmurs extend beyond the second sound into diastole. Arrhythmias are most often observed during deep sleep. The nurse will need considerable practice with the stethoscope to make accurate observations [7, pp 7—11].

The heart rate of a newborn varies with crying, activity, sleeping, and feeding. However, a persistent rate below 100 or above 180 beats per minute is abnormal and should be investigated.

An instinctive feeling that "something is not quite right about the baby" may be a first indication of a problem, causing the nurse to reappraise certain areas.

Cyanosis or pallor are often the first signs of heart disease. If cyanosis increases with crying, this is much more suggestive of heart disease than of a respiratory problem, which crying usually helps. Other signs of heart disease may include tachypnea, failure to feed well, breathlessness during or after feeding, irritability, tachycardia (gallop rhythm), edema of the face and feet, enlarged heart (cardiomegaly on x-ray), hepatomegaly (liver more than 3 cm below the right costal margin), abnormal electrocardiogram, and abrupt and unexpected weight gain of several ounces.

Peripheral pulses should always be examined by simultaneously palpating the brachial and femoral pulses. A strikingly prominent brachial pulse, coupled with a weak or absent femoral pulse, suggests coarctation of the aorta. In congestive heart failure the femoral pulses will be feeble or absent; infants with patient ductus arteriosus or aortic valve insufficiency will have bounding pulses [3].

Taking the blood pressure is usually not considered routine in examination of the newborn. However, if any condition that might affect the blood pressure is suspected, pressure should be taken in both an arm and a leg. The cuff should cover two-thirds of the upper arm or leg. The method used may be the ausculation, palpation, or the flush method. The neonate's pulse may be difficult to palpate. In the flush method;

Apply but do not inflate the cuff. Elevate the extremity and massage to produce blanching. Then raise the cuff pressure to above the expected systolic pressure. Lower the extremity to heart level and slowly lower the pressure in the cuff. The point at which a flush appears in the limb is the approximate systolic pressure. (Normal is 60 mm Hg at birth and 80 mm Hg after one week [2].)

Abdomen

The contour of the abdomen is noted first. Ordinarily it is cylindrical and slightly protuberant. Some gross abnormalities such as distention, localized bulging, or congenital absence of abdominal musculature are apparent on inspection alone. The umbilicus is routinely inspected for the healing of the cord. A scaphoid or turnip-shaped abdomen is suggestive of a diaphragmatic hernia and requires immediate surgery.

Percussion may help localize masses in the abdomen and may demonstrate gaseous distention of the bowel. Palpation should be gentle (only one to two fingers may be required in a premature). The best findings will be obtained when the infant is quiet and relaxed. The following may be palpated:

1. Xiphoid process — prominent.
2. Liver — 2 cm below costal margin.
3. Spleen — usually not felt, but the tip at the costal margin may be felt.
4. Kidneys — found deep at the lower poles (larger flank masses: hydronephrosis, Wilms' tumor, neuroblastoma).
5. Umbilical or inguinal hernia.
6. Bladder — distention: pressure on pubic area may force male to urinate so that you can observe for a forceful stream.

Other points of importance to note are vomiting, excessive mucus (TEF), eating habits, first stool by 24 hours after birth, and normal color, consistency and odor of stools. A rectal examination is done with the little finger (or catheter) to rule out imperforate anus and pelvic masses.

Genitalia

It is important to recognize ambiguity of sex in the genitalia so that a mistaken gender is not assigned. The neonate should void within 48 hours of birth. Uric acid crystals may normally be found in the neonate's urine and appear as a dusty red, clay-colored stain on the diaper. It should not be mistaken for hematuria. Normally, the urine is not concentrated, cloudy, or hematuric. In a breech presentation, the genitalia may be bruised and edemateous for several days after birth. The following are observations to be made:

Female . Gaping vulva; labia minora more prominent than labia majoria; clitoris varies in size; hymenal tag; clear milky and bloody vaginal discharge; one fingertip length between anus and introitus (question ambiguity of sex if not present).

Male . Penis and scrotum vary in size; prepuce covers entire glans of penis; testis is in the scrotum or can be induced there; forceful urinary stream; healing of circumcison if performed. Watch for hypospadias, hydrocele (transilluminates well), and torsion of testes (firm, swollen, discolored).

REFERENCES

1. Arnold, H., et al. The Newborn: Transition to extrauterine life. *Am. J. Nurs.* 65:77, 1965.
2. Avery, G., Kraybill, E., and Mullick, U. Examination of the newborn infant. *G. P.* 36:78, 1968.
3. Black, J. A. *Neonatal Emergencies — and Other Problems.* New York: Appleton-Century-Crofts, 1972.
4. Damoulaki-Sfakianaki, E., Robertson, A., and Cordero, L. Skin creases on the sole of the foot as a physical index of maturity: Comparison between Caucasian and Negro infants. *Pediatrics* 50:483, September, 1972.
5. Dubowitz, L. M. S., Dubowitz, V., and Goldberg, C. Clinical assessment of gestational age. *J. Pediatr.* 77:1, 1970.
6. Korones, S. B. *High-Risk Newborn Infants. The Basis for Intensive Nursing Care.* St. Louis: Mosby, 1972.
7. Nadas, A., and Fyler, D. *Pediatric Cardiology* (3rd ed.). Philadelphia: Saunders, 1969.
8. Shimek, M. L. Screening newborns for hearing loss. *Nurs. Outlook* 19:115, 1971.

SUGGESTED READINGS

Blake, F. *Nursing Care in Children* (8th ed.). Philadelphia: Lippincott, 1970.

Cochran, W. Guide to visual diagnosis in the newborn. *Hosp. Med.* 8:38, 1972.

Fitzpatrick, E., Reeder, S., and Mastroianni, L. *Maternity Nursing* (12th ed.). Philadelphia: Lippincott, 1971.

Harding, P. G. R. The metabolism of brown and white adipose tissue in the fetus and newborn. *Clin. Obstet. Gynecol.* 14:685, 1971.

Hodgemen, J. E. Clinical evaluation of the newborn infant. *Hosp. Pract.* 4:70, 1969.

Hott, K. S. Neurological examination of the newborn. *Hosp. Med.* 8:86, 1972.

Hurlock, E. *Child Development* (4th ed.). New York: McGraw-Hill, 1964.

Kelley, V. (Ed.). *Brennemann's Practice of Pediatrics* (vol. 1, part 2) Maryland: Prior, 1972. Chaps. 80 and 83.

Moore, M. L. *The Newborn and the Nurse.* Philadelphia: Saunders, 1972.

Mussen, P., Conger, J., and Kagan, J. *Child Development and Personality* (3rd ed.). New York: Harper & Row, 1969.

Nelson, W. E. (Ed.). *Textbook of Pediatrics* (9th ed.). Philadelphia: Saunders, 1969.

Parmelee, A. H. *Management of the Newborn* (2nd ed.). Chicago: Year Book, 1959.

Roach, L. Color changes in dark skins. *Nursing '72* 2:19, 1972.

Smart, M., and Smart, R. *Infants: Development and Relationships.* New York: Macmillan, 1973.

Ziegel, E., and Van Blarcom, C. C. *Obstetric Nursing* (6th ed.). New York: Macmillan, 1972.

INFANCY, CHILDHOOD, AND ADOLESCENCE

15

Barbara A. Sachs
Anne L. Sharpe
Carolyn P. Stoll

GLOSSARY

amblyopia Subnormal vision, usually in one eye, without a detectable lesion on physical examination "Lazy eye."

bruxism Grinding of teeth.

clubbing Rounding of the fingernails or toenails, progressing to thickening and shininess of the terminal phalanx.

croup Acute obstruction of the larynx caused by allergy, foreign body, infection, or new growth and characterized by resonant barking cough, hoarseness, and persistent stridor.

cryptorchidism Failure of one or both testes to descend into the scrotum.

cyanosis Bluish discoloration of specific surfaces of the body due to inadequate oxygenation of the blood.

dentition Process which moves the tooth from its developmental· position into the oral cavity in occlusion with its antagonist; tooth eruption.

development Maturation of systems, acquisition of skills, adaptability, responsibility, and creative expression.

dyspnea Deep, labored, difficult respirations.

encopresis Incontinence of feces in a child who has achieved bowel control previously, not caused by organic defect or physical illness.

epiglottitis Inflammation of the lidlike structure which covers the entrance to the larynx.

exstrophy of the bladder Failure of fusion in the anterior walls of the abdomen and bladder.

fusion Development of binocular vision by cerebral combination of the two retinal images to produce a single image.

hydrocele Scrotal cystic mass filled with clear fluid.

hypoxia Inadequate amount of oxygen.

macule Discolored spot on the skin that is not elevated above the surface.

nodule Small, solid node which can be palpated.

papule Small, circumscribed solid elevation of the skin.

paradoxical respirations Respirations in which a lung or portion of a lung is deflated during inspiration and inflated during expiration.

pustule Small elevation of epidermis filled with purulent fluid.

regurgitation Nonforceful expulsion of small quantities of food or liquid.

rumination Voluntary or habitual regurgitation of previously swallowed food.

squatting Bending of the knees so that the buttocks are close to or rest on the heels.

strabismus Tendency of the eye to deviate due to poor muscle control.

stuttering Speech disorder in which rhythm and continuity of diction is broken by spasms of muscles used in the speech mechanism.

vesicle Small, cystlike circumscribed elevation of the epidermis containing fluid.

vomiting Forceful expulsion of gastric contents accompanied by contractions of the abdominal muscles.

wheal Edematous, short-lived elevated area on the skin which can vary greatly in size.

PEDIATRICS

> We approach all problems of children with affection. Theirs is the province of joy and good humor. They are the most wholesome part of the race, for they are freshest from the hands of God.
>
> Charles Stewart Mott
> C. S. Mott Children's Hospital Plaque
> Ann Arbor, Michigan

The purpose of this chapter is to present highlights of the child's physical and psychosocial development, with emphasis on the differences between the physical appraisal of the child and the adult. Detailed information pertaining to adult body systems has been presented in the preceding chapters. It is assumed that the pediatric nurse will already have a basic understanding of the physical examination of the adult.

Approaches to interviewing techniques and the characteristics of development are discussed separately for infants, toddlers through school age, and adolescents. Body systems and miscellaneous topics are summarized for children of all ages, with points of concern mentioned for children of specific ages when indicated. It is not the writers' intent to cover all aspects of physical diagnosis but rather to focus on essentials of practice, with the recommendation that the nurse pursue standard medical references and resources for information of greater depth on specific systems.

Those involved in the health care of children of all ages must be direct and truthful in communications with both child and parent and should provide time for questions and anticipatory guidance. There is immeasurable satisfaction in assisting parents not only to cope with the various stages of development but also to anticipate and enjoy their child's growth toward independence. Each age has its special characteristics, which can bring pleasures that outweigh the frustrations of developmental problems. Nurses can help parents discover the joy that children bring to those around them.

INFANCY

Interview

Interviewing during the infancy period will naturally involve only the parent directly. However, considerable information can be obtained by observing the parent-infant relationship as the history is obtained. The nature of touch, holding, and body contact between parent and child will provide significant clues to the parents' security with a new infant and to the degree of trust the infant has in them.

A history of specific developmental achievements and behavior as well as of sleeping, feeding, and play habits is essential. When feeding problems are a major concern, the parent can be asked to offer a feeding in the nurse's presence, thereby providing an opportunity to assess the parent's comfort and skill, as well as the infant's response.

Whenever possible, it is desirable to have both parents present for interviewing and examination. Concerns expressed by the father are often different from those voiced by the mother. If the infant is restless or fussy, the father can be asked to comfort him in an outer room, allowing the mother to be more relaxed and attentive for the interview. When the infant is ill, however, the nurse should proceed directly to the examination, obtaining essential information during the procedure.

Examination

The entire examination for the infant under 6 months of age can be completed on the examining table. Parents can assist with undressing the infant, with provisions for safety, and with restraining measures for examination of ears, nose, and throat. The nurse will need to be attuned to the interaction of the parent and child to determine the quality of the infant-parent relationship. Observations and skillful questioning will reveal developmental achievements.

The infant over 6 months of age who has learned to sit up can be better examined while held in his parent's arms, or by sitting on the examining table with the parent beside him. He is apt to be frightened of the examining instruments, and will be more cooperative if allowed to handle them briefly, or if the nurse makes a game out of using them. Since infants of 6 months and older usually experience anxiety when separated from their mothers or when confronted by strangers, a familiar toy, blanket, or bottle may be helpful in distracting attention to permit a quiet period for auscultation. Development is more accurately assessed after the infant demonstrates acceptance of the nurse and no longer seems fearful of the strange environment.

Development

Parents may express concern about the normalcy of their baby's growth and development during the first year. Questions and anxiety levels of experienced and inexperienced mothers vary. Parents need information about the demanding behavior of infants and need to have outlets to release their own feelings appropriately, since controlled anger or permissiveness can be frightening to the child seeking limits. The nurse must be aware of the wide latitude of normal behavior, and the pattern of each child's growth and development over an extended period of time, thereby focusing on factors that influence his development.

The crucial developmental task of the first year is the development of a sense of trust. The infant, who begins life as an individual with reflexive behavior, gradually learns that his cries of hunger, discomfort, or need for attention are answered by his mother. As his needs are met, he gradually associates pleasure and security with his mother's care and begins to develop his sense of trust. This trust is further developed as he learns to move about his environment, to do things for himself, and to interact with significant persons in his life.

During the first year (especially in the first 6 months) physical growth and maturation is rapid (see Fig. 15-1), with increasing adequacy of physiologic processes, and particularly rapid development of the nervous system. Birth weights for full-term infants usually double by 5 months and triple in one year. Length increases from a range of 18 to 21 in. (45.7 to 53.3 cm) to a range of 27 to 31 in. (68.6 to 78.7 cm). Head circumference increases rapidly to accomodate growth of the brain. Average head circumference at birth is 35 cm, increasing to between 46 and 47 cm at 1 year.

Development throughout infancy and childhood is orderly and sequential, proceeding in a cephalocaudal direction. For example, head control precedes control of the upper extremities, followed by control of the lower extremities. Also, development in the extremities progresses in a proximal-distal direction, with control of the arms preceding finger control.

The gross motor skills of an infant advance on a continuum: from lifting and gradually controlling his head to lifting head and chest; rolling over; sitting with support; sitting steadily without support; creeping; pulling to a stand; standing alone; and walking.

The fine motor skills of an infant advance through stages of eye-hand coordination: following objects with the eyes; bringing the hands together at the midline; grasping offered objects; reaching for objects; swiping at objects; transferring objects from hand to hand; radial-palmer grasp and pincer grasp.

Language, which begins at birth with the infant's first cry, progresses to small throaty sounds, coos, laughs, squeals, and repetitive sounds; then, by the end of the first year, to several words, mostly names.

In the personal-social realm, the infant progresses from staring at his surroundings to smiling (first responsively, then spontaneously) and to having some separation anxiety when his parents leave him with others. He plays "peekaboo," waves "bye-bye," and begins to feed himself finger foods and drink from a cup.

The Denver Developmental Screening Test (Fig. 15-2) is a useful tool for assessment of specific infant developmental milestones, giving norms for their attainment.

Developmental Concerns

Nutrition. Nutrition is a major concern for mothers of young infants. Frequency and amounts of bottle or breast feedings vary with the growth pattern of the infant. Feeding schedules need to be flexible, allowing time for the infant to satisfy sucking needs. Additional information on infant feeding is presented in the section on the gastrointestinal system.

Weaning. The infant can usually be weaned directly to the cup for juices between 4 and 8 months. Cup feedings can then gradually replace breast or bottle feedings. The bedtime feeding is usually the last bottle to be relinquished and may need to be given as late as 14 to 15 months of age.

Sleeping Patterns (1 to 3 Months). Sleeping patterns in the first three months are as follows:

At 1 month. Sleeps most of the time. Sleep not always quiet. May make sucking motions; opens and closes eyes; breathes unevenly.

At 2 months. Awake for portions of day; sleeps most of night; beginning to give up night feeding; requires late evening and early morning feeding.

At 3 months. Sleeps well when wakeful times have been interesting. Likes bright toys hanging over crib. Enjoys social attention; likes to hear voices and see household activities.

Nap Patterns. Nap patterns evolve in the following manner.

At 1 to 6 months. Has 2 to 3 naps per day, with range of 1 to 4 hours.

From 6 to 10 months. Has 2 naps per day.

From 10 months to 2 years. Has 1 nap per day, usually in the afternoon.

Teething. The infant may be irritable and fussy and have increased salivation as teeth erupt. A clear nasal discharge, reddened gums, and, occasionally, a nonspecific facial rash may be noted. Fever is not usually present. Chewing on a blunt, firm object or cracked ice wrapped in a cloth may relieve pain.

Eyes. *Strabismus* is present to varying degrees in many infants during the neonatal period. The infant's eyes can focus accurately when he is awake and alert, and slight deviations of eye movement may occur when the infant is tired. Should irregular movements persist, the parents should consult an ophthamologist.

Handling the genitals. Around 6 months of age, infants discover their genitals and handle them in the same way they handle their fingers and toes. Curiosity and exploration are aspects of healthy learning and should not be forcefully prohibited. Distracting the infant with a toy is possible and allows completion of dressing procedures.

Immunizations. Only healthy children should receive immunizations. Children with acute infection or skin infections should be immunized after the problem has cleared up. Those with seizures, blood or lymph diseases, or those receiving

PERCENTILE CHART FOR MEASUREMENTS OF INFANT BOYS

THIS CHART provides for infant boys standards of reference for body weight and recumbent length by month from birth to 28 months and for head circumference by week from birth to 28 weeks. It is based upon repeated measurements at selected ages of a group of more than 100 white infants of North European ancestry living under normal conditions of health and home life in Boston, Mass. The distribution of the measurements obtained from the infants at each age is expressed in percentiles, each percentile giving a value which represents a particular position in the normal range of occurrences. The number of the percentile refers to the position which a measurement of the given value would hold in any typical series of 100 infants. Thus, the 10th percentile gives the value for the tenth in any hundred; that is, 9 infants of the same sex and age would be expected to be smaller in the measurement under consideration while 90 would be expected to be larger than the figure given. Similarly the 90th percentile would indicate that 89 infants might be expected to be smaller than the figure given while 10 would be larger. The 50th percentile represents the median or midposition in the customary range. Here, the 10th and 90th percentiles are presented in heavy lines to show the limits within which most infants remain. The lighter lines in the graphs divide the distributions into segments for ready recognition and description of individual differences as well as of the "regularity" of progress. The 3rd and 97th percentiles represent unusual though not necessarily abnormal findings.

In line with common usage in the United States, the charts are ruled on a scale in pounds to represent weight. They are ruled, however, in centimeters to represent length and head circumference, because this scale facilitates accuracy in measuring and recording and centimeter rules and tapes are readily available. For the convenience of those preferring them, scales for kilograms and inches are placed outside of the principal scales and paralleling them. Therefore, if weights are taken in kilograms and lengths and head circumferences in inches, they may be plotted directly without conversion by placing a ruler at the appropriate points on the outer scales of the charts.

To determine the percentile position of any measurement at a given age, the vertical age line is located and a dot is placed where this intersects the horizontal line representing the value obtained from the measurement. Vertical lines give age by one-month intervals for weight and length and one-week intervals for head circumference; horizontal lines give ½-pound, 1-cm. and 0.5-cm. intervals respectively. This permits by interpolation accurate placement for age to weeks, for weights to 2 ounces and for centimeters to 0.5 cm. Recognition of the position within or outside of the range held by an infant in respect to each measurement recorded calls attention to the relative size and build of the individual at the time. More importantly, comparisons of percentile positions held by these measurements at repeated periodic examinations indicate adherence to or possibly significant deviation from previous percentile positions. Under normal circumstances, one expects an infant to maintain a similar position from age to age — that is, on or near one percentile line or between the same two lines. Occasional sharp deviations or gradual but continuing shifts from one percentile position to another call for further investigation as to their causes. In all cases, readings of measurements should be checked and care should be taken to secure the same position of the infant at all examinations. The following procedures were used in obtaining these norms and therefore are recommended:

Body Weight — The infant is weighed without clothing, preferably on special infant scales.

Recumbent Length — The infant lies relaxed on a firm surface parallel to a centimeter rule or on a special infant measuring board which permits the following procedure. The soles of the feet are held firmly against a fixed upright at the zero mark on the rule, and a movable square is brought firmly against the vertex. Care must be taken to secure extension at the knees, and the head should be held so that the eyes face the ceiling.

Head Circumference — This measurement is more satisfactory if taken with the infant lying on his back. The tape is passed around the head from above and placed anteriorly over the lower forehead just above the supraorbital ridges. With the position of the tape thus fixed anteriorly, the largest circumference is obtained by passing it posteriorly over the most prominent part of the occiput.

FIGURE 15-1. Anthropometric charts. (Courtesy Children's Hospital Medical Center, Boston.)

INFANT BOYS

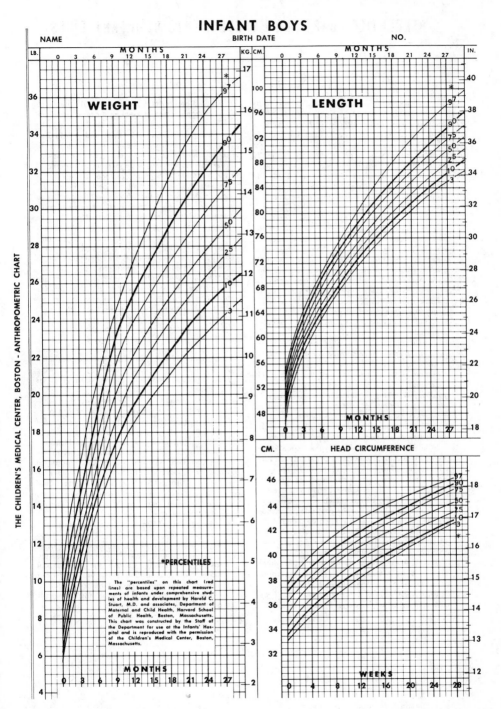

NAME   BIRTH DATE   NO.

WEIGHT

LENGTH

HEAD CIRCUMFERENCE

*PERCENTILES

The "percentiles" on this chart (red lines) are based upon repeated measurements of infants under comprehensive studies of health and development by Harold C. Stuart, M.D. and associates, Department of Maternal and Child Health, Harvard School of Public Health, Boston, Massachusetts. This chart was constructed by the Staff of the Department for use at the Infants' Hospital and is reproduced with the permission of the Children's Medical Center, Boston, Massachusetts.

THE CHILDREN'S MEDICAL CENTER, BOSTON - ANTHROPOMETRIC CHART

PERCENTILE CHART FOR MEASUREMENTS OF INFANT GIRLS

THIS CHART provides for infant girls standards of reference for body weight and recumbent length by month from birth to 28 months and for head circumference by week from birth to 28 weeks. It is based upon repeated measurements at selected ages of a group of more than 100 white infants of North European ancestry living under normal conditions of health and home life in Boston, Mass. The distribution of the measurements obtained from the infants at each age is expressed in percentiles, each percentile giving a value which represents a particular position in the normal range of occurrences. The number of the percentile refers to the position which a measurement of the given value would hold in any typical series of 100 infants. Thus, the 10th percentile gives the value for the tenth in any hundred; that is, 9 infants of the same sex and age would be expected to be smaller in the measurement under consideration while 90 would be expected to be larger than the figure given. Similarly the 90th percentile would indicate that 89 infants might be expected to be smaller than the figure given while 10 would be larger. The 50th percentile represents the median or midposition in the customary range. Here, the 10th and 90th percentiles are presented in heavy lines to show the limits within which most infants remain. The lighter lines in the graphs divide the distributions into segments for ready recognition and description of individual differences as well as of the "regularity" of progress. The 3rd and 97th percentiles represent unusual though not necessarily abnormal findings.

In line with common usage in the United States, the charts are ruled on a scale in pounds to represent weight. They are ruled, however, in centimeters to represent length and head circumference, because this scale facilitates accuracy in measuring and recording and centimeter rules and tapes are readily available. For the convenience of those preferring them, scales for kilograms and inches are placed outside of the principal scales and paralleling them. Therefore, if weights are taken in kilograms and lengths and head circumferences in inches, they may be plotted directly without conversion by placing a ruler at the appropriate points on the outer scales of the charts.

To determine the percentile position of any measurement at a given age, the vertical age line is located and a dot is placed where this intersects the horizontal line representing the value obtained from the measurement. Vertical lines give age by one-month intervals for weight and length and one-week intervals for head circumference; horizontal lines give ½-pound, 1-cm. and 0.5-cm. intervals respectively. This permits by interpolation accurate placement for age to weeks, for weights to 2 ounces and for centimeters to 0.5 cm. Recognition of the position within or outside of the range held by an infant in respect to each measurement recorded calls attention to the relative size and build of the individual at the time. More importantly, comparisons of percentile positions held by these measurements at repeated periodic examinations indicate adherence to or possibly significant deviation from previous percentile positions. Under normal circumstances, one expects an infant to maintain a similar position from age to age — that is, on or near one percentile line or between the same two lines. Occasional sharp deviations or gradual but continuing shifts from one percentile position to another call for further investigation as to their causes. In all cases, readings of measurements should be checked and care should be taken to secure the same position of the infant at all examinations. The following procedures were used in obtaining these norms and therefore are recommended:

Body Weight — The infant is weighed without clothing, preferably on special infant scales.

Recumbent Length — The infant lies relaxed on a firm surface parallel to a centimeter rule or on a special infant measuring board which permits the following procedure. The soles of the feet are held firmly against a fixed upright at the zero mark on the rule, and a movable square is brought firmly against the vertex. Care must be taken to secure extension at the knees, and the head should be held so that the eyes face the ceiling.

Head Circumference — This measurement is more satisfactory if taken with the infant lying on his back. The tape is passed around the head from above and placed anteriorly over the lower forehead just above the supraorbital ridges. With the position of the tape thus fixed anteriorly, the largest circumference is obtained by passing it posteriorly over the most prominent part of the occiput.

FIGURE 15-1. (Continued)

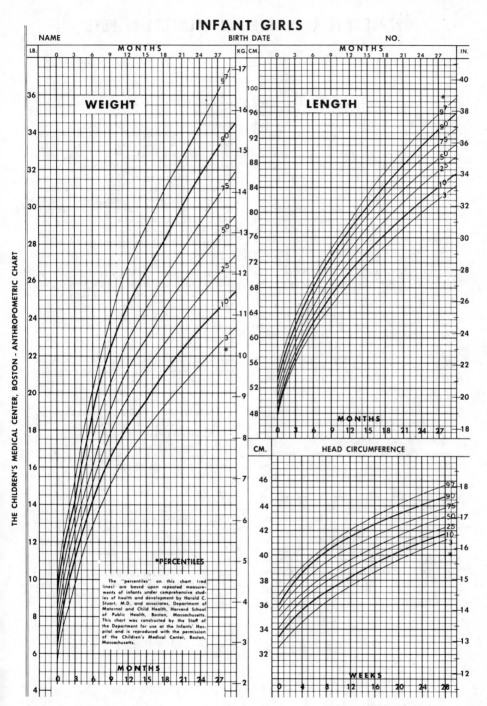

INFANT GIRLS

NAME   BIRTH DATE   NO.

WEIGHT

LENGTH

HEAD CIRCUMFERENCE

*PERCENTILES

The "percentiles" on this chart (red lines) are based upon repeated measurements of infants under comprehensive studies of health and development by Harold C. Stuart, M.D. and associates, Department of Maternal and Child Health, Harvard School of Public Health, Boston, Massachusetts. This chart was constructed by the Staff of the Department for use at the Infants' Hospital and is reproduced with the permission of the Children's Medical Center, Boston, Massachusetts.

THE CHILDREN'S MEDICAL CENTER, BOSTON - ANTHROPOMETRIC CHART

PERCENTILE CHART FOR MEASUREMENTS OF BOYS

THIS CHART provides for boys standards of reference for body weight and recumbent length at ages between 2 and 6 years and for weight and standing height from 6 to 13 years. It is based upon repeated measurements at selected ages of a group of more than 100 white boys of North European ancestry living under normal conditions of health and home life in Boston, Mass. The distribution of the measurements obtained from these children at each age is expressed in percentiles, each percentile giving a value which represents a particular position in the normal range of occurrences. The number of the percentile refers to the position which a measurement of the given value would hold in any typical series of 100 children. Thus, the 10th percentile gives the value for the tenth in any hundred; that is, 9 children of the same sex and age would be expected to be smaller in the measurement under consideration while 90 would be expected to be larger than the figure given. Similarly the 90th percentile would indicate that 89 children might be expected to be smaller than the figure given while 10 would be larger. The 50th percentile represents the median or midposition in the customary range. Here, the 10th and 90th percentiles are represented in heavy lines to show the limits within which most children remain. The lighter lines in the graphs divide the distribution into segments for ready recognition and description of individual differences as well as of the "regularity" of progress. The 3rd and 97th percentiles represent unusual though not necessarily abnormal findings.

In line with common usage in the United States, the charts are ruled on a scale in pounds to represent weight. They are ruled, however, in centimeters to represent length under 6 years and height thereafter, because this scale facilitates accuracy in measuring and recording and centimeter rules and tapes are readily available. For the convenience of those preferring them, scales for kilograms and inches are placed outside of the principal scales and paralleling them. Therefore, if weights are taken in kilograms and lengths and heights in inches, they may be plotted directly without conversion by placing a ruler at the appropriate points on the outer scales of the chart.

To determine the percentile position of any measurement at a given age, the vertical age line is located and a dot is placed where this intersects the horizontal line representing the value obtained from the measurement. Vertical lines give age by 2-month intervals and horizontal lines by 2-pound and 2-cm. intervals. This permits by interpolation accurate placement for age to ½ month and for measurements to ½ pound or 0.5 cm. Recognition of the position held by a child within or outside of the range in respect to each measurement recorded calls attention to the relative size and build of the individual at the time. More importantly, comparisons of percentile positions held by these measurements at repeated periodic examinations indicate adherence to or possibly significant deviation from previous percentile positions. Under normal circumstances, one expects a child to maintain a similar position from age to age — that is, on or near one percentile line or between the same two lines. Occasionally encountered sharp deviations or more gradual but continuing shifts from one percentile position to another call for further investigation as to their causes. In all cases, readings of measurements should be checked and care should be taken to secure the same position of the child accurately at all examinations. The following procedures were used in obtaining these norms and therefore are recommended:

Body Weight — The child is weighed without clothing except light undergarments.

Recumbent Length — The child lies relaxed on a firm surface parallel to a centimeter rule. The soles of the feet are held firmly against a fixed upright at the zero mark on the rule, and a movable square is brought firmly against the vertex. The head is held so that the eyes face the ceiling.

Height — The child's heels should be near together, and heels, buttocks and occiput should be against a firm vertical upright mounting the measuring stick. The eyes should be horizontal and approximately in the same plane as the external auditory canals. A right angle triangle or other movable device should be placed firmly on the head at right angles to the measuring stick and the measurement read after a satisfactory position has been adopted.

FIGURE 15-1. (Continued)

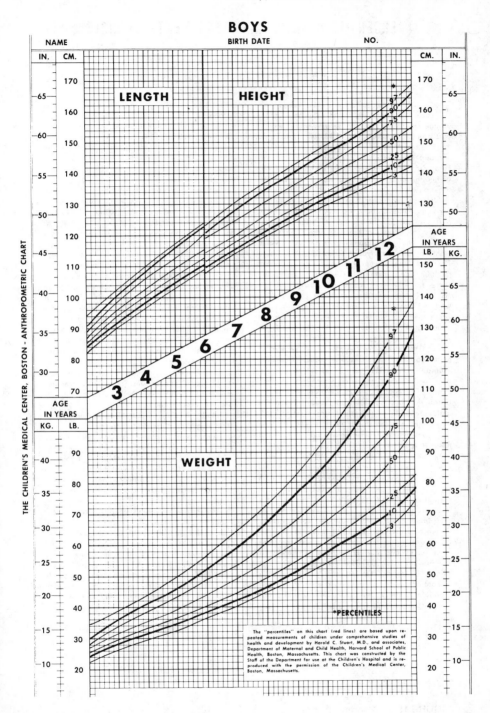

PERCENTILE CHART FOR MEASUREMENTS OF GIRLS

THIS CHART provides for girls standards of reference for body weight and recumbent length at ages between 2 and 6 years and for weight and standing height from 6 to 13 years. It is based upon repeated measurements at selected ages of a group of more than 100 white girls of North European ancestry living under normal conditions of health and home life in Boston, Mass. The distribution of the measurements obtained from these children at each age is expressed in percentiles, each percentile giving a value which represents a particular position in the normal range of occurrences. The number of the percentile refers to the position which a measurement of the given value would hold in any typical series of 100 children. Thus, the 10th percentile gives the value for the tenth in any hundred; that is, 9 children of the same sex and age would be expected to be smaller in the measurement under consideration while 90 would be expected to be larger than the figure given. Similarly the 90th percentile would indicate that 89 children might be expected to be smaller than the figure given while 10 would be larger. The 50th percentile represents the median or midposition in the customary range. Here, the 10th and 90th percentiles are represented in heavy lines to show the limits within which most children remain. The lighter lines in the graphs divide the distribution into segments for ready recognition and description of individual differences as well as of the "regularity" of progress. The 3rd and 97th percentiles represent unusual though not necessarily abnormal findings.

In line with common usage in the United States, the charts are ruled on a scale in pounds to represent weight. They are ruled, however, in centimeters to represent length under 6 years and height thereafter, because this scale facilitates accuracy in measuring and recording and centimeter rules and tapes are readily available. For the convenience of those preferring them, scales for kilograms and inches are placed outside of the principal scales and paralleling them. Therefore, if weights are taken in kilograms and lengths and heights in inches, they may be plotted directly without conversion by placing a ruler at the appropriate points on the outer scales of the chart.

To determine the percentile position of any measurement at a given age, the vertical age line is located and a dot is placed where this intersects the horizontal line representing the value obtained from the measurement. Vertical lines give age by 2-month intervals and horizontal lines by 2-pound and 2-cm. intervals. This permits by interpolation accurate placement for age to ½ month and for measurements to ½ pound or 0.5 cm. Recognition of the position held by a child within or outside of the range in respect to each measurement recorded calls attention to the relative size and build of the individual at the time. More importantly, comparisons of percentile positions held by these measurements at repeated periodic examinations indicate adherence to or possibly significant deviation from previous percentile positions. Under normal circumstances, one expects a child to maintain a similar position from age to age — that is, on or near one percentile line or between the same two lines. Occasionally encountered sharp deviations or more gradual but continuing shifts from one percentile position to another call for further investigation as to their causes. In all cases, readings of measurements should be checked and care should be taken to secure the same position of the child accurately at all examinations. The following procedures were used in obtaining these norms and therefore are recommended:

Body Weight — The child is weighed without clothing except light undergarments.

Recumbent Length — The child lies relaxed on a firm surface parallel to a centimeter rule. The soles of the feet are held firmly against a fixed upright at the zero mark on the rule, and a movable square is brought firmly against the vertex. The head is held so that the eyes face the ceiling.

Height — The child's heels should be near together, and heels, buttocks and occiput should be against a firm vertical upright mounting the measuring stick. The eyes should be horizontal and approximately in the same plane as the external auditory canals. A right angle triangle or other movable device should be placed firmly on the head at right angles to the measuring stick and the measurement read after a satisfactory position has been adopted.

FIGURE 15-1. (Continued)

GIRLS

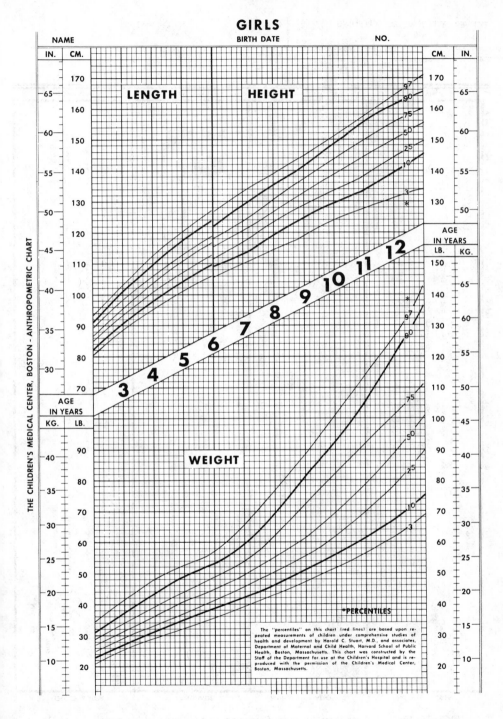

NAME   BIRTH DATE   NO.

LENGTH   HEIGHT

THE CHILDREN'S MEDICAL CENTER, BOSTON - ANTHROPOMETRIC CHART

AGE IN YEARS

WEIGHT

*PERCENTILES

The "percentiles" on this chart (red lines) are based upon repeated measurements of children under comprehensive studies of health and development by Harold C. Stuart, M.D. and associates, Department of Maternal and Child Health, Harvard School of Public Health, Boston, Massachusetts. This chart was constructed by the Staff of the Department for use at the Children's Hospital and is reproduced with the permission of the Children's Medical Center, Boston, Massachusetts.

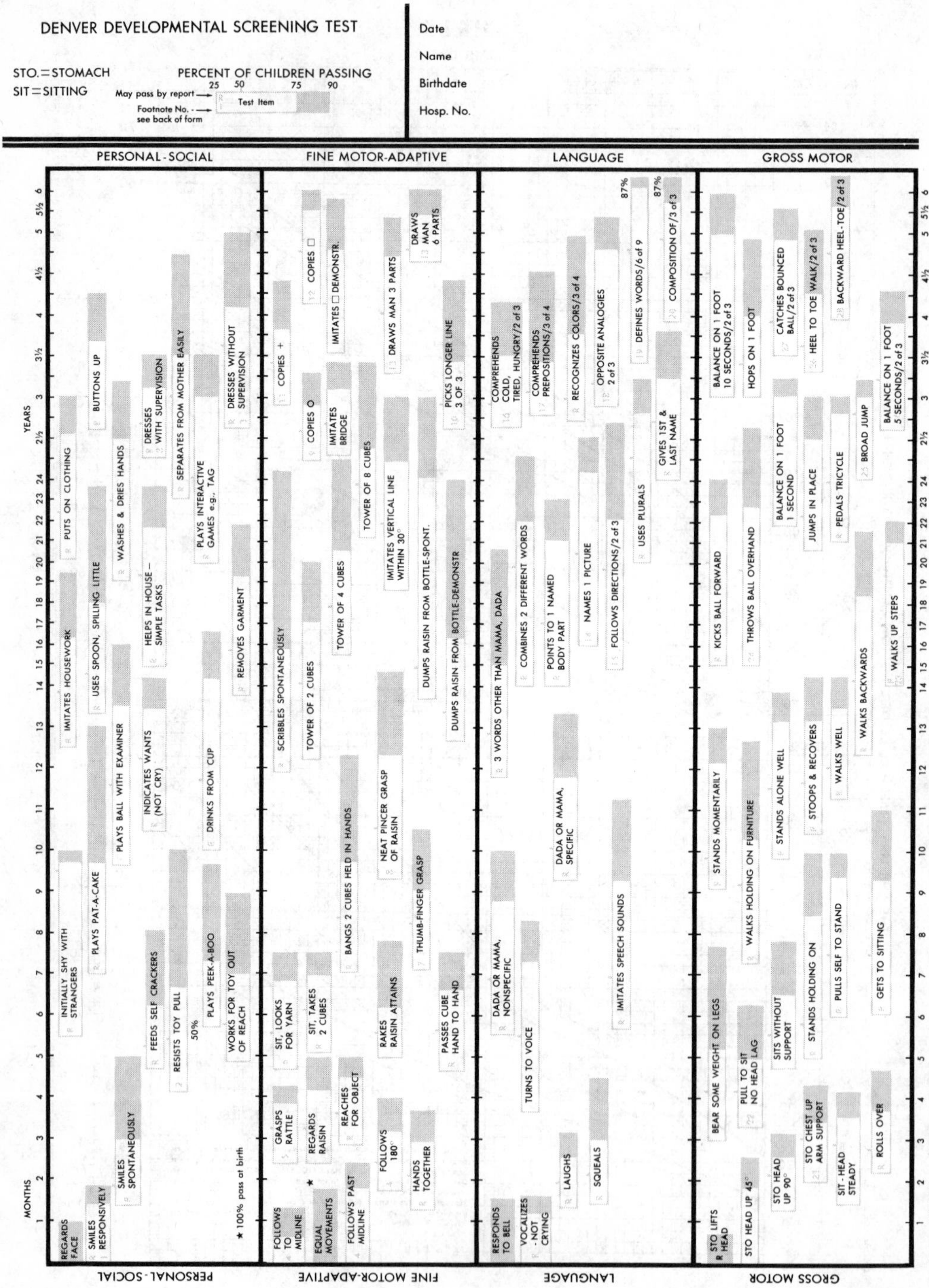

FIGURE 15-2. Denver Developmental Screening Test. (Reprinted by permission of Dr. William K. Frankenburg, University of Colorado Medical Center.)

1. Try to get child to smile by smiling, talking or waving to him. Do not touch him.
2. When child is playing with toy, pull it away from him. Pass if he resists.
3. Child does not have to be able to tie shoes or button in the back.
4. Move yarn slowly in an arc from one side to the other, about 6" above child's face.
   Pass if eyes follow 90° to midline. (Past midline; 180°)
5. Pass if child grasps rattle when it is touched to the backs or tips of fingers.
6. Pass if child continues to look where yarn disappeared or tries to see where it went. Yarn
   should be dropped quickly from sight from tester's hand without arm movement.
7. Pass if child picks up raisin with any part of thumb and a finger.
8. Pass if child picks up raisin with the ends of thumb and index finger using an over hand
   approach.

  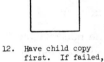

9. Pass any en-
   closed form.
   Fail continuous
   round motions.
10. Which line is longer?
    (Not bigger.) Turn
    paper upside down and
    repeat. (3/3 or 5/6)
11. Pass any
    crossing
    lines.
12. Have child copy
    first. If failed,
    demonstrate

   When giving items 9, 11 and 12, do not name the forms. Do not demonstrate 9 and 11.

13. When scoring, each pair (2 arms, 2 legs, etc.) counts as one part.
14. Point to picture and have child name it. (No credit is given for sounds only.)

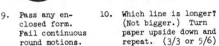

  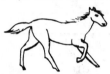

15. Tell child to: Give block to Mommie; put block on table; put block on floor. Pass 2 of 3.
    (Do not help child by pointing, moving head or eyes.)
16. Ask child: What do you do when you are cold? ..hungry? ..tired? Pass 2 of 3.
17. Tell child to: Put block on table; under table; in front of chair, behind chair.
    Pass 3 of 4. (Do not help child by pointing, moving head or eyes.)
18. Ask child: If fire is hot, ice is ?; Mother is a woman, Dad is a ?; a horse is big, a
    mouse is ?. Pass 2 of 3.
19. Ask child: What is a ball? ..lake? ..desk? ..house? ..banana? ..curtain? ..ceiling?
    ..hedge? ..pavement? Pass if defined in terms of use, shape, what it is made of or general
    category (such as banana is fruit, not just yellow). Pass 6 of 9.
20. Ask child: What is a spoon made of? ..a shoe made of? ..a door made of? (No other objects
    may be substituted.) Pass 3 of 3.
21. When placed on stomach, child lifts chest off table with support of forearms and/or hands.
22. When child is on back, grasp his hands and pull him to sitting. Pass if head does not hang back.
23. Child may use wall or rail only, not person. May not crawl.
24. Child must throw ball overhand 3 feet to within arm's reach of tester.
25. Child must perform standing broad jump over width of test sheet. (8-1/2 inches)
26. Tell child to walk forward, heel within 1 inch of toe.
    Tester may demonstrate. Child must walk 4 consecutive steps, 2 out of 3 trials.
27. Bounce ball to child who should stand 3 feet away from tester. Child must catch ball with
    hands, not arms, 2 out of 3 trials.
28. Tell child to walk backward, toe within 1 inch of heel.
    Tester may demonstrate. Child must walk 4 consecutive steps, 2 out of 3 trials.

DATE AND BEHAVIORAL OBSERVATIONS (how child feels at time of test, relation to tester, attention
span, verbal behavior, self-confidence, etc,):

corticosteriods or immunosuppressive drugs should be referred to their physician for advice. Patients with a history of allergy to egg or fowl should not receive vaccines prepared with these tissues. A schedule approved by the American Academy of Pediatrics for active immunization and tuberculin testing of normal infants and children appears in Table 15-1.

TODDLER, PRESCHOOL, AND SCHOOL AGE CHILD

Interview

The nurse should be sensitive to individual differences and plan the interview and examination sequence accordingly. Accurate appraisal may be obtained by conducting the health interview with the parent and assessment of the child over

Table 15-1.   Recommended Schedule for Active Immunization of Normal Infants and Children*

Age	Type of Immunization	
2 mo	DTP[1]	TOPV[2]
4 mo	DTP	TOPV
6 mo	DTP	TOPV
1 yr	Measles[3]	Tuberculin test[4]
	Rubella[3]	Mumps[3]
1½ yr	DTP	TOPV
4–6 yr	DTP	TOPV
14–16 yr	Td[5]	and thereafter every 10 years

*Modified from American Academy of Pediatrics, Committee on Infectious Diseases, 1974. Used by permission of the Academy.

[1]DTP—diphtheria and tetanus toxoids combined with pertussis vaccine.

[2]TOPV—trivalent oral poliovirus vaccine. This recommendation is suitable for breast-fed as well as bottle-fed infants.

[3]May be given at 1 year as measles-rubella or measles-mumps-rubella combined vaccines (see Rubella, section 9, and Mumps, section 9, for further discussion of age of administration).

[4]Frequency of repeated tuberculin tests depends on risk of exposure of the child and on the prevalence of tuberculosis in the population group. The initial test should be at the time of, or preceding, the measles immunization.

[5]Td—combined tetanus and diphtheria toxoids (adult type) for those more than 6 years of age in contrast to diphtheria and tetanus (DT) which contains a larger amount of diphtheria antigen. *Tetanus toxoid at time of injury:* For clean, minor wounds, no booster dose is needed by a fully immunized child unless more than 10 years have elapsed since the last dose. For contaminated wounds, a booster dose should be given if more than 5 years have elapsed since the last dose.

Storage of Vaccines

Because biologics are of varying stability, the manufacturers' recommendations for optimal storage conditions (e.g., temperature, light) should be carefully followed. Failure to observe these precautions may significantly reduce the potency and effectiveness of the vaccines.

several visits. Usually, interviewing begins after rapport is established between the nurse, child, and parent. Engaging the child in simple play or allowing him to explore some of the examining equipment helps promote his cooperation and provides an opportunity to begin assessing his growth and development and his relationship with his parents.

The initial interview is concerned with essential information. Additional history should be delayed until after the examination. Conduct the detailed interview without distractions from the child, if possible. Because the "parenting person" will possess the most detailed information about the child, it is important to interview that person. The history obtained during the interview should include the prenatal and neonatal information mentioned in Chapter 14, general development, immunizations received, and communicable diseases contracted.

The school age child can comprehend more detailed verbal explanations of the nurse examiner's purpose. The 6-year-old has a short attention span but can be expected to sit quietly or play while a cursory history is obtained. In the later school years it may be beneficial to interview the child separately from the parents to gain additional insights into the history and assessment, including school adjustment and achievement.

Examination

Because of the young child's fear of the unfamiliar and his normal inclination toward activity, it is often preferable to examine the child soon after establishing rapport. (The acutely ill child should be examined immediately, beginning with the chief complaint and obtaining essential information as the examination progresses.) The purpose of the examination should be explained in simple terms. Anxiety that is aroused when the toddler is separated from his mother may be alleviated by performing as much of the physical appraisal as possible on her lap, or in her presence if an examining table is used. Abdominal examination must be done with the child lying on a flat surface.

The parent of the young child can be utilized to assist the nurse examiner in a manner similar to that described for the infant. The child should not be unnecessarily exposed, since modesty is pronounced in the preschooler. Because children may retain a rigid abdomen out of fear or sensitivity to tactile stimuli, Caporaro [2] suggests that the examiner place the patient's hand in the palm of his own hand and ask the child to help palpate. This helps to achieve muscle relaxation and to avoid a ticklish sensation. Intrusive procedures (entering body orifices) are especially frightening to the young child, and time should be taken to explain candidly the necessity of performing them. Pelvic examinations, when indicated in the school age child, should be done by a gynecologist.

Further evaluation of developmental milestones and history continues throughout the examination and affords the nurse an opportunity to discuss normal growth and development with the parent. Usually, the school age child can be examined without the parents present, but the nurse needs to be alert to the child's needs and permit the parents' in the room if the child wishes.

Development

Although physical growth slows after the first six months of life, development continues at a rapid pace. The major task of the second and third years is development of autonomy, which leads to the familiar toddler, "No." The child generally first develops bowel control, then bladder control. He learns to feed himself, to undress and dress himself, and to walk, climb, ride a tricycle, and throw objects. He expresses his needs and desires through a rapidly expanding vocabulary, used with increasing skill. The 4-year-old is developing his sexual identity and shows an intense attraction for the parent of the opposite sex. A helpful tool for evaluating development of the infant through the age of 6 is the Denver Developmental Screening Test (see Fig. 15-2). When the test is administered, the child's parents should be informed that it is a screening instrument and that no child is expected to accomplish every item. The nurse must be thoroughly familiar with the manual describing its use.

Developmental Concerns from One to Five. As the child matures and new behavior patterns develop, parents express additional concerns.

Nutrition. Nutrition is a major developmental concern for parents of children between 1 and 5 years of age. With the normal decrease in physical growth during these years, appetite diminishes. Parents who have been providing for the nutritional needs of the rapidly growing infant often become anxious over seeming anorexia in the toddler. Problems are exaggerated by forcing intake or creating struggles at meals. Reassurance can be offered that a decreased appetite is normal and that an active toddler who demonstrates a weight gain of several pounds and skeletal growth of several inches each year is progressing satisfactorily. Parents with children who are chronically ill or have acute infections also need to understand that illness further decreases appetite.

Sleep disturbances. Sleep disturbances are usually exhibited in children between 2 and 6 years of age and may be related to the frequent occurrence of nightmares in this period. The child needs both reassurance and limits. The child should be comforted when he awakens, and the nature of the nightmares should be explored. A night light or an open door may be helpful, but parents should avoid having the child sleep with them. Children who have recently experienced emotional trauma may also show exacerbation of sleeping problems. The possibility of pinworms should be investigated if sleeping disturbances accompanied by rectal itching and bruxism occur.

Nocturnal Enuresis. Nocturnal enuresis occurs in many 3- and 4-year-olds who have good bladder control when awake. This occurs most frequently in males and often has an emotional basis. Sleep reduces inhibitions, and tension and aggression toward parents may be expressed through enuresis. Poor bladder training, anomalies of the urinary system, developmental lag, and regression should also be considered. Recommendations include: limiting the child's fluids for several hours before bedtime; thoroughly awakening him at several intervals during the night and helping him to the bathroom; attempting to reduce the child's anxiety; and putting less pressure on him in the form of high expectations. Soiled linen should be changed without a punitive attitude.

Bowel Training. Bowel training is accomplished much earlier than bladder control because myelinization of the spinal cord innervating rectal sphincters occurs earlier than in the portion innervating bladder sphincters. Constipation can develop between the ages of 2 and 3 years as a part of the negative behavior of the toddler. While striving for autonomy, he expresses his independence by withholding his "gift" from his parents. Encopresis may indicate developmental lag or serious behavioral disturbances.

Thumbsucking. Thumbsucking usually occurs between 12 and 18 months and is related to unsatiated oral need, boredom, or anxiety. Prolonged thumbsucking in the preschool years can cause some alteration in jaw formation and minor dental problems. Parents should attempt to establish reasonable expectations for the anxious child and provide him with appropriate attention.

Temper Tantrums. Temper tantrums begin around 1 year of age, reaching a peak at about 18 months of age. They are usually symptoms of frustration which the preverbal child cannot adequately express. Relief of immediate frustration and direction of the child toward more acceptable expressions of emotions are recommended. Retaliation or appeasement are not workable means of coping with this behavior.

Masturbation. Masturbation may be marked during the fourth and fifth years (oedipal period). A second period of frequent genital play occurs in the preadolescent years. No damage results from masturbation. Shaming the child and making him feel guilty should be avoided. He can be taught to seek privacy when engaging in this normal behavior.

Stuttering. Stuttering is a common speech disorder which may appear at various intervals in the life cycle but occurs primarily during the preschool years, at the time of entry into school, and at puberty. Its cause is believed to be anxiety. The severity of the problem may be increased by overly concerned parents. The child may feel rejected and unworthy and avoid contact with others. Management should be directed toward relieving anxiety, reducing the parents' concern, and helping them develop a patient, accepting, nonstressful approach toward their child.

During the school age years, appetite gradually returns, muscle mass increases, and fine motor skills become developed to a degree that permits greater manual dexterity. Hormone changes stimulate skeletal growth and the development of secondary sexual characteristics.

Table 15-2.   Developmental Charts for Ages 3 to 15 years*

AGES 3 TO 4 YEARS

Activities to be observed:
Climbs stairs with alternating feet.
Begins to button and unbutton.
"What do you like to do that's fun?"
  (Answers using plurals, personal
  pronoun, and verbs.)
Responds to command to place toy
  in, on, or *under* table.
Draws a circle when asked to draw
  a man (girl, boy).
Knows his sex. ("Are you a boy or
  a girl?")
Gives full name.
Copies a circle already drawn. ("Can
  you make one like this?")

Activities related by parent:
Feeds self at mealtime.
Takes off shoes and jacket.

AGES 4 TO 5 YEARS

Activities to be observed:
Runs and turns without losing balance.
May stand on one leg for at least 10
  seconds.
Buttons clothes and laces shoes. (Does
  not tie.)
Counts to 4 by rote.
"Give me 2 sticks." (Able to do so
  from pile of 4 tongue depressors.)
Draws a man. (Head, 2 appendages,
  and possibly 2 eyes. No torso yet.)
"You know the days of the week. What
  day comes after Tuesday?"
Gives appropriate answers to: "What
  must you do if you are sleepy?
  Hungry? Cold?"
Copies + in imitation.

Activities related by parent:
Self care at toilet. (May need help with
  wiping.)
Plays outside for at least 30 minutes.
Dresses self except for tying.

AGES 5 TO 6 YEARS

Activities to be observed:
Can catch ball.
Skips smoothly.
Copies a + already drawn.
Tells his age.
Concept of 10 (eg., counts 10 tongue
  depressors). May recite to higher
  numbers by rote.
Knows his right and left hand.
Draws recognizable man with at least
  8 details.
Can describe favorite television pro-
  gram in some detail.

Activities related by parent:
Does simple chores at home. (Taking out
  garbage, drying silverware, etc.)
Goes to school unattended or meets school
  bus.
Good motor ability but little awareness of
  dangers.

AGES 6 TO 7 YEARS

Activities to be observed:
Copies a △.
Defines words by use. ("What is an
  orange?" "To eat.")
Knows if morning or afternoon.
Draws a man with 12 details.
Reads several one-syllable printed words.
  (My, dog, see, boy.)
Uses pencil for printing name.

AGES 7 TO 8 YEARS

Activities to be observed:
Counts by 2s and 5s.
Ties shoes.
Copies a ◇.
Knows what day of the week it is (not
  date or year.)
Reads paragraph #1 Durrell:

Reading:
"Muff is a little yellow kitten. She drinks
milk. She sleeps on a chair. She does not
like to get wet."

Corresponding arithmetic:

$$7 \quad\quad 6 \quad\quad 6 \quad\quad 8$$
$$+4 \quad\quad +7 \quad\quad -4 \quad\quad -3$$

No evidence of sound substitution in speech
  (eg; *fr* for *thr*).
Adds and subtracts one-digit numbers.
Draws a man with 16 details.

AGES 8 TO 9 YEARS

Activities to be observed:
Defines words better than by use. ("What
  is an orange?" "A fruit.")
Can give an appropriate answer to the
  following:
  "What is the thing for you to do if. . .
    —you've broken something that belongs
      to someone else?"
    —a playmate hits you without meaning
      to do so?"
Reads paragraph # 2 Durrell:

Reading:
"A little black dog ran away from home. He
played with two big dogs. They ran away
from him. It began to rain. He went under

a tree. He wanted to go home, but he did not know the way. He saw a boy he knew. The boy took him home."

Corresponding arithmetic:

```
        45
  67    16     14      84
 + 4   + 27    − 8    − 36
```

Is learning borrowing and carrying processes in addition and subtraction.

AGES 9 TO 10 YEARS

Activities to be observed:
Knows the month, day, and year.
Names the months in order. (Fifteen seconds, one error.)
Makes a sentence with these 3 words in it: (One of 2. Can use words orally in proper context.)
1. work . . . . money . . . . men
2. boy . . . . river . . . . ball
Reads paragraph # 3 Durrell:

Reading:
"Six boys put up a tent by the side of river. They took things to eat with them. When the sun went down, they went into the tent to sleep. In the night, a cow came and began to eat grass around the tent. The boys were afraid. They thought it was a bear."

Corresponding arithmetic:

```
  5204    23     837
 − 530    X3     X 7
```

Should comprehend and answer question: "What was the cow doing?"
Learning simple multiplication.

AGES 10 TO 12 YEARS

Activities to be observed:
Should read and comprehend paragraph # 5 Durrell:

Reading:
"In 1807, Robert Fulton took the first long trip in a steamboat. He went one hundred and fifty miles up the Hudson River. The boat went five miles an hour. This was faster than a steamboat had ever gone before. Crowds gathered on both banks of the river to see this new kind of boat. They were afraid that its noise and splashing would drive away all the fish."

Corresponding arithmetic:

```
 420
 X 29      9⟌72      31⟌62
```

Answer: "What river was the trip made on?"
Ask to write the sentence: "The fishermen did not like the boat."
Should do multiplication and simple division.

AGES 12 TO 15 YEARS

Activities to be observed:
Reads paragraph # 7 Durrell:

Reading:
"Golf originated in Holland as a game played on ice. The game in its present form first appeared in Scotland. It became unusually popular and kings found it so enjoyable that it was known as "the royal game." James IV, however, thought that people neglected their work to indulge in this fascinating sport so that it was forbidden in 1457. James relented when he found how attractive the game was, and it immediately regained its former popularity. Golf spread gradually to other countries, being introduced in America in 1890. It has grown in favor until there is hardly a town that does not boast of a private or public course."

Corresponding arithmetic:

```
 536 ⟌4762     1/3        7 1/6
              + 1/3      − 3/4
```

Reduce fractions to lowest forms.

Ask to write sentence: "Golf originated in Holland as a game played on ice."
Answers questions:
"Why was golf forbidden by James IV?"
"Why did he change his mind?"
Does long division, adds and subtracts fractions.

---

*Modified from S. R. Leavitt, H. Gofman, and D. Harvin, in Kempe et al. [6], by permission of the authors and publishers.

Developmental Concerns in the School Age Child

The tasks of middle childhood are successful school adjustment, development of a time-space concept, and a development of a sense of justice and morality (superego). Intellectual development with abstract thinking and reasoning ability is an important part of the school child's mental processes. He also develops more independence and begins to feel secure while away from home and parents for extended periods of time. Use of charts like the one shown in Table 15-2 is a simple way to assess the child's development.

Nail-biting is one of the developmental problems occurring in the school age child. It usually indicates anxiety and has no serious consequence. *Tics* most commonly occur between the ages of 5 and 10 years. Although usually a sign of emotional problems, they are sometimes caused by local irritation. Treatment should be specific for cause. *Ritualistic behavior* occurs frequently between six and eight years when the school age child is developing a conscience. Peer group play is organized by strict rules. The child with poorly controlled conscience may develop elaborate rituals in an attempt to repress socially unacceptable feelings. If these rituals interfere with normal activities, professional consultation is indicated.

Aggression/withdrawal may result from sibling rivalry, feelings of inferiority, or inconsistent parenting. Careful determination of the cause should precede education directed at more acceptable expression of feelings. *Excessive fear or dependency* may result from a child's being urged toward too much independence too early or from overprotection. *School phobias* most frequently occur in girls in the early school years. A wide variety of symptoms may be presented, but the origin can often be traced to school pressures and social maladjustment (mutual dependency of mother and child). Careful evaluation should be done to rule out organic disease.

Delinquency is more than the occasional petty larceny that occurs during the middle school years when gang influence is strong. It is the ongoing illegal activities of a child or adolescent. The incidence of delinquency is increasing in America, and the crimes committed by children are similar to those of adults.

If a child exhibits illegal behavior, his ego strength, relationship to authority, neurotic guilt, and need for punishment require evaluation. Parents' fluctuation between overindulgence and high expectations should also be noted. The child usually harbors feelings of depression and of being unloved and has low self-esteem. Management is directed toward developing consistent external controls to assist the weak internal controls (conscience, or superego) of the child.

ADOLESCENCE

Interview and Examination

Approaches to interviewing the adolescent patient require the same sensitivity to individuality as in other age groups. Since the adolescent can be classified neither as a child nor an adult, emphasis should be placed on understanding development during this period, including fluctuations between dependent and independent behavior.

It is imperative that the interviewer convey sincere interest in the adolescent and his problems. A sense of trust between the practitioner and the patient is essential and will require varying lengths of time to establish. Direct, truthful responses to his questions and assurance that all information will remain confidential will assist in the development of trust and rapport.

Unlike the adult, the adolescent does not usually present orderly information about his illness or complaints. He may not even recognize his specific problem, or he may be reluctant to reveal or discuss his concerns. The adolescent is usually resentful of individuals who have an authoritative manner, and he sometimes appears angry or withdrawn when coping with feelings of fear and discomfort. There may even be rejection of the nurse for several visits. Occasionally, a patient may openly and instantly share his feelings and problems. It is important to allow extended time during such an interview in order to gain significant information that may not be repeated at a later visit. The patient may find anxiety-provoking subjects difficult to talk about directly and then suddenly bring up a sensitive topic for discussion during the physical examination, when less attention is focused on verbal communications.

There are a number of areas of psychosocial development that should be explored with each adolescent. They include his self-concept, body image, manner of coping with life stresses, relationships with peers, feelings for others, with particular attention to heterosexual relationships, future vocational goals, and progress toward independence from his family. Adolescents attempt to conform to their peer group in appearance and actions, and they are very much concerned with how they appear to others compared with their self-image. Varying degrees of hypochondriasis may occur because the adolescent is concerned with physical perfection. Nevertheless, it is essential for the practitioner to complete a careful history and examination to determine the presence of any specific disease.

When interviewing adolescents, it is important to be attentive, avoid interrupting and interruptions, and particularly to avoid offering advice unless solicited. Careful observations of the adolescent are essential throughout the interview. Mannerisms, tics, restlessness, and a variety of signs of uneasiness may be apparent when specific subjects are discussed. A rigid posture, grimaces, stuttering, excessive modesty, and inability to face the interviewer are all signs of anxiety and insecurity to be considered in the appraisal of the patient. Finally, the manner in which the adolescent expresses himself is critical. Depth of feeling and choice of words is as important as the content of the conversation.

Parents accompanying adolescents for health care visits may be invited to join their child for the initial interview. Interaction between the parent and child should be carefully observed. At the time of examination, however, it is advisable to see the adolescent alone, allowing him sufficient opportunity to discuss his symptoms and problems privately. Whenever possible, parents should be invited to visit the practitioner a day or two in advance of their child's visit.

Rapid acceleration of growth and body changes coupled with newly aroused sexual drives may stimulate a variety of fantasies and fears in an adolescent who previously felt comfortable with his physical self. It is helpful to review developmental changes, stressing the advent of the secondary sex characteristics and the accompanying changes in impulses and desires that occur. Adolescents often feel lonely and uncertain but mask their insecurity with bold, aggressive behavior. Parents can also be helped to evaluate their child more favorably when provided with information about developmental progression during adolescence.

Developmental Concerns

Acne Vulgaris. Acne vulgaris is present in varying degrees in 75 to 90 percent of adolescents under 18 years of age [8, p. 305]. The seriousness of acne for this age group cannot be overestimated, for even mild acne can affect popularity and self-confidence at a time when attractiveness and friendships are essential. Acne is related to overproduction of oil from sebaceous glands controlled by hormones which are predominantly androgenic. Other causes include infection, familial predisposition, endocrine gland imbalance, poor diet, lack of sleep or exercise, excessive sweating, and emotional conflicts. Frequent thorough cleansing of the face with a detergent soap in the morning, afternoon, and at bedtime is the recommended treatment. Adolescents with severe acne should be referred to a dermatologist.

Obesity. Obesity is seen throughout childhood, with peaks during the first four years of life and between 7 and 11 years of age. It is a difficult problem in adolescence, a time when children are most sensitive to appearance and approval from peers. Lowrey [8, p. 415] suggests that any child who weighs 20 percent or more above the mean for his height and age should be considered obese.

Obesity in adolescence is usually caused by poor dietary habits, frequently related to emotional stress. Eating becomes a source of satisfaction and comfort when coping with anxiety and tension. Treatment is often difficult and prolonged and consists of a counseling program in exercise and dietary restriction. Results are entirely dependent on the adolescent's degree of motivation and frequently are disappointing. When the problem is severe, referral for psychiatric counseling may be necessary.

Dysmenorrhea. Dysmenorrhea is a common adolescent problem and may be severe enough to cause frequent absences from school. Complaints vary considerably and may include cramping, lower abdominal fullness, headache, nausea, vomiting, irritability, and, frequently, constipation and diarrhea. A careful history, physical, and pelvic examination should be completed to rule out a pathological condition of the pelvis. In adolescence, psychogenic factors associated with menstrual pain are prevalent and may be due to fears and fantasies based on misconceptions and misinformation. A detailed explanation of the menstrual cycle is essential for the premenarchial girl, as is information on other aspects of puberty, including anticipated secondary sexual developments.

Veneral Disease. It is most important that examinations and cultures for venereal disease be done on patients thought to be sexually active. There appears to be no satisfactory explanation of the increased incidence in venereal disease among adolescents. Lack of adequate sex education has been mentioned as a possible influence, as well as the preoccupation with sex in our society, evident in films, television, and advertising. The availability of abortions, decreased parental supervision, increased emancipation of females, and a changing morality are other possible contributing factors.

Adolescents may refuse to seek treatment because of the sensitive nature of the problem and because they fear their parents will be notified. In many states the law requires parental approval prior to diagnosis and treatment. Some states have recently passed legislation permitting the usual requirements of parental consent to be waived. The nurse will need to be informed of regulations governing her practice but should maintain respect for confidentiality whenever possible. It is essential that sufficient time be allowed for education and counseling during such clinic visits.

Drug Abuse. The incidence of drug use in adolescents has been increasing, even among the very young teen-ager. A variety of treatment centers have been established, predominantly in larger cities. Education for parents and teachers about early symptoms of drug use is very much needed. Nurses can help parents appraise their child's behavior more objectively by emphasizing the clues suggestive of drug abuse. The reader is referred to Suggested Readings for resources providing a discussion of this subject.

GENERAL INDICES OF HEALTH STATUS

Behavior

The child's general appearance must be observed quickly but carefully. In the preverbal or seriously ill child, pertinent observations can assist in rapidly determining the degree of illness. The smiling playful child is usually not acutely ill. Strength, pitch, frequency, and duration of cry, as well as general behavior and posture, are valuable indices of health status. Table 15-3 provides suggestions for consideration in assessment of types of cries.

Table 15-3. Interpretation of Cries

Cry	Position/Behavior Activity	Indication
Strong	Rubbing body part Doubled up Wincing	Pain Anxiety Sudden injury
Frequent, constant, prolonged		Seriously ill Severe pain
Low-pitched		Laryngeal abnormalities Thyroid dysfunction Mental retardation
High-pitched	Persistent or resistant body position Restlessness	Central nervous system pathology Emotional problems
With movement only	Persistent or resistant body position	Central nervous system pathology Fracture
Infrequent, short, weak	Quiet Little movement Staring	Debilitated condition
Irritable	Restless, hyperactive Apprehensive	Respiratory distress Central nervous system involvement Emotional problems

Nutritional State

The symptoms of abnormal nutritional states are sometimes different in children than in adults, although they are evaluated similarly. Acute dehydration is manifested by parched tongue, sunken, tearless eyes, a weak or absent cry, and a lethargic to semicomatose state. The anterior fontanelle in the infant will also appear sunken. Children with chronic malnutrition have protuberant abdomens (a classical sign not to be confused with the normal pot-bellied appearance of young children), flat buttocks, and prominent sucking pads in the cheeks. Poor muscle tone, muscular atrophy, and a slow response to stimuli are additional findings.

Temperature

The temperature is usually taken prior to starting the physical examination. Axillary or rectal temperatures are taken in infants and young children. Reliable oral temperatures can usually be obtained from children above age 5 who can understand instructions. Fever may occur in children with many illnesses, as well as during periods of excitement, vigorous play, and following meals. Children in the younger age periods (infancy through 8 years) frequently have very high fevers (104° F [40° C]) with bacterial, viral, and protozoan infections and dehydration.

Convulsions may accompany high temperature elevations in children between the ages of 6 months and 5 years, especially when the rate of temperature elevation is rapid. In this age group, 5 percent of the children have at least one seizure, with approximately 40 percent of the group suffering their first convulsion with fever [11]. Febrile convulsions, if prolonged and accompanied by significant hypoxemia, may result in brain damage. Therefore, children who experience repeated seizures should be referred to a physician for anticonvulsant therapy. Additional treatment should be directed toward fever control and prevention.

Skin

The skin of children differs from that of adults in several ways. The infant's epidermis is thin, poorly developed, and susceptible to irritation and infection. Sweating is scanty or may be absent. During childhood, the cohesion of epidermal cells is weak, resulting in blistering following minor trauma or staphylococcal infections. The skin is dry and susceptible to chapping due to scanty sebaceous secretions. The final transitional phase to adult skin occurs in adolescence and is accompanied by acne vulgaris [1].

Assessment of dermatologic health includes obtaining a history of family allergy, information about the occupations of family members, presence of pets, the health of family members and playmates, and knowledge of the patient's hygiene and habits.

Examination. Although a detailed history is valuable, there is no substitute for exposure of the skin and direct examination. A pocket magnifier may be useful to the examiner. As in the adult, the child's skin should be examined for color, texture, petechiae, ecchymoses, turgor, scars, and nevi. The degree of sweating is noted and may be present after 1 month of age, especially in the crying, vigorously active, or overly warm infant. The nails of the child are examined for evidence of poor hygiene, nail-biting, and bacterial or fungal infections. Normally, hair is found only on the scalp, eyebrows, and lashes from early infancy until near puberty. If there is variation from this pattern, familial characteristics and potential disease should be investigated. Pubic hair appears between the ages of 8 to 12 years, followed by axillary hair about six months later. Facial hair in boys appears about one year after pubic hair development. Sparse or excessive hair may indicate disease conditions.

Lymph node enlargement occurs readily in children with infections; therefore an attempt should be made routinely to palpate the following lymph nodes: occipital, postauricular, anteroposterior cervical, parotid, submaxillary, sublingual, axillary, epitrochlear, and inguinal. Frequently, discrete, shotty, nontender, cool nodes up to 3 mm in diameter are normal findings in children and usually indicate previous infections. In the inguinal and cervical regions, nodes up to 1 cm in diameter are considered normal until puberty. Warm, large, tender, or isolated nodes, as well as lymphadenopathy, require medical investigation. The child should be observed for edema, and, fluid retention due to systemic disease will be most pronounced as periorbital edema.

The incidence of skin problems in infants and children is second only to that of respiratory problems. Accurate examination of skin lesions includes noting distribution, configuration, topography, type of lesion (macule, papule, vesicle, pustule, nodule, wheal), nature of the lesion (hemorrhage, inflammation, tumor), and evidence of modification due to secondary infection or self-medication. The stage of lesion development is noted also, although one stage may be superimposed on another. Frequently, one skin area looks inflamed and edematous, signs of the acute stage, with other areas showing the improvement of the subacute stage, and still other skin areas having the dry, leathery appearance of chronic dermatitis.

Skin Problems.   Good skin care includes keeping the epidermis clean, dry, and free of oils and ointments which obliterate pores. Powders are soothing and help absorb moisture. They should be applied as a fine film to avoid forming lumps when wet. Although used extensively by parents, cornstarch tends to cake and irritate skin [1].

Transient *heat rashes* (*miliaria rubra*), caused by mechanical obstruction of excretory ducts in the epidermis, occur most commonly on the face, neck, trunk, and in the diaper areas of infants. Treatment is directed toward keeping the infant cool by bathing, removing excessive clothing, and placing in a cool environment. *Intertrigo,* characterized by raw, denuded areas resulting from rubbing of skin surfaces in moist body areas, may predispose the patient to *Candida* infection. The child should be kept cool with loose fitting clothing. *Candidiasis* (*thrush*), appears as white, curdlike lesions on inflamed oral mucosa or as satellite lesions with sharp margins in the diaper area. In the newborn it is caused by *Candida* infections of the mother, but in older infants and children it may be a complication of disease or of drug therapy. *Seborrhea,* relatively common in infancy and childhood, is caused by excessive secretions of the sebaceous glands. A scaling, erythematous rash covered with yellowish scales occurs over the scalp, forehead, eyebrows, eyelids, behind the ears, and on the back of the neck. This condition, known as "milk crust" or "cradle cap" in infancy, is called dandruff in older children. *Contact dermatitis* may be a reaction to products such as powders, soap, or bubble bath. Discontinuing their use usually results in improvement of the condition. *Roseola,* characterized by acute onset of high fever and a delayed erythematous macular or maculopapular rash, primarily on the neck and trunk, is common to infants and young children. Treatment is symptomatic.

In older children, skin problems include food and drug allergies, athlete's foot, and ringworm of the scalp or body. Children and adolescents are susceptible to such viral skin problems as *herpes simplex, herpes zoster, viral exanthema,* and, especially, *warts.* As children begin to explore the outdoors, *contact dermatitis* from insecticides, fertilizers, and poison oak and poison ivy may cause severe skin eruptions. *Sunburn* often results from extended periods of sun exposure during outdoor activities. Although children of any age may suffer *insect bites,* school age boys are the most frequent victims of stinging insects. Children, however, rarely suffer the severe anaphylatic reactions to bites which are seen in adults.

School age children are susceptible to *contagious impetigo,* a bacterial infection of the face, extremities, and exposed body surfaces, and may infect their peers. *Anal itching,* caused by poor hygiene, contact or atopic dermatitis, or pinworms, may be a childhood complaint. *Atopic dermatitis (eczema),* caused by allergies, irritants, and other agents, is fairly common. Characterized by erythema and a thin vesicular rash, it is usually found on the flexor surfaces of the extremities and often becomes secondarily infected from scratching.

Many communicable disease of childhood are accompanied by skin rashes. Familiarity with rash distribution and other symptoms of common communicable diseases assists with differential diagnosis. The rashes of *measles* (rubeola), *scarlet fever,* and *roseola* are macular, while exanthema causes papular rashes. *Chicken pox* (varicella) in its early stages may resemble impetigo but later develops into vesicles. Other vesicular conditions are herpes and sunburn. Impetigo and adolescent acne are pustular skin eruptions.

Relief of the itch, scratch, secondary infection cycle is the primary treatment goal for most skin problems. Skin manifestations of systemic diseases must be considered by the nurse examiner when assessing dermatologic problems.

EYES, EARS, NOSE, THROAT

Early detection of sensory deficits is dependent on an accurate history of development and on direct observations during physical examinations.

Eyes

Eye growth parallels central nervous system growth and is summarized in Table 15-4.

Examination. In addition to revealing ocular health and visual acuity, eye examination may be an important source of information about systemic diseases, especially central nervous system problems. Because few young children are cooperative during ocular examination, skillful use of the left hand is helpful in attracting the child's gaze. Eye examinations are usually delayed until the end of the assessment because they are frightening to the young child. Children over 5 are usually more cooperative.

Observations of the child's eyes are similar in most respects to those in the adult evaluation. Differences include the need to focus attention on the presence of amblyopia, or strabismus. Early therapy is essential, since treatment results are discouraging after age 4. Head tilting or turning similar to that seen in torticollis may indicate problems with ocular muscle coordination, while photophobia and tearing may be signs of infant glaucoma.

Table 15-4. Ocular Development from Birth to Age 4

Age	Development and Behavior
Birth	Infant resists lid opening; small pupils; soft pliable lens; doesn't cry tears, although eyes are bathed in tears; awareness of dark and light; closes eyes in bright light; blurred central vision because of incomplete macular development; peripheral vision; pseudostrabismus due to facial shape; nystagmus because of poorly developed muscle control.
1 month	Follows movement of large, conspicuous objects.
2 months	Jerky ocular movement when following moving objects.
4 months	Macula matures enough to permit fixation. Infant inspects own hands. Fixates immediately on small block brought within 12—24 inches of eye.
6 months	Pseudostrabismus disappearing; accommodation reflex present; hand-eye coordination developing; follows dropped object; fixates well in presence of competing stimuli.
1 year	Fusion developing; discriminates shapes; vision 20/180.
18 months	Convergence well established. Depth perception poor—runs into objects.
4 years	Vision 20/20. Can be screened with Snellen E Chart.

Children complaining of eyestrain require careful refraction. If corrective lenses are indicated, the child should determine the wearing time during the adjustment period. Prior to the decision, he should wear the glasses long enough to appreciate what corrected visual acuity can reveal.

Screening. Visual testing for young children is difficult. Gross evaluation of visual acuity can be obtained by noting interest in light or bright objects and by the pupillary reaction to light. The 1- or 2-year-old can be tested by placing an assortment of brightly colored, different-sized objects about him and observing which are noticed and picked up. The child over 2 years of age usually cooperates with illiterate E testing by indicating the direction of the bars of the letter, or the direction of the legs on the animal pictures. A child over 4 years of age can be tested with the Snellen test cards. School age children and adolescents are evaluated similarly to adults.

Ears

Normal infants can hear immediately after birth. Table 15-5 summarizes ear growth and auditory development.

Examination. Ear examinations tend to be uncomfortable for children and are usually postponed until the end of the physical appraisal. The external ear is observed for shape, position on the head, and the presence of sinuses in front of the ear. The mastoid is palpated for tenderness. The otoscope is fitted with the largest possible speculum and should not enter the ear canal more than 0.25 to 0.5 in. External canals are checked for furuncles, vesicles, drainage, and foreign bodies. The direction of the infant's ear canal is upward, so the auricle is pulled downward to visualize the drum, while the older child's auricle is pulled up and

Table 15-5.   Auditory Development from Birth to Age 5

Age	Development and Behavior
Birth	Eye blinking and Moro reflex response to sounds; subcortical response to sounds because of lack of myelinization of cortical auditory pathways; anatomic maturity of auditory mechanism.
2 months	Voluntary muscle response to sound.
6 months	Infant localizes direction of sound.
5 years	Final development of auditory function; eustachian tube becoming longer and more curved; incidence of otitis media decreasing.

back because of the anatomic differences of the more mature ear canal. Tympanic membranes are observed for color, light reflex, retraction or bulging, perforation, and mobility. Immediate medical therapy is required if infection is present, since untreated otitis media can lead to more severe infections, including abscesses of the neck and lymph nodes, mastoiditis, and meningitis. Chronic otitis media can also cause hearing loss.

Screening.   Hearing can be measured with instrumentation that utilizes an acoustical signal. Infants will react to the sound by eye blink, Moro reflex, arousal response (stirring, eye opening, limb movement), head turn, sucking activity, and cessation of movement or vocalization. By 3 months the infant begins to turn his head and eyes toward the source of sound, and by 6 months he fixates on the source of a soft sound. Children 2 to 5 years of age respond well to play techniques in which, when a sound is transmitted through earphones, they place a peg in a board, or a small toy in a box. A 5-year-old will lift his finger when hearing a sound through earphones if the examiner makes a game of it. Gross measurements of hearing can be made using noisemakers. A small child will blink when he hears a sharp noise made at each ear separately and out of his range of vision. An older child can hear a whispered question or simple command at 8 feet.

These testing procedures should be done at birth, and at each visit during the first year, to detect hearing deficits early. Treatment should be instituted before critical developmental periods are reached. For children who respond poorly to office testing, screening materials may be given to the parents for use in the home, where the child may be more relaxed and cooperative. Results should be reported to the nurse. Speech development can be assessed utilizing the Denver Development Screening Test (Fig. 15-2). Speech problems or failures may be caused by lack of desire or need to communicate. Muscle coordination difficulties, hearing loss, emotional disturbances, or mental retardation may also cause communication difficulties.

Nose Examination

External nasal examination includes observation of shape and flaring and for evidence of the child's ability to breathe nasally. The lower half of the child's nasal septum is composed of cartilage and is more flexible than the adult septum, with the ability to absorb more trauma. Sinuses are percussed for tenderness after 2 years of age. Examination of the interior of the nose is done with a light to observe the color of the mucosa, the presence and characteristics of secretions, polyps, swollen turbinates, signs of hemorrhage, or the presence of foreign bodies.

Oral Examination

During the oral examination, number, condition, texture, and position of the teeth are carefully noted. Occlusion, lip chewing, mouth breathing, and the size, condition, and markings of the tongue are also observed.

At the time of primary tooth eruption, many children have nasal congestion and discharge, slight temperature elevation, loose stools with or without diaper rash, are irritable, and drool excessively.

Excessive bottle feeding and a high carbohydrate diet markedly increase the incidence of dental caries. Brushing of the teeth should be started about the time of the child's first dental visit (at 2½ to 3 years of age). Children continue to require assistance and supervision of oral hygiene practices until they are 6 or 7 years of age and need reinforcement again during adolescence.

Tooth eruption is related to genetic factors, rather than to jaw growth, bone, or chronological age (see Table 15-6). Primary teeth erupt earlier in boys, while girls experience earlier eruption of secondary teeth. Premature infants generally experience later eruption than full term infants. Sequence and site of tooth eruption are more important than the child's age, and gross deviations should be carefully evaluated. Children who experience early tooth loss because of trauma should be evaluated carefully for spacing of remaining teeth and possible malocclusion.

Throat Examination

Throat examinations are sometimes difficult for young children who resist the intrusion or gag on the tongue depressor. If the child does not gag spontaneously, the gag reflex should be elicited and its characteristics noted. In young children, the examiner must become skilled at noting the presence, size, and condition of the tonsils, color of the pharyngeal mucosa, and presence of exudate or abscesses in one quick glance. Older children can cooperate with the examiner, permitting more time for this appraisal.

Respiratory System

General appraisal of the child's respiratory status encompasses such observations of the chest as shape, circumference, expansion, symmetry, retraction, scapular position, masses, and tenderness. The infant's chest has a greater anteroposterior

Table 15-6.   Dental Growth and Development[a]

	Primary or Deciduous Teeth					
	Calcification		Eruption[b]		Shedding	
	Begins at	Complete at	Maxillary	Mandibular	Maxillary	Mandibular
Central incisors	4th fetal month	18–24 months	6–10 months (2)	5–8 months (1)	7–8 years	6–7 years
Lateral incisors	5th fetal month	18–24 months	8–12 months (3)	7–10 months (2)	8–9 years	7–8 years
Cuspids	6th fetal month	30–39 months	16–20 months (6)	16–20 months (6a)	11–12 years	9–11 years
First molars	5th fetal month	24–30 months	11–18 months (5)	11–18 months (3)	9–11 years	10–12 years
Second molars	6th fetal month	36 months	20–30 months (7)	20–30 months (7a)	9–12 years	11–13 years

	Secondary or Permanent Teeth			
	Calcification		Eruption[b]	
	Begins at	Complete at	Maxillary	Mandibular
Central incisors		3–4 months	9–10 years	7–8 years (3)	6– 7 years (2)
Lateral incisors	Maxilla: Mandible:	10–12 months 3–4 months	10–11 years	8–9 years (5)	7– 8 years (4)
Cuspids		4–5 months	12–15 years	11–12 years (11)	9–11 years (6)
First premolars		18–24 months	12–13 years	10–11 years (7)	10–12 years (8)
Second premolars		24–30 months	12–14 years	10–12 years (9)	11–13 years (10)
First molars		Birth	9–10 years	5½–7 years (1)	5½– 7 years (1a)
Second molars		30–36 months	14–16 years	12–14 years (12)	12–13 years (12a)
Third molars	Maxilla: Mandible:	7–9 years 8–10 years	18–25 years	17–30 years (13)	17–30 years (13a)

[a]Modified from Kempe, C. et al. [6, p. 27], by permission of the authors and the publisher.
[b]Figures in parentheses indicate order of eruption. Many otherwise normal infants do not conform strictly to the stated schedule.

than transverse diameter, giving it a round appearance. Some degree of concavity or convexity may be present and is considered normal. The chest circumference usually is measured and compared with the head circumference in children under 2 years of age; after 2 years of age, the head circumference is surpassed by that of the chest, and only gross deviations are measured and recorded. A round chest configuration after 6 years of age is a significant sign of chronic pulmonary obstruction.

Respirations in the infant and child are abdominal, with little chest movement until about age 6, when respirations become thoracic. Rates vary greatly (see Table 15-7) and should be noted when the child is quiet. Note also the rhythm and depth of respirations. Excitement, respiratory disorders, fever, poisonings, acidosis, and cardiac failure will increase the rate. Causes of slow respiratory rates (bradypnea) are similar for children and adults.

Table 15-7.   Respiratory Rates*

Age	Rate
Premature	40—90
Newborn	30—80
3 Years	20—30
5 Years	20—25
10 Years	17—22
15 Years	15—20

*Modified from Lowrey, G. H.   *Growth and Development of Children* (6th ed.). Copyright © 1973 by Year Book Medical Publishers, Inc., Chicago. Used by permission.

Dyspnea.   Dyspnea may be symptomatic of cardiac disease, anemia, hypothyroidism, or respiratory tract obstruction, although exercise, pain, or emotional factors also may cause difficulty in breathing. The nurse examiner should attempt to determine the cause of dyspnea. Forcing infants to cry, asking young children to run, and requesting older children to breathe deeply, forcibly exhaling a few times, helps indicate the amount of exertion which precipitates dyspnea. Respiratory effort should be evaluated at intervals during the examination to determine whether or not the degree of dyspnea decreases as the child's apprehension diminishes. The position in which the child experiences the least dyspnea may be significant in determining the location of the difficulty. Young children with high airway obstruction, for example, will assume a knee-chest position and cannot tolerate lying supine. Paradoxical respirations usually indicate neuromuscular disorders, necessitating more extensive diagnostic evaluation.

Cough.   The frequency and characteristics of any cough are noted, and the cough reflex is tested. Infants may have a weak or poorly developed reflex, and it may be difficult to clear mucus from the airway. Normally, infants are not mouth breathers, so nasal passages must be kept clear. Mouth breathing in older children may indicate infection, allergy, or obstruction.

Respiratory Sounds.   Because pitch depends on diameter of the passageway, the small airway size in infants and young children causes unique pediatric respiratory sounds. Expiratory wheezes are relatively frequent, but other sounds offer the nurse examiner clues about the location of airway obstruction. A gargling, snoring sound indentifies postpharyngeal distress, such as a tumor.

Laryngeal stridor is usually inspiratory, high-pitched, harsh, and noisy, as is extrathoracic tracheal distress. The stridor of croup can be described as a crowing sound. Intrathoracic tracheal distress and bronchial difficulties cause a prolonged expiratory phase with wheezing, like that occurring in asthma.

Examination. The positioning of the child for the chest examination is similar to that of the adult. Palpation of the chest is done with the examiner's hand placed lightly but firmly on the chest wall. Masses, tenderness, and nodes are confirmed by using palm and fingertips. Tactile fremitus is a tingling feeling over the entire chest. Coarse fremitus indicates mucus in the upper respiratory tract, while decreased fremitus is a sign of obstruction or disease. Percussion of the child's chest is performed by tapping with the index or middle finger over every half inch of the chest and axillary region. Posteriorly, the nurse examiner begins at the shoulder and percusses down to the diaphragm, comparing right and left sides at every level. Anteriorly, percussion begins above the clavicle and proceeds downward to the level of dullness. Percussion usually includes the diaphragm and liver. The axillary regions are percussed down to the level of the eighth rib. Because the small chest size in the infant makes it difficult to note all areas of dullness and obstruction, percussion is less helpful than careful observation of respiratory rate and effort.

Because of the small chest size, a bell-shaped stethoscope should be fitted tightly to the chest wall and in the intercostal spaces for adequate auscultation. The chest is examined bilaterally, comparing right and left pulmonary findings for each area of the thorax, proceeding as for percussion. It may be necessary to restrain the child's fingers to avoid noise artifacts. The thinness of the chest wall causes breath sounds to be harsh and loud, making quality difficult to differentiate until a child is 5 or 6 years of age. A loud slapping sound may indicate a tracheal foreign body. Loud, rapid, "swishy" breath sounds may be heard in children who have been exercising. Peristalsis heard over the lower left anterior chest is usually due to the proximity of the bowel but may be a sign of diaphragmatic hernia.

Infections. Infections of the respiratory tract are the most common illnesses of children, occurring with great frequency through school age. Viruses cause the majority of illnesses, and treatment is symptomatic. Children should be taught proper use of tissues to prevent droplet spread of infection. Foreign bodies in the toddler, croup or epiglottitis in the preschooler, and allergies in children of any age may cause severe respiratory distress.

CIRCULATORY SYSTEM

Basic information to include in examination of the heart is size, shape, rhythm, quality of sounds, thrills, and murmurs. Measurement of heart size is an important indication of heart disease, and although difficult in children, estimation of size can be made with careful inspection, palpation, and percussion. As in the newborn and in the adult, the point of maximum impulse (PMI) usually indicates the location of the apex of the heart. In 2- to 5-year-old children it is generally found at the nipple line, at the fourth interspace; in children over 5 years, within the nipple line at the fifth interspace. Although usually not visible, the cardiac impulse may be noted in the thin, excited, or hyperactive child. A diffuse impulse may indicate cardiac enlargement or failure but also can be a normal finding.

Heart sounds should be sharp and clear. During childhood, heart sounds are of a higher pitch and shorter duration than in adult life. Slurred or "mushy" heart sounds are generally characteristic of severe heart disease. In the newborn, the first sound (mitral and tricuspid valve closure) and the second sound (aortic and pulmonic valve closure) are approximately equal in intensity. In later childhood, the apical first sound is louder than the second, and the pulmonic second sound is louder than the first.

It is often difficult to be certain of the presence of murmurs. They are classified as innocent or organic and should be described in terms of the following: position in the cardiac cycle, location and point of maximum intensity, and response to exercise and change of position. Systolic murmurs come at or after the first sound and before the second; diastolic murmurs come at or after the second sound and before the first. Many children have murmurs without heart disease; however, patients presenting with murmurs should be referred to the pediatrician for diagnosis and treatment. Sinus arrhythmia (phase variation in the heart rate, usually associated with the respiratory cycle) is a normal finding in many children over age 3 and is especially prominent in young adolescents. Occasional premature beats or extrasystoles may be noted in children but have no clinical significance.

Signs and Symptoms of Cardiovascular Disease

Cyanosis may be due to pulmonary disease or to cyanotic congenital heart disease. In heart disease, cyanosis may be limited to nail beds and mucous membranes or may be generalized. Cyanotic and hypoxic spells may be a frequent symptom in infants and children with specific congenital cardiac defects (e.g., tetralogy of Fallot). Characteristics of hypoxic spells include irritability, sudden increase in cyanosis, and marked dyspnea, which may progress to unconsciousness, convulsions, and coma. Clubbing of fingers and toes suggests severe cyanotic heart disease and is usually not apparent until the child is 1 year of age.

The following signs revealed by the history may be indicative of congenital heart disease: poor weight gain; feeding problems; fainting (hypoxia) spells; difficulty in swallowing, with frequent regurgitation of curdled milk; respiratory difficulty, with increased comfort in a position of hyperextension; fatigue on exertion; and squatting (characteristic of some types of heart disease).

Signs of heart failure in young children differ from those seen in an adult. Weight gain, rapid respirations, and dyspnea in the supine position are early signs. An enlarged liver, venous engorgement, orthopnea, and gallop cardiac rhythm may or may not be present. Pulmonary and peripheral edema are late signs of cardiac failure.

Pulse Rate and Rhythm

Cardiac rate varies markedly during infancy and childhood, especially during activity. When possible, heart rate in infancy should be obtained during sleep to lessen activity and distractions. Heart rate in the older child may also be affected by emotional factors, such as fear and anxiety during examination. As with the newborn and the adult, pulses in both the upper and lower extremities should always be examined and compared.

Average heart rates for infants and children are presented in Table 15-8.

Table 15-8.   Resting Heart Rates (per minute) at Different Ages*

Age	Lower Limits of Normal	Upper Limits of Normal	Average
Newborn	70	160	120
1—12 months	80	140	110
1—5 years	80	110	95
5—10 years	70	100	85
10—15 years	55	90	75

*Reprinted, by permission from Kelminson and Nora [5].

Blood Pressure

Using the correct size of the blood pressure cuff is imperative, or readings will be inaccurate. The width of the cuff should cover approximately two-thirds of the length of the child's upper arm or upper leg and at least three-fourths of the circumference of the extremity. Infant blood pressure may be obtained by a flush technique, which is performed as follows: Wrap the extremity in a pressure dressing. Raise the pressure in the blood pressure cuff slightly above the anticipated reading, and note the systolic reading at the time of flush, as normal color returns when the dressing is removed and cuff pressure released. Normal blood pressures at various ages are listed in Table 15-9.

GASTROINTESTINAL TRACT

A careful history of feeding and bowel habits is essential to the appraisal of the gastrointestinal tract of infants and children. Persistent regurgitation, vomiting,

Table 15-9. Normal Blood Pressures for Various Ages (mm Hg)[a]

Age	Systolic	2 S.D.	Diastolic	2 S.D.
Infants[b]				
1st day	52			
4th day	70			
10th day	80			
2nd month	95			
8th month	95			
1year[c]	96	30	65	25
2 years	99	25	65	25
4 years	99	20	65	20
6 years	100	15	60	10
8 years	105	15	60	10
10 years	110	17	60	10
12 years	115	19	60	10
14 years	118	20	60	10
16 years	120	16	65	10

[a]Modified from Lowry, G. H. *Growth and Development of Children* (6th ed.). Copyright © 1973 by Year Book Medical Publishers, Inc., Chicago. Used by permission.
[b]The figures for infants represent averages by the flush method described in the text.
[c]From 1 year on, the figures in the columns represent the average for systolic and diastolic pressure and 2 standard deviations. Diastolic pressure is indicated by the first change in auscultatory sound.

colic, diarrhea, or constipation may indicate the parents' need for information and education or may be a presenting sign of a serious illness. General guidelines for infant feedings should be reviewed with all parents even though they have had experience with other children.

Infant Feeding
Selection of a formula should be consistent with that recommended by the pediatrician. The infant should be held for feedings whenever possible. Bottles should not be propped, although babies are generally able to hold their own bottle by the age of 6 to 7 months. Although burping in mid-feeding may be sufficient, in the younger infants especially, more frequent opportunities to burp may be necessary to prevent colic, restlessness, and regurgitation. After feeding, the infant should be placed on his right side or abdomen. Orange juice may be introduced after the second or third month and can be an adequate source of vitamin C if the infant takes up to 3 or more ounces daily. Mothers should avoid warming orange juice, since heat destroys vitamin C. Although many pediatricians prefer to depend on daily multivitamin preparations as a source of vitamin C, it is important for parents to develop the habit of offering citrus fruits to their children daily. A few ounces of water can be offered during excessively hot weather if desired.

Opinions vary regarding the proper time to introduce solid foods into the infant's diet. Knowledge of the feeding program recommended by the physician caring for the child is necessary. As a general principle, it is important to introduce one food at a time, advancing to a selection of cereals, vegetables, meats, and fruits over a period of months. Should an infant consistently reject the introduction of solid foods, it may be wise to discontinue the attempt for several days. As the infant grows, he will show interest in feeding himself and should be permitted to use his fingers in an effort to explore food consistency as well as taste.

The following is a general guide to feeding habits during the first year:

Age 1 to 3 months.   Flexible feeding plan; instinctive need to suck, even after hunger is satisfied.

Age 3 to 6 months.   Solid foods started; offer one at a time in small amounts initially to determine possible allergies and dislikes. May push food from mouth in beginning.

Age 5 to 6 months.   Sips from cup. Let infant handle empty cup at 6 months; will gradually acquire skill with addition of milk.

Age 6 months.   Appetite decreases due to slowing of body growth. Let appetite be guide to quantities offered.

Age 9 to 12 months.   Begins to feed self. Messy at first, with gradual increase in coordination and skill.

Dietary Requirements in Childhood and Adolescence

The need for nutritional education for parents and older children can not be overemphasized. Caloric requirements vary for each child according to his age, sex, and activity. Charts and nutritional pamphlets with specific requirements are readily available and should be carefully explained to the parent. Table 15-10 provides a summary of some of the essential nutrients.

Increased calories are required during periods of infancy and adolescence when activity, growth, and development are accelerated. Periods of concern for the mother generally occur during the preschool years, when her child's appetite is diminished, and during adolescence, when eating habits are sporadically poor due to the child's desire to be thin and attractive.

Gastrointestinal Problems

Vomiting.   Vomiting is frequently seen in children in association with acute infections, faulty feeding techniques, fear and anxiety, and a wide range of disturbances of varying severity. Characteristics of the vomitus (color, volume, force, consistency, and time of occurrence) should be determined. It is important that the nurse ascertain whether nausea precedes or follows vomiting. In newborns, vomitus containing bile material suggests bowel obstruction. Other conditions meriting consideration when vomiting occurs at various ages are: pyloric stenosis (infancy), central nervous system disturbance, food poisoning, surgical conditions, allergies, and cardiac disease.

Examination of the abdomen can be accomplished best on a flat surface with

Table 15-10. Approximate Daily Dietary Requirements of Children at Different Ages Under Ordinary Conditions (adapted from recommendations of the Committee on Growth and Development of the White House Conference on Child Health and Protection, the Food and Nutrition Board of the National Research Council, and other sources)[a]

Age	Water ml./Kg.	Water oz./lb.	Calories per Kg.	Calories per lb.	Protein Gm./Kg.	Protein Gm./lb.	Minerals[b] Ca (Gm.)	Minerals[b] P (Gm.)	Minerals[b] Fe (mg.)	Vitamins[c] A (I.U.)	Vitamins[c] B1 (mg.)	Vitamins[c] B2 (mg.)	Vitamins[c] Niacin (mg.)	Vitamins[c] C (mg.)	Vitamins[c] D (U.S.P.)
3 days	80–100	1.2-1.5			3.5-4	1.8	0.6	1.5	6	1500	0.4	0.6	7	35	400
10 days	125-150	1.9-2.3			3.5-4										
3 months	140-165	2.1-2.5	100-130	45-60	3.5										
6 months	130-155	2-2.3					0.7		7	1500	0.4	0.6	7	35	
9 months	125-145	1.9-2.2							8	1500	0.5	0.8	8	35	
1-3 years	115-135	1.7-2	90-100	41-45	2.5	1.6	0.8	1.5	8	2000	0.5	0.8	8	40	400
4-6 years	90-110	1.3-1.7	80-90	36-41	2.2	1.4	0.8	1.5	10	2500	0.6	1.0	11	40	400
7-9 years	70-90	1.1-1.3	70-80	32-36	2.2	1.1	0.8		12	3500	0.8	1.3	13	40	400
10-12 years	60-85	0.9-1.3	60-70	27-32	1.8	0.9	1.1	1.5+	14	4500	1.0	1.4	16	40	400
13-15 years	50-65	0.75-1	50-60	23-27	1.7	0.7	1.4	1.5+	15	5000	1.2	1.8	18	45	400
15 + years	45-55	0.67-0.8	40-50	18-23	1.4	0.5 +	1.4	1.5+	15	5000	1.4	2.0	16	50	400
Adult	40-50	0.6-0.75	40-45	18-21	1	0.5	0.8	1.5+	10-15	5000	1.0	1.6	16	55	400

[a]Modified from Silver et al. [12] by permission of the authors and publisher.

[b]Other minerals (all ages):
Magnesium 200-400 mg/day
Potassium 1-2 gm/day
Sodium 1-2 gm/day
Chloride 2-3 gm/day
Iodine Trace

[c]Other vitamins:
Folacin Under 6 months, 0.05 mg.; 6 months to 10 years, 0.1-0.3 mg.; over 10 years, 0.4 mg.
B6 Levels similar to thiamine up to 12 years; over 12 years, 1.6-2 mg.
B12 Under 1 year, 1-2 µg.; 1 to 8 years, 2-4 µg.; over 8 years, 5 µg.

the child in a supine position with knees slightly flexed. It is important to palpate the abdomen for masses and to note whether it is tense, soft, hard, or tender. Initially, palpation should be superficial, followed by more extensive examination as the child becomes less fearful and more relaxed. A tense abdomen may indicate a surgical emergency, necessitating immediate referral to the physician. The abdomen is a particularly good site to determine dehydration by checking skin turgor.

Abdominal Pain.   Episodes of abdominal pain are frequent in childhood and are often a manifestation of functional gastrointestinal illness; however, pain as a response to emotional stress should be considered. Examination during and between attacks of abdominal pain is desirable. In the young child the complaint of a "stomachache" is used to indicate a variety of symptoms usually located in the abdominal area. Frequently, the child points directly to the umbilicus when referring to a general area of abdominal discomfort.

Bowel Habits and Stool Characteristics.   Information on bowel habits and stool characteristics (consistency and color) should be obtained with the history on all infants and children. The reader is referred to the Ross Laboratories publication, *Infant Stool Cycle* [4] for charts and a description of normal and abnormal stools in infancy. Diarrhea associated with systemic infections is common in children [4].

GENITOURINARY SYSTEM

Urinary System

Kidneys are more easily palpated in infants and young children than in adults. The lower portion of the right kidney and the upper portion of the left usually can be palpated, but in some instances they cannot be. Tumors, polycystic kidneys, congenital anomalies, infection, or renal vein thrombosis may cause enlargement of the kidney. The bladder can be percussed and palpated 1 to 4 cm above the symphysis pubis. Bladder enlargement may be due to urinary tract obstruction, voluntary retention of urine, or low spinal cord disease [10].

The force and location of the urinary stream should be determined by history and observation. In the male the position of the urethral orifice is normally at the tip of the glans. In hypospadias, the opening is on the ventral surface; in epispadias, it is on the dorsal surface. Both conditions necessitate referral to a urologist. The prepuce should be examined for infection and phimosis. If urinary tract infection is suspected, a midstream specimen is required for culture or bacterial count. The finding of 100,000 or more organisms per milliliter in a clean-voided, midstream specimen indicates infection but should be repeated [10]. Catheterization is seldom necessary and is generally avoided to prevent the possibility of trauma or introduction of infection. When a sterile urine sample is desired, suprapubic percutaneous bladder aspiration is the method of choice but should be attempted only when the bladder is full. In all instances, urine samples are examined when fresh, since bacteria grow rapidly in vitro in a urinary culture medium, and red cells disintegrate within an hour at room temperature.

Abnormal Findings. In children, the most common abnormal findings are urinary tract infections and hematuria.

Urinary tract infections. The incidence of urinary tract infections is second only to respiratory infections in childhood and may have serious consequences if untreated. Male infants are more frequently affected than females, but in childhood and adolescence, such infections are overwhelmingly more common in girls. *Escherichia coli* is the most common infecting organism, with the *Klebsiella* group being the next most common. Other contributing factors in females are pinworms, masturbation, the use of bubble bath, and constipation. In the adolescent female, the incidence of urinary tract infections may be associated with sexual intercourse.

Urinary tract infections may be manifested by abrupt onset of fever as high as 104°F (40°C), or may be absent in chronic infections. Infants may have vomiting, weight loss, failure to thrive, lethargy, and jaundice. Manifestations in children include urgency, frequency, dysuria, and pain or tenderness over the costovertebral angle. Toddlers are more apt to complain of abdominal pain or scream violently on urination. Fatigue and headache may occur in chronic infections. Urethral discharge indicates the presence of infection somewhere in the urinary tract.

Hematuria. Painless urinary tract bleeding may be evident in a number of children and can be benign. Treatment is usually not indicated, but referral to a urologist is required to rule out tumors, tuberculosis, and chronic glomerulonephritis.

Genitalia

The female child is inspected for vaginal discharge, adhesions, hypertrophy of the clitoris, and pubertal changes. The labia minora atrophy following the neonatal period and enlarge at puberty due to the production of estrogens. A large clitoris, though usually a normal finding, may indicate adrenal hyperplasia or precocious puberty. Infants and young children are referred to a gynecologist for vaginal examination. Examination of the male child's genitalia includes inspection of the meatal opening, the circumcision and the foreskin, determination of the size of the testes, and notation of pubertal changes. Presence of phimosis, hydrocele, hernia, and cryptorchidism will require extensive examination and referral. The penis of the obese boy often appears abnormally small; however, size can be appropriately evaluated by pushing the fat away.

Examination of the scrotum should be carried out when the child is not cold or frightened. Testes and cords can be palpated, and the scrotum appears loose. Hernia and hydrocele should be considered when the scrotum appears enlarged. In suspected cases of cryptorchidism, the boy should be examined while sitting in a chair holding his knees with his heels on the seat, since increased intraabdominal pressure may force the testes into the scrotum. The size of the testis is approximately 2 cm after puberty; the left testis is usually lower than the right. Hydroceles are usually not tender and may often be found in children under age 2.

Pubertal Change

Pubertal changes vary considerably between sexes and among individuals. Growth and sexual development follows a sequential pattern, with extensive physical, psychological, and endocrine changes. The first signs of sexual maturation appear between 8 and 14 years of age. The development of secondary sex characteristics in females (Table 15-11) precedes that in males (Table 15-12) by about two years.

Table 15-11   Average Time of Appearance of Sexual Characteristics in American Girls*

Pelvis	Female contour evident in early childhood and becomes well established by 8—10 years
Breasts	I. Preadolescent
	II. Bud stage: nipple and areola enlarged, small mound beneath, 9—11 years
	III. Nipple enlarged and areola forms mound above the surrounding skin of breast, pigmentation apparent. 12—13 years
	IV. Nipple projects but aerola level with surrounding skin, glandular tissue palpable, histologic maturity. 14—17 years
Vagina	Some thin milky secretion often begins a year before menarche; glycogen content in cells and epithelial changes on smear, 11—12 years
Pubic hair	I. Initial appearance, 11—12 years
	II. Mainly labial, darker and coarser than body hair, 12—13 years
	III. Well-formed triangle, curly and dark, 13—14 years
	IV. Thick, spreads to thighs
Menarche	13 years.
Axillary hair	Initial appearance, 12—14 years
	Increases in amount until early adulthood
Acne	Varies in severity and duration, usually precedes menarche

*Modified from Lowrey, G. H. *Growth and Development of Children* (6th ed.). Copyright© 1973 by Year Book Medical Publishers, Inc., Chicago. Used by permission.

Precocious Puberty

True precocious puberty refers to sexual maturation before age 8 in girls and age 10 in boys; that is, the hypothalamic-pituitary mechanism initiates sexual development with the potential for production of mature sperm or ova. The onset of precocious puberty may be at any age and has been found to be far

Table 15-12.　Average Time of Appearance of Sexual Characteristics in American Boys

Breasts	Some hypertrophy often assuming a firm nodularity, 12—14 years. Disappearance of hypertrophy, 14—17 years.
Testes and penis	Increase in size begins, 10—12 years. Rapid growth, 12—15 years.
Pubic hair	Initial appearance, 12—14 years. Abundant and curly, 13—16 years.
Axillary hair	Initial appearance, 13—16 years.
Facial and body hair	Initial appearance, 15—17 years.
Acne	Varies considerably, 14—18 years.
Mature sperm	Average, about 14—16 years.

more common in girls than in boys. Breast development is usually the first sign of this condition in females, but general patterns vary.

NEUROMUSCULOSKELETAL SYSTEM

The nervous system of the infant is relatively mature at birth and is completely mature by the age of 5 years. Neurologic evaluation of the infant or child begins with some general observations of head size and shape, level of consciousness, position of the body, especially of the head and neck, spontaneous activity, coordination of movements, muscle tone and resistance, sensation, irritability, vigor and pitch of cry, and the presence of tremors or twitching.

The infant's sucking, grasping, Moro, and Babinski reflexes and the position of the thumb are appraised as for the newborn. Head positioning, tonic neck reflex, nuchal rigidity, hyperextension of the neck (opisthotonos) and the fullness and tenseness of fontanelles should be noted. Because the open fontanelles allow for skull expansion, intracranial bleeding or other causes of slowly increasing intracranial pressure are difficult to determine early in infants.

At birth there are six fontanelles, the anterior, posterior, two mastoid (posterolaterals), and two sphenoids (anterolaterals). Only the anterior remains palpable after several months. Normal fontanelle closures are as follows: posterior, birth to 8 weeks; anterolateral, 12 weeks; anterior, 18 months or earlier; posterolateral, 12 months.

It is difficult to examine cranial nerves in the uncooperative or preverbal child, and the results are unreliable. General appearance, responsiveness, and abilities are good indications of the intactness of the child's nervous system. Neurologic examination in the older child and adolescent is similar to that in the adult.

Evaluation of mental development is an important part of the neurologic appraisal. A careful developmental and behavioral history of the child may provide early clues about the neurologic status of the child.

In the toddler and preschool child, observation of play and use of the Denver Developmental Screening Tool (Fig. 15-2) are helpful in evaluating satisfactory mental development. Prior to the time the child begins school, his mental development must be determined to plan for appropriate educational experiences. If the child's progress appears unsatisfactory, psychological testing should be conducted. The quality of nurturing must also be investigated. Intensive stimulation often dramatically improves the functioning of a slightly retarded child. Whenever possible, the retarded child should receive vocational training to prepare him for a useful, self-supporting life.

In the past, mental retardation has been categorized by apparent degrees of severity. Seemingly, the current trend is to diagnose children as retarded without assigning categories [9]. This trend is controversial and is not yet widely practiced.

Generally, muscle development corresponds to the state of nutrition and activity. Increase in muscle mass follows increased skeletal growth with the weight of muscle compared with total body weight nearly doubling between infancy and adulthood. At birth muscle forms about 20 to 25 percent of the infant's total weight. Muscle examination in infants and children is the same as in adults. Pain, deformity, and limitation of function are carefully noted.

The child's posture is dependent on his age, health, and physique. As the child grows, the flexibility of the spine, the vertebral curves, and the center of gravity change. The pot-bellied appearance of the young child is less pronounced by age 6, when the center of gravity becomes subumbilical.

The preadolescent growth spurt is due to androgen stimulation of bone and is usually experienced earlier by girls than by boys. Sexual maturation is related more closely to bone age than to chronological age. As calcification of the bones continues, the incidence of fractures increases. At puberty the center of gravity is at the ilium, and the child's posture resembles the adult's.

Pediatric skeletal examination is similar to that in adults. Deformities may indicate congenital anomalies or skeletal trauma and should be investigated thoroughly by radiography. Infants and toddlers often have a flat-footed appearance due to fat pads along the longitudinal arch. These pads disappear with the exercise of the muscles of the foot that occurs with walking and are no longer noticeable by about 3 years of age. Urging the child to stand before he displays an interest in the upright position can strain the arch and should be discouraged. Although infants have an inward bowing of the legs from knee to ankle, usually attributable to uterine position, the bowlegged appearance is most noticeable in the 2-year-old. This is a self-correcting condition and should not be confused with the deformities of rickets.

Selection of children's shoes is usually of concern to parents, and opinions about the ideal shoe vary. The main purpose of shoes is foot protection. Shoes should be nonrestrictive, allowing approximately one-half inch extra in the width and three-eighths to three-fourths inches extra in the length. The shoes should be high enough to hold the heel in place and should have enough depth for the toes. The heel should not be elevated. Flexible soles provide for natural exercise of the foot muscles. If care is taken to prevent trauma, walking barefoot as much as possible on soft surfaces in the toddler and preschool years is helpful in developing a strong foot.

COMMON PEDIATRIC EMERGENCIES

Accidents are the leading cause of death in children and adolescents. Every year, 15,000 children under fifteen years of age die in accidents, and another 17 million (1 in 3) are injured. Many suffer severe permanent injury [7]. The nurse's role in childhood accident prevention includes investigation of causes and provision of anticipatory guidance to parents about preventive measures.

Among the factors relating to accidents and injuries are troubled family relationships, stress, environmental hazards, the specific developmental stages of the child, and family safety attitudes [13]. Parents need to be informed about these factors and impressed with the need to remain calm and seek help in emergency situations. Community assistance is usually available from fire and rescue squads, hospital emergency units, poison control centers, and physicians.

Because of the active, curious nature of the child, falls are a common cause of pediatric injuries and often result in fractures and head injuries. The nurse must be skilled in obtaining specific information and in advising distraught parents via telephone. For example, on hearing a report of a toddler fall involving head trauma, the nurse should question the parents regarding the level of consciousness, respiratory distress, evidence of headache, irritability, nausea, vomiting, dizziness, gait disturbances, and the presence and character of nasal or ear discharge. Parents need to be instructed to report changes promptly.

Burns are another significant cause of childhood trauma. Many could be prevented by vigilant supervision of children's activities, so that they do not play with matches, flammable liquids, or electrical equipment. One of the most hazardous rooms in the home is the kitchen, where spilled cooking liquids can and do cause severe burns in children. Care must also be taken with bath-water temperatures.

Another common pediatric emergency involves ingestion of toxic or caustic substances. Improved packaging of aspirin has reduced salicylate intoxications, but ingestions of other drugs and common house and garden sprays and cleaning compounds have increased. Syrup of ipecac, an emetic available at drugstores without prescription, should be kept in every home, along with a first aid chart indicating when vomiting should be induced. Additional skill in management of childhood emergencies can be obtained from a formal first aid course. Parents should be encouraged to enroll in these classes.

To prevent bites, children should be taught to avoid unfamiliar pets, small wild animals, and snakes. Increasing numbers of small animals have been reported to be rabid and pose a real threat to the unsuspecting child.

Although some children appear to be accident-prone, accidents usually result from impulsive behavior. There may be several reasons for this: Children sustaining injuries are often impulsive, aggressive, tense, and obstinate and suffer from disturbed relationships with authority figures (parents), a situation which can produce guilt. To relieve the unconscious guilt, the child may punish himself for unacceptable feelings by sustaining injuries, or he may seek to attract his parents' attention and concern by wounding himself.

Children who present with frequent injuries, multiple bruises, old scars, radiologic evidence of healed fractures, or discrepancies between the description of the accident and the injuries observed require thorough investigation. Child abuse occurs in every social stratum and is inflicted most often on one child in the family by young parents who are isolated from sources of emotional support. Frequently, these parents have been abused by their own parents. Suspected child abuse is to be reported to the local child protective service agency or appropriate authorities.

The nurse's responsibility in childhood accidents is to investigate their psychosocial components, emphasizing the child's need for love and supervision and obtaining psychiatric consultation for families with disturbed relationships and frequent accidents.

TELEPHONE COMMUNICATIONS IN PEDIATRIC PRACTICE

Parents often rely on telephone communications with health professionals for reassurance about their children and their own parenting abilities. Calls frequently relate to behavior, nutrition, elimination, or sleeping habits, although concerns change as children develop. The nurse must develop a calm, patient approach to telephone callers. The parents must feel that the nurse understands the concerns expressed and is not rejecting them because of the nature or frequency of their calls.

The nurse must be able to elicit history and symptomatology quickly and in chronological sequence through skilled questioning via telephone. Responses to problems and concerns should be directed at reducing parental anxiety. Some brief anticipatory guidance and health teaching may be done during the telephone conversation. The nurse should try to determine whether the parent's call represents a family crisis, a high anxiety level, or a child with a health problem. Although telephone communication with a health professional can be reassuring to anxious parents, it should not become a substitute for seeing the patient when indicated, or for deeper involvement in the family's health concerns.

REFERENCES

1. Adams, R. M.   Principles and practice of topical therapy. *Pediatr. Clin. North Am.* 18:686,1971.
2. Caporaro, V. J. Gynecologic examination in children and adolescents. *Pediatr. Clin. North Am.* 19:515, 1972.
3. Frankenburg. W. K., and Dodds, J. B.   Denver Developmental Screening Test. University of Colorado Medical Center, Denver, Colorado.
4. *Infant Stool Cycle*. Clinical Education Aid. (No. 3). Columbus, Ohio: Ross Laboratories, 1963.
5. Kelminson, L., and Nora, J. Heart and Great Vessels. In C. H. Kempe, H. K. Silver, and D. O'Brien (Eds.), *Current Pediatric Diagnosis and Treatment* (2nd ed.). Los Altos, Calif.: Lange Medical Publishers, 1972 P. 277.
6. Kempe, C. H., Silver, H. K., and O'Brien, D. (Eds.). *Current Pediatric Diagnosis and Treatment* (2nd ed.). Los Altos, Calif.: Lange Medical Publishers, 1972.
7. Levine, M. I.   A pediatrician's view. *Pediatr. Ann.* 2 (1):5, 1973.
8. Lowrey, G. H. *Growth and Development of Children* (6th ed.). Chicago: Year Book, 1973.
9. Mercer, J. R. *Labeling the Mentally Retarded; Clinical and Social System Perspectives in Mental Retardation.* Berkeley, Calif.: University of California Press, 1973.
10. Moon, J. B., and O'Brien, D. Kidney and Urinary Tract. In C. H. Kempe, H. K. Silver, and D. O'Brien (Eds.), *Current Pediatric Diagnosis and Treatment* (2nd ed.). Los Altos, Calif.: Lange Medical Publishers, 1972. P. 437.
11. Nelhaus, G. Neuromuscular Disorders. In C. H. Kempe, H. K. Silver, and D. O'Brien (Eds.), *Current Pediatric Diagnosis and Treatment* (2nd ed.). Los Altos, Calif.: Lange Medical Publishers, 1972. p. 493.
12. Silver, H. K., Kempe, C. H., and Bruyn, H. B. *Handbook of Pediatrics* (10th ed.). Los Altos, Calif.: Lange Medical Publishers, 1973. p. 48.
13. Wheatley, G. Childhood accidents. *Pediatr. Ann.* 2 (1):10, 1973.

SUGGESTED READINGS

Barness, L. A. *Manual of Pediatric Physical Diagnosis* (4th ed.). Chicago: Year Book, 1972.
Barnwell, E., et al. *Infant and Preschool Assessment and Counseling Guide for Nurses.* Lansing, Mich. Bureau of Maternal and Child Health, Michigan Department of Public Health, 1972.
Behrman, H. T. *Practitioner's Illustrated Dermatology.* New York: Grune and Stratton, 1972.
Brazelton, T. B. *Infants and Mothers.* New York: Dell, 1969.
Childhood accidents. *Pediatr. Ann.* 2:1, 1973 (entire issue).
Coffin, P. *1,2,3,4,5,6.* New York: Macmillan, 1971.
Cooke, R. *Biological Basis of Pediatric Practice.* New York: McGraw-Hill, 1968.
Child Study Association of America, Inc. *You, Your Child and Drugs.* New York: Child Study Press, 1971.
Daniel, W. A. Common problems of adolescence. *Pediatr. Ann.* 2:14, 1973.
Daniel, W. A. *The Adolescent Patient.* St. Louis: Mosby, 1970.
Fraiberg, S. H. *The Magic Years.* New York: Scribner's Sons, 1959.
Frykman, J. H. *A New Connection. An Approach to Persons Involved in Compulsive Drug Abuse,* San Francisco: C/J Press, 1970.
Gallagher, J. R., et al. *Medical Care of the Adolescent* (2d ed.). New York: Appleton-Century-Crofts, 1966.

Green, M., and Haggerty, R. *Ambulatory Pediatrics.* Philadelphia: Saunders, 1968.

Kempe, C. H., and Helfer, R.   *Helping the Battered Child and His Family.* Philadelphia: Lippincott, 1972.

Kestenbert, J., et al.   *The Adolescent: Physical Development, Sexuality and Pregnancy.* New York: MSS Information Corporation, 1973.

Krugman, S., and Ward, R. *Infectious Diseases of Children.* St. Louis: Mosby, 1968.

Kunin, C. M.   Epidemiology and natural history of urinary tract infection in school age children. *Pediatr. Clin. North Am.* 18:509, 1971.

Lampe, M. *Drugs: Information for Crisis Treatment.* Beloit, Wis.: Stash Press, 1972.

Liebman, S. D., and Gellis, S. S. (Eds.). *Pediatrician's Ophthalmology.* St. Louis: Mosby, 1966.

Marks, M. B. Stinging insects: Allergy implication. *Pediatr. Clin. North Am.* 16:177, 1969.

McDonald, R. *Dentistry for the Child and Adolescent.* St. Louis: Mosby, 1969.

Overdose Aid. Department of Social Services, [Michigan Department of Public Health,] Lansing, Michigan. Copyright 1972, Russell F. Smith.

Palensky, N., Desoix, C., and Sharlin, S. *Child Neglect: Understanding and Reaching the Parent.* New York: Child Welfare League of America, Inc., 1972.

Siffert, R. S.   Orthopedic check list for neonates and infants. *Hosp. Pract.* 5:66, 1970.

Stancil, J. B.   The other ingredient of health care. *Pediatr. Ann.* 2:14, 1973.

Stuart, H., and Prugh, D. (Eds.)   *The Healthy Child.* Cambridge, Mass.: Harvard University Press, 1964.

U.S. Department of Health, Education, and Welfare, Office of Child Development. *Infant Care.* Children's Bureau Publication. Washington D.C.: U. S. Government Printing Office, 1973.

THE ELDERLY

16

Josephine M. Sana

GLOSSARY

aged Having lived or existed long; old.
aging Progressive changes produced with the passage of time.
elderly * Pertaining to people in later life; between middle age and old age.
geriatrics Branch of medicine concerned with the pathology and treatment of the aged ill.
gerontology Scientific study of the problems of aging in all their aspects — clinical, biologic, historical, sociological, pschological.
later maturity† Years from 65 to 74; characterized by the onset of major changes in life circumstances and patterns; physiologic changes usually occur gradually.
middle age The turning point of maturity; time of self-assessment and preparation for new and modified life patterns.
old age The final stages of the normal life span, usually 75 years or older, and a period of life with marked dependencies.

The clinical assessment of elderly adults necessitates consideration of multiple factors uniquely related to their age and the aging process. Knowledge of the changes characteristically associated with growing old, and of their functional implications, is essential and is the primary focus of this chapter. It is important, however, that the nurse be aware of other salient factors affecting the health and welfare of the elderly and, consequently, her practice of nursing.

POPULATION TRENDS AND IMPLICATIONS FOR NURSING

One of the most significant outcomes of the scientific advances in the health field is the extension of life expectancy. A person born in the United States at the beginning of this century had a life expectancy of less than 50 years. In 1970, the average life expectancy at birth was about 75 years for the female and somewhat lower for the male [3]. Persons age 65 and older numbered under 4 million in 1900, constituting 4.1 percent of the total population. By 1970, this age group had increased more than five times, to number over 20 million, and represented 9.9 percent of the population of the United States [9]. Population

---

*This term is used throughout the chapter in effort to avoid ambiguity for the reader. The life periods are not absolutes and their definitions must be regarded flexibly.
†New stage in the adult life cycle defined by the noted gerontologist, Clark Tibbitts, Director, Training Grant Staff, Administration on Aging, Department of Health, Education, and Welfare [7].

projections indicate that there may be as many as 30 million people 65 years and older in the year 2000. It is estimated that this group will continue to constitute about 10 percent of the total population [1, 8].

The impact of this changing population profile on nursing is already apparent. The relatively circumscribed field of geriatric nursing is growing rapidly and developing as an important specialized area of practice. Custodial and ritualistic nursing practices are being replaced by more diversified, scientifically based nursing care approaches and interventions. To assist nurses in making these practice transitions, nurse practitioner and continuing education programming has expanded.

The sheer magnitude and scope of the needs influencing the health and welfare of the elderly, and ultimately of the total population, mandated a priority of national attention and action. Intensified research into the problems of aging by the health professions, particularly in the field of gerontology, generated much new knowledge. Clinical translation of relevant new knowledge into current nursing practice is now in progress, and the numbers of nurses specializing in gerontological nursing is increasing.

Nurses caring for adults in other than gerontological or geriatric settings are also more frequently involved with the elderly. There is a concerted effort to maintain the elderly in their community and home environments as long as possible. This imposes more and more complex demands on nurses practicing in home care programs, health maintenance organizations, and community or hospital-based outpatient clinics.

COMMON MISCONCEPTIONS ABOUT THE ELDERLY

Some of the terms frequently associated with the elderly are "senile," "sick," "disabled," "dependent," and "alone." All of these terms are stereotypes and their use is often inspired by limited professional and personal experiences with the elderly. The existing data show that only about 4 percent of persons in the 65 and older age group are institutionalized for care [6]. Less than 1 percent can be appropriately described as "senile." Actually, the majority enjoy relatively good health up to the age of 70. Of those 65 years of age and older, 7 of every 10 either reside with their spouses, relatives, or friends or function as the head of the household. Generally, they are active, contributing members of society, maintaining themselves independently in their own homes or apartments and paying taxes. In many instances, they are productively employed [4].

NURSE ORIENTATIONS AND VALUES
ABOUT AGING AND THE ELDERLY

It is especially important that the nurse working with older people be aware of her orientations and feelings about aging and the elderly. Close personal contacts with older people during the nurse's formative years, and the positive or negative nature of these experiences, influence the professional orientations and the attitudes she expresses in her practice. Evidence of the youth orientation of our society is overwhelming. This emphasis on youth and youthfulness is undeniably devaluative of age and aging. The demeaning effects on the elderly, and on their self-concept and functional well-being, are amply documented in the literature and will not be detailed further. It is of cardinal importance for the nurse to recognize that the elderly are particularly sensitive to expressions of these attitudes and values. However unintentional and subtle their reflection in the nurse's practice, the process and outcomes of the appraisal and other care interactions with the elderly will be adversely affected.

Insight into the value systems operant in our professional endeavors as nurses is but one dimension deserving our careful consideration. As products of our culture, we need to examine our value systems in terms of their effects on society as a whole. As producers of our culture, we need to recognize our potential to impact on it, both as individuals and in our collective roles and to become responsible forces for social change. It is somewhat ironic, that as a society, we bury "trinkets" of our time in time capsules, so those in the future will be sure to be informed about their heritage, yet attach so little value to the elderly in our midst who *are* our heritage.

HEALTH AND AGING

Some health problems are generalized as characteristic of the older population. Although knowledge of these problems is most useful to the nurse appraising the elderly, their relevance to individual patients is highly variable. Generalizations must be applied with caution, since the elderly differ as much one from another, as individuals vary in the population at large. As Fritz [4], describing one group of older people, said, "They [have] the interesting mixture of virtues and faults we find at every age."

Characteristically, the health problems of the elderly are chronic in nature and very often multiple. Commonly, the functional disabilities observed in the elderly are much less incapacitating than the examining nurse would expect in view of the extent and the seriousness of the diseases they have. Causes for many chronic diseases are unknown or poorly understood, limiting preventive or corrective approaches. Data obtained during appraisal, however, can contribute to the early detection of these health problems and the implementation of measures to arrest or slow their progression. Disease exacerbation and complications tend to stress the old more severely than the young; recuperative abilities are less, and recovery is usually slower and less complete. The nurse assessing the elderly should fully appreciate the importance of her role in preventing or minimizing these crises states as well as promoting the patient's fullest functional and coping potentials. Although serious disease may develop insidiously in older people, presenting disruptive symptoms only in late stages, many chronic problems are revealed in readily observable ways.

Generally, aging is accompanied by a decrease in the ability of an individual's body system to perform efficiently. Reserve capacities are also decreased, and there are fewer and slower reactions to stimuli from within and outside the body. The onset and rate of change occurring in different body systems will vary with the system as well as with the person's life experiences and heredity. Environmental, economic, and psychological stresses often counter hereditary influences, altering the rate and nature of the aging process.

The fact that the elderly are adults warrants explicit restatement here, for it is fundamental to interacting effectively with older people in the appraisal situation. The content of the chapters directly concerned with adult assessment (Section II) should be viewed as generally appropriate and applicable to the appraisal of the elderly. The guides to observation, palpation, percussion, and auscultation are employed essentially as described in the preceding section. The nurse will need to adapt these appraisal approaches to meet the particular needs and responses of the older person. Interpretation of clinical findings will need to be modified to take into account the changes normally occurring with increased age. Adult norms will therefore have to be used flexibly and adjusted to incorporate age-related changes and individualistic aging patterns in the appraisal.

INTERVIEWING THE ELDERLY

The interview with an elderly person will be facilitated if the nurse examiner takes sufficient time to assure adequate orientation and make the patient comfortable. The use of informal forms of address or given names may be distasteful to the older person, who may view it as disrespectful and demeaning. The nurse should therefore determine and respect the patient's preference.

Of prime importance is the nurse's skill in preparing the older person for the appraisal in an *unhurried* manner. Time pressures experienced by the nurse are often great, and the desire to avoid undue time entrapments is understandable. The ability of the older person to respond intelligently and cooperatively, however, can be materially impaired by being rushed. Nonverbal communications indicating that the nurse "is very busy" and "does not have much time" are quickly received by the patient. A patient's attempts to accommodate to the nurse's time frame and expectations usually conflict with his best interests and welfare. Physical findings may be inadvertently induced or intensified by unspoken demands placed on the older patient to move about and change positions quickly.

Appraisal activities need advance explanation to avoid surprise and unnecessary anxiety. Instructions should be concise and uncomplicated. Questions should be clearly phrased, brief, and devoid of potentially confusing technical terminology. Sufficient time for a response must be provided; experiences accumulated over years of living may not be recalled immediately in the detail required by the nurse's questions. In other instances, the elderly may engage in extensive review, giving a great deal of information extraneous to that sought by the interviewing nurse. Unless the nurse deals sensitively with the informant, important data may be lost or withheld in the communication exchange.

Mental Performance and Aging

Early in the appraisal interview, the nurse examiner should begin assessing the elderly person's ability to comprehend and respond reliably. Tentative impressions of mental functioning can be formulated while eliciting the initial social data. Specific information should be obtained routinely about the patient's family and friends, home environment, current employment or retirement status, educational background, and recreational interests and activities. During this data-gathering process, the nurse not only gains an understanding of the patient as an individual, but also evaluates his language ability, coherency, and comprehension. The patient's attention span and ability to recall and relate past and recent events are also noted. Patient reliability as an informant is validated by periodic rechecking of dates, times, events, and other selected data.

The following considerations should guide the nurse in assessing the mental status of elderly individuals. The older person responds less often and more slowly than a younger person and needs more time to collect and interpret information. This slowing of reaction time with aging indicates less efficiency rather than qualitative impairment.

Learning ability and intelligence are maintained well into later years of life. Generally, the learning process takes more time in the elderly because learnings, amassed over years of living and experiencing must be modified or replaced by new information and ideas.

It is essential for the aging person to continue to exercise his mental abilities. Functional loss is great and rapid when the brain is not used. The consequent mental deterioration and incapacitation can be catastrophic to the total well-being of the elderly patient.

Characteristically, memory impairment with aging is for recent events, while past memory remains essentially intact. Frequently, the older person soon recognizes this memory change in himself even though the difficulty may be transient and mild. Some patients will verbalize their concern or embarrassment freely but anxiously. When asked to recall recent occurrences, others may protect against their insecurity by dwelling on past memories.

Mental functioning declines more slowly than physical functioning. Ordinarily, marked alterations are not observed until the very advanced years. However, repetitive assaults by disease and illness are not tolerated well by the elderly and hasten the deterioration of mental functioning.

The nurse should find the methods for testing orientation, memory, and other cognitive functions described in Chapter 13 helpful in appraising the mental status of the elderly. Findings need to be carefully recorded, for functional alterations may be indicative not only of the aging process but also of serious psychological problems or organic disease.

Sensory Perception

Impairments of hearing or sight will have direct bearing on the patient's ability to comprehend and respond appropriately during the appraisal interview and examination. The nurse appraising the elderly must ascertain whether or not auditory or visual acuity impairments are present and, if so, obtain a gross estimate of their extent. This can be accomplished with little difficulty during the interview and assessment of mental status. A thorough appraisal of the special sensory modalities includes investigation of the status of the patient's sight, touch, taste, smell, pain, temperature, and position sense.

Hearing. Loss of hearing severely handicaps the overall functional ability of the elderly. The ease and safety with which the older person can move about outside his home boundaries is usually decreased markedly. Work and recreational options are more limited. Adaptive behaviors are easily misinterpreted as age-related alterations in personality and mental functioning, masking the generic problem. The social isolation associated with this sensory impairment is of significant magnitude in itself. When added to the other significant changes in the life situation generally experienced in later maturity, the effects on the individual can be overwhelming.

The incidence of hearing defects is probably much greater in the older population than available statistics indicate. Impairments of hearing present less overtly than impairments of sight and are less easily detected by others. Often, the older person is not immediately or acutely aware of the onset and insidious progression of hearing loss.

Difficulties experienced in hearing may be denied by some. Others may recognize the problem but rationalize it as an aspect of aging they must accept without recourse. Too often, appropriate medical help is not sought, and the problem remains undiagnosed until other concerns bring the older person to the health care facility. The nurse testing the patient's auditory acuity may be the first to detect a hearing disorder.

The two most common hearing disorders are presbycusis and otosclerosis. *Presbycusis,* a perceptive hearing loss associated with aging, involves damage to and deterioration of the neural structures of the inner ear, the auditory nerve, or both. Initially, the ability to hear high-frequency tones is lost; hearing of low frequency tones is affected last. The patient's ability to distinguish between spoken words is diminished and further compromised by noisy environments.

The onset of *otosclerosis,* a conductive hearing loss due to changes in the structure and function of the ossicles (small bones) of the middle ear, is generally in the younger or middle years of life. Surgical correction is often possible for this hearing disorder. Neural involvements may develop over time, and the older person may demonstrate a mixed hearing loss. Audiologic testing and physician referral is arranged to determine the precise nature of the hearing deficit and the potential usefulness of a hearing aid, surgery, or other therapy.

Vision. Numerous changes in the eye and its function accompany the aging process, with great impact on the quality of life of the elderly. Visual acuity, as does hearing acuity, decreases with age, and the psychosocial effects of this sensory deprivation are as wide-ranging and complex. Depending on the severity of visual impairment, new constraints may be experienced by the older person. Independence and safety in ambulation and driving is often lessened. Diversional and occupational activities are more restricted, and self-care demands new and difficult adjustments. It must be remembered that many older people have excellent vision. However, those who have severe visual fields defects and severe defects in macular vision may be eligible for special financial and tax benefits. The nurse needs to be aware of the nature of these benefits and of the criteria for eligibility so that she can counsel patients appropriately (see Chap. 7).

In addition to the problem of impaired macular vision, the two other eye conditions most frequently seen with aging are glaucoma and visual field defects. The potential for blindness associated with untreated glaucoma mandates routine examination for increased intraocular pressure in adults over 40 years of age. Particular attention to the patient's family history and symptomatology is warranted, since glaucoma has a familial tendency and presents alerting symptoms (see page 112).

Lens opacities (cataracts) develop with aging and eventually interfere with vision. Well-developed cataracts may be observed by the nurse without added illumination. The patient will need to be referred for precise diagnosis and evaluation for surgery.

The ophthalmoscopic examination has particular significance for the elderly. The high incidence of diabetes and vascular disease in later years is well recognized. Consequently, fundoscopic examination should be done routinely to detect changes indicative of vascular changes and retinal damage (see pages 117-118).

Other Senses. Perception of taste, smell, touch, temperature and pain and proprioception (movement and position) alters with aging. In general, the nature of change is one of blunting and loss.

After age 45 the number of taste cells gradually decreases, and sensitivity to tastes is correspondingly less. This loss, combined with the decreasing ability to sense and differentiate odors, often affects the older person's eating habits and nutrition. Previous desires for and satisfaction with various foods are lost, and appetite is diminished.

The highly interrelated sensory mechanisms of touch, temperature, and pain are dulled. Consequently the older person's alerting system to environmental danger and tissue injury is impaired. The value of pain as a signal of disease and damage is great, and the seriousness of reduced pain perception and response to pain should not be underestimated. It is not uncommon for the elderly to frequently sustain cuts, burns, and bruises; these should be noted carefully and the circumstances of their occurrence clarified.

Adaptation to external temperature changes is diminished, and extremes of heat and cold are poorly perceived and tolerated. Body temperature adjusts more slowly in illness, and fever may appear later than normally expected. For this reason, fever in the elderly patient has added significance as a finding and should be evaluated medically for its underlying cause. Metabolism is slowed in the elderly, and temperature-regulating mechanisms function less efficiently.

The person with altered proprioception is less secure about his body positioning in space. This impairment of position-sensing ability is compensated for by slower, more cautious body movement. The slowing of movement allows the patient added time for sensory input, so that more information about the environment can be gathered and processed by the nervous system. The nurse examiner may be cued to this problem by the patient's notable tendency to use visual input as a substitute for the impaired position sense. This is demonstrated by the older person who looks down to watch the placement of his feet when walking. Specific testing methods to be used are detailed in Chapter 13.

Skin Changes

As with other biologic aspects of aging, changes in the skin will vary greatly from one older person to another. However, alterations in the skin are among the most readily discernible changes in the aging process.

In the aging skin, subcutaneous fat and water are lost, and there is decreased turgor. As a result, the skin becomes lined and wrinkled. Skin folds hang loosely, giving the appearance of flabbiness. Diminished glandular function and dehydration result in skin dryness. Elasticity is reduced; the skin is more friable, subject to excoriation, and easily traumatized. The skin becomes less vascular, and healing time is prolonged. Alterations in skin pigmentation are noticeable in the blotchy, spotty patterning. Both skin and hair thin, the latter losing pigment and becoming gray. Some skin areas become thickened, and keratotic lesions may be observed on the face and body.

Elderly persons may be distressed by generalized itching, commonly caused by excessive dryness of the skin. However, if the itching is localized, there is greater likelihood of other causes. Dermatitis and fungal infections are among the more common skin problems in aging and should be considered in the appraisal. Skin cancer is a major problem, and the lesions are generally found on skin areas exposed to the sun and weathering.

Appraisal of the skin of the elderly must include careful examination of the feet. The examining nurse should make a special point of inquiring about any foot problems the elderly person is experiencing and should be attentive to any complaints. Ability "to get around" is crucial to independence in self-care activities. Ambulation may be compromised by the discomfort of foot conditions amenable to improvement, if not to actual prevention or correction. The older person may have special problems in caring for the skin and nails of the feet. These problems are to be identified and appropriate instruction and assistance provided. At times assistive equipment is indicated, and consultation with a physical or occupational therapist will need to be arranged. Excessive sweating and foot odor may pose an embarrassing and troublesome problem, necessitating special foot care and treatment. Cuts, blisters, and fissures are easily infected and treatment should not be delayed. The presence of calluses and corns should be noted and an attempt made to determine and remedy their cause. Because these conditions may become painful and incapacitating, referral to a dermatologist or podiatrist may be indicated.

Motor Performance and Musculoskeletal Considerations

Loss of muscle mass and strength is a major change with aging. Energies are depleted more quickly, and tolerance for physical activity is lowered. The complaint of not being able to do as much as before is commonly heard from the elderly. Muscles move with less smooth coordination, and speed of muscle movement is decreased, resulting in poorer performance of motor activities. The change is generally noticed first in loss of motor skills for more complex tasks and for activities demanding precise, coordinated movement.

Osteoarthritic changes in the joints with associated pain on movement is particularly debilitating. Joint stiffening and impaired range of motion may be severly incapacitating and distressful. The nurse will have to examine the patient's joint function with special care and gentleness to minimize discomfort and anxiety. Decreased range of motion should be quantitated whenever possible and measurements recorded for making comparisons and noting changes.

Intervertebral disc changes occur with the "wear" of years, and normal spinal curvatures are exaggerated. The stooping posture is apparent in many older people.

Hormonal changes with aging are important in assessing older women. Postmenopausal females, particularly Caucasians, are predisposed to osteoporosis. This loss of minerals from bone increases the elderly person's vulnerability to fractures, and a careful history of recent trauma, no matter how slight, should be elicited.

Cardiovascular and Respiratory Function

Heart disease is a health problem common to the elderly and is the major cause of death in people over 65. Changes in cardiovascular functioning in the older person are usually the result of a combination of factors, the aging process being only one [2].

The ability of the heart to function efficiently decreases with advancing years. Usually, there is some degree of fibrosis of the myocardium, with a decrease in its contractility. Cardiac output is less at rest, and the heart's ability to respond to increased work demands by increasing its output is decreased. The decrease in cardiac reserve in the elderly person has significant implications for their ability to adapt to sudden stresses, either physical, mental, or emotional [2]. The nurse's understanding of what these stresses might be for the patient she is examining should guide her in providing care and counsel. Elderly patients frequently need help in identifying what and how to make modifications in their life-style to minimize or prevent stress. Available community services are often unused because the older person is unaware of them or does not know how to arrange for them. The nurse can be extremely helpful in facilitating the patient's use of these resources.

When examining the older patient for peripheral vascular function, several facts should be kept in mind. Vessel lumens may become narrowed and partially occluded by the deposit of fatty substances. Symptoms of circulatory insufficiency may be experienced by the older patient but not be considered sufficiently important to mention unless he is asked about them. Fibrotic changes also occur in the vessel walls, making them hard and pipelike. These can be seen and palpated easily. With the loss of elasticity in arteries, there is an increased peripheral resistance to blood flow and the systolic blood pressure usually becomes elevated.

Care must be exercised by the nurse when having the elderly change position during the appraisal. Usually, older people do not compensate well for the effects of gravity on the circulatory system and may readily experience orthostatic hypotension.

Two of the most common cardiac symptoms found in the elderly are chest pain (angina) and dyspnea. The nature and circumstances surrounding either of these symptoms must be explored thoroughly with the patient. He should be asked specifically whether or not the dyspnea occurs at night, has an acute onset, is accompanied by chest pain, is precipitated by exertion, and if so, with what kind and how much exertion. If exertional dyspnea is the complaint, it is important to clarify whether or not this has been previously experienced with the activities described.

Cardiovascular changes affecting pulmonary circulation will influence the respiratory status of the older patient. Much of the comprehensive descriptions of the respiratory and cardiovascular examinations given in Chapters 9 and 10 will have relevance for the nurse appraising the elderly. It may be helpful to the nurse appraiser to examine these two areas of patient function in sequence.

Ordinarily, respiratory function is adequate in the elderly unless pathology is present. However, it should be recalled that the loss of elasticity in the body musculature of the elderly also pertains to the respiratory muscles and chest wall, and some impairment of respiratory excursion may be present. The patient's history of smoking and exposure to occupational and other dangerous pollutants should be documented by the nurse. The elderly are more susceptible to respiratory infections than younger patients and often suffer more serious consequences from them. Any indication of a recent need to curtail activities should be probed for respiratory function implications.

Throughout the assessment process the nurse working with older adults will find rich guidance in this principle [5] :

"...there are distinctions to be made between the state of being old, the process of becoming old and changing potentials for the future old."

Mindful of these distinctions, the nurse in her appraisal role will contribute in some knowledgeable and planned way to the quality of each for her patient ... and herself.

REFERENCES

1. Busse, E. W., and Pfeiffer, E. (Eds.). *Behavior and Adaptation in Late Life* (1st ed.). Boston: Little, Brown, 1969.
2. Chinn, A. B. (Ed.). *Working With Older People: A Guide To Practice*. Vol. IV. *Clinical Aspects of Aging*. Washington, D.C.: Department of Health, Education, and Welfare, Public Health Service, Publication No. 1459, June, 1971.
3. Facts on Aging. In *Aging*. Washington, D.C.: Department of Health, Education, and Welfare, Administration on Aging, Publication No. 146. Reprinted from May, 1970. Pp. 2–11.
4. Fritz, D. B. *Growing Old is A Family Affair*. Richmond, Virginia: John Knox Press, 1972.
5. Riley, M. W., Riley, J. W., and Johnson, M. E. (Eds.). *Aging In Society*. New York: Russell Sage Foundation, 1969.
6. Scott, F. G. Overview and An Orientation to Aging. In, *Perspectives in Aging II: Operational Focus*. A Continuing Education Book. Corvallis, Ore.: 1971. Chap. 2, Pp 5–7.
7. Tibbitts, C. Middle-Aged and Older People in American Society. In F. G. Scott and R. M. Brewer (Eds.), *Perspectives in Aging II: An Operational Focus*. A Continuing Education Book. Corvallis, Ore.:, 1971. Chap. 3, Pp. 13–21.
8. Shanas, E. Health status of older people. *Am. J. Public Health*. 64:261, 1974.
9. *Stat. Bull. Metropol. Life Ins. Co.* 54:4, 1973.

SUGGESTED READINGS

Brantl, V. M., and Brown, Sr. Marie. *Readings in Gerontology*. St. Louis: Mosby, 1973.
Burnside, I. M. *Psychosocial Nursing Care of the Aged*. New York: McGraw-Hill, 1971.
Butler, R. N., and Lewis, M. I. *Aging and Mental Health* St. Louis: Mosby, 1973.
de Beauvoir, S. *The Coming of Age*. New York: J. P. Putnam's Sons, 1972.
Jaeger, D., and Simmons, L. *The Aged Ill*. New York: Appleton-Century-Crofts, 1970.
Kimmel, D. C. *Adulthood and Aging*. New York: Wiley, 1974.
Neugarten, B. L. *Middle Age and Aging*. Chicago: University of Chicago Press, 1973.
Pastalan, L., and Carson, D. (Eds.). *Spatial Behavior of Older People*. Ann Arbor, Mich.: University of Michigan Institute of Gerontology, 1970.

INDEX

INDEX